Neurologic Disease

Michael Andrew Meyer

Neurologic Disease

A Modern Pathophysiologic Approach to Diagnosis and Treatment

Springer

Michael Andrew Meyer, M.D.
Department of Neurology
Guthrie Clinic
Corning, NY, USA

ISBN 978-3-319-39579-1 ISBN 978-3-319-39581-4 (eBook)
DOI 10.1007/978-3-319-39581-4

Library of Congress Control Number: 2016943316

Printed on acid-free paper

This Springer imprint is published by Springer Nature
The registered company is Springer International Publishing AG Switzerland

Preface

We all want to know this answer: How does our brain work?

"…I am conscious… but how?" is a question every person asks at some time…

"… I think, therefore I am" said Descartes in the seventeenth century—but how does the brain actually think?

How does a highly interconnected mass of nerve cells process information, and simultaneously is aware of itself and surroundings in the form of consciousness?

As neurologists, we unfortunately see patients slip away into a world of unconsciousness from which they may never return, despite our best efforts to save them. We can define what is lost and how—we know that the absence of higher cortical functions leaves patients in an irretrievable state of brain death with only the most primitive brain stem and/or spinal reflexes, but how exactly does a viable network of interconnected areas of cerebral cortex generate consciousness and meaningful human existence?

"… I think, therefore I am." These seventeenth-century words of Descartes remind us how the brain defines who we are. Without proper functioning of the brain, our very sense of who we are can disappear—without a functioning brain, there is no quality of life, and we have come to measure life as just that. For the unfortunate ICU patient who has suffered a prolonged cardiac arrest and then revived, a pumping heart alone, without the brain being active and living as well, offers no life value.

This book examines all diseases of the nervous system and explores the central and peripheral nervous system in health and disease and the rapid diagnosis and treatment of an illness that affects the patient in profound ways and can make the difference between having a good long quality of life or being paralyzed and bedridden with diminished quality of life. In neurologic emergency cases, it is important to remember that the brain needs oxygen continuously and any deprivation of the circulation can lead to lifelong disability. Therefore, the astute physician must be aware of the clues to form a proper diagnosis and the subsequent need to find and implement therapy as soon as possible. The fundamentals of neuroscience are emphasized here as the root of knowledge for clinical neurology—once the basic science is grasped, the pathophysiology behind clinical neurology becomes readily apparent.

This book is also written to inspire the physician who wants to find new cures for untreatable illnesses—many illnesses in neurology are not treatable at the current time, and an exciting field lies before the inspired neurologist to find cures to these devastating illnesses. In this regard, the inspired neurologist is invited to learn as much as possible about the molecular working of the nervous system, with the hopes that genetic therapies can intervene with the disease process.

Although this book is intended to train the next generation of physicians, it hopefully will also guide other established physicians in understanding the complexities of neurological disease as many may not be specialists in neurology. The book is written from the perspective of an initial inquiry into symptoms and goes forward from a simple set of symptoms into the actual possibilities and how a diagnosis is linked to a possible treatment plan that could be formed.

The approach to diagnosis is timeless and involves not only skills acquired by physicians through years of training but what could arguably be the most important skill of all, good, basic communication. The doctor and the patient must communicate effectively: the patient must clearly communicate their problem to the best of their ability, and the doctor must carefully listen and ask the right questions. Frequently patients with neurological disease may simply not be able to give any history. Consider the patient arriving in the emergency room with a sudden occlusion of the main artery leading to the left side of the brain where language takes place. In such a case, a left middle cerebral artery occlusion will leave the patient speechless and powerless on the right side of the body—history from another person who witnessed the event is critical in this case to know the time of onset—is this of great importance when considering intravenous medications to break up the clot (tPA must be used within 180 min of symptom onset). At the other end of the time spectrum, the patient may have incurred a slowly progressive aphasia—clues and details from others are essential in the classification of the problem as being likely of a degenerative nature. Without a clear and accurate history, the neurologist may only have a few clues to the underlying problem.

Although the approach to diagnosis in taking a careful history and physical examination may be timeless and involve skills doctors have employed for hundreds of years, the technology with which we explore these diseases has evolved in a dramatic way that is constantly being updated, as is the ever-expanding breadth of knowledge we have about neurological disease mechanisms.

Corning, NY Michael Andrew Meyer, M.D.

Contents

1 Introduction to Differential Diagnosis in Neurology

To understand the brain is an awesome task that is not easily accomplished from any one vantage point. The neuroscientist working on the mechanics of synapses shuttling back and forth sees things from one aspect, whereas the clinical neurologist sees thing from another. To comprehensively understand the brain and its workings, knowledge from many vantage points is needed; although one can focus on a singular part, it is the global action of many interrelated parts that creates the challenge.

Our knowledge of the brain is at an exponential stage of growth at the moment—it is a very exciting time to be part of this growth phase and to understand the inner workings of the most complicated and most important thing in the entire universe—our brain!

Life is nothing without a functional brain … . there is meaningful existence with just a functioning brain stem and spinal cord—there is no level of consciousness within those structures without the higher regions of the brain (i.e., cerebral cortex) being intact.

The challenge to every clinical neurologist is to understand and treat diseases of the brain, spinal cord and peripheral nerves and muscle—to treat illness and disease of the nervous system presupposes a sound knowledge of how these regions normally work in the healthy individual.

A greater challenge is to undertake a commitment to understand the process of disease and then come up with a practical cure for the illness. Unfortunately, many neurological illness are irreversible but to make progress in this area would be of such benefit to patients … . imagine the benefit of findings a cure for spinal cord paralysis, or perhaps finding a way to halt programmed cell death after hypoxic injury to the brain, as may occur after cardiac arrest or with stroke.

This book is dedicated to the mission of inspiring both young and old in health care to do the absolute best for their patients—whether the contribution is at the bench, or the bedside, keep the patient and their plight as the focal point to your efforts. Learn as much as you can about the nervous system and how it works at a basic science level—*Knowledge is Power*!

1.1 General Principles

Neuronal functioning was a mystery to the Greeks and Romans—later on, Descartes was to hypothesize that the Pineal carried the secret to the soul. It was not only until the 1700s that Galvani performed the most basic studies on nerves and the electrical nature of neural conduction with additional studies by Thomas Hunter on the electric torpedo drawing the connection between neural fiber functioning and electrical phenomenon. It was the subsequent pioneering studies of electrophysiologists in the mid-1900s on giant nerve fibers of the squid that the molecular basis of conduction of impulses became apparent. In one of the most amazing accomplishments in the area of neuroscience, two

M.A. Meyer, *Neurologic Disease*, DOI 10.1007/978-3-319-39581-4_1

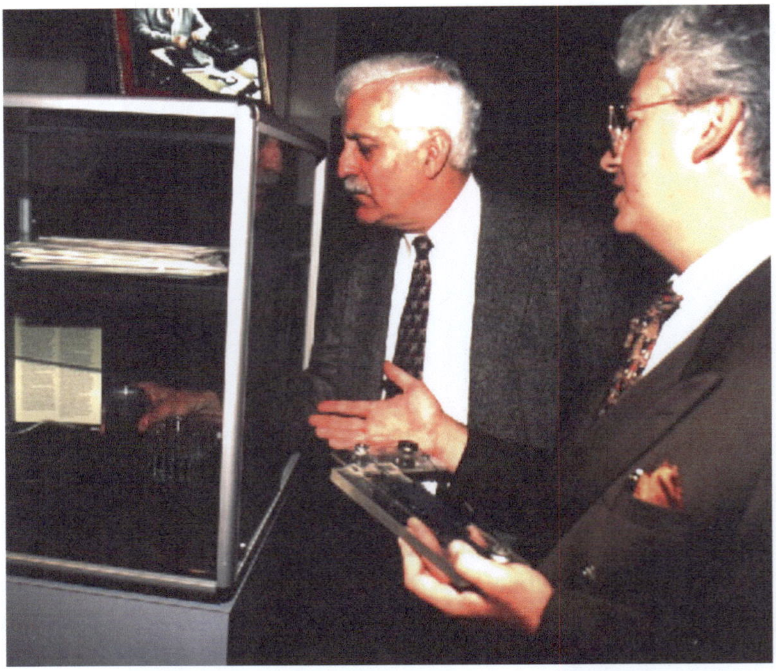

Fig. 1.1 The author is shown above with Dr. Raymond Damadian, inventor of MRI—both are inspecting the original mock-up for the first CT scanner design concept created by Neurologist William Oldendorf. © 2014 by Michael Meyer, MD. With permission from Raymond V. Damadian

British scientists (Hodgkin and Huxley), armed with only a slide rule and oscilloscope, were able to better define internal versus external currents across the nerve fiber membrane. With the help of the squid giant nerve fiber, these two brilliant scientists came up with a way to clamp the voltage at certain intervals and measure the resultant currents at each step; their plots of current versus time under various conditions that include the use of tetrodotoxin allowed them to understand that inward current of sodium ions obeyed third order exponential kinetics with an inactivation phase; these had molecular implications about the how the molecular gate or channel worked, as outward current carried by potassium ions obeyed fourth order kinetics. Mathematical formulas were subsequently constructed with the use of only a slide rule to model how an action potential occurs and then propagates down a nerve fiber. This can now be imaged with fluorescent dyes sensitive to voltage changes (e.g. cerebellar Purkinje neurons, see Chap. 11; axonal electrical currents are portrayed later on in Chap. 2).

The next quantum leap advancement in clinical neuroscience has come with the advent on noninvasive imaging modalities to visualize the brain and its function with the use of CT, MRI, and PET scanning. In the 1970s, the introduction of CT was an amazing advancement and was quickly followed by MRI in the early 1980s (Fig. 1.1) with advent of PET imaging of brain metabolic activity as well.

In Fig. 1.1, the author is shown above with Dr. Raymond Damadian, inventor of MRI—both are inspecting the original mock-up for the first CT scanner design concept created by neurologist William Oldendorf, who created this at home in his kitchen in 1960 by heating metal to fashion a lead shield to contain a radioactive source that passed gamma rays through the test object (carried on a toy train track, as above!) and assay for differential absorption dependent on density. In the basement labs of Downstate Medical Center, Dr. Damadian devised the first MR scanner dating back to the early 1970s.

1.2 Organizational Principles

The most fundamental unit of neuronal functioning is the neuron—everything else is subservient around the functioning and existence

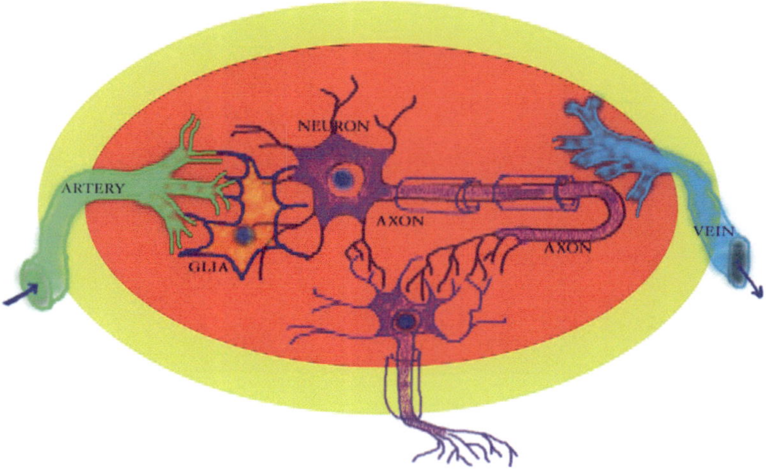

Fig. 1.2 The basic organization principle of neuronal functioning. © 2014 by Michael Meyer, MD

of the neuron and its dendritic and axonal processes. The neuron and its fibrous extensions are enveloped by a capsule of glial cells that have nutrient and supportive functions for the neuron.

The basic organization principle can be summarized as follows:

Artery → capillaries → glial → neuron

The flow of information is as follows:

Dendrite → neuron cell body → axon → synapse

The basic organization principle can likewise be illustrated as shown in Fig. 1.2.

An important aspect of the above model is the concept of circulation: proper circulation of oxygenated blood through arterial channels is vital to neuronal health; blood must exit in an unobstructed manner through venous channels or otherwise incur symptomatic venous hypertension (acute obstruction to venous outflow with superior sagittal sinus thrombosis can be a life-threatening event—please see case example in Chap. 3). The yellow envelope in the model shown above also reflects the fact that the brain literally is floating in cerebrospinal fluid (CSF), with circulation of CSF occurring in an unobstructed manner [any acute obstruction can cause headache and other severe symptoms, whereas chronic slowly developing obstruction induces dysfunction through pathologic stretch and strain upon long fiber tracts, as in normal pressure hydrocephalus (NPH)].

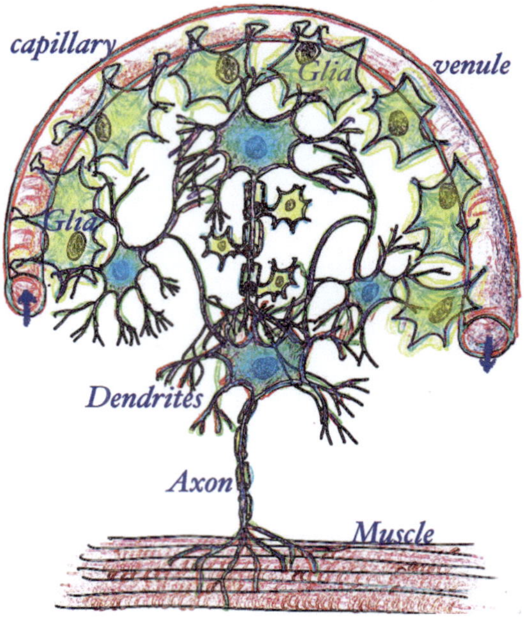

Fig. 1.3 A schematic that captures the anatomy of the ventral horn of the spinal cord, where spinal motor neurons directly connect to muscle via axonal branches. © 2014 by Michael Meyer, MD

This fundamental unit can be transformed into a schematic that captures the anatomy of the ventral horn of the spinal cord, where spinal motor neurons directly connect to muscle via axonal branches (see Fig. 1.3).

A key part of the model is the fact that glial cells make up a substantial fraction of cellular

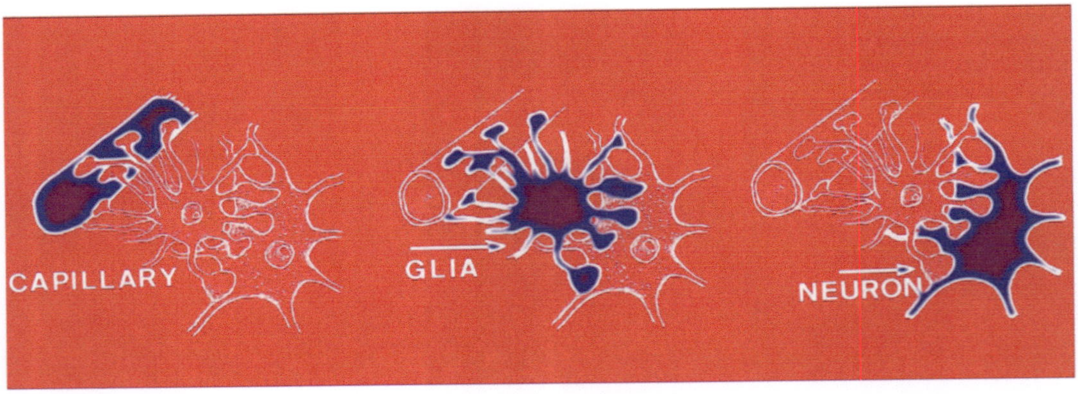

Fig. 1.4 A key part of the model is the fact that glial cells make up a substantial fraction of cellular elements within the brain and play vital roles in protecting the nerve cells they envelop and also serve nutritive and supportive roles. © 2014 by Michael Meyer, MD

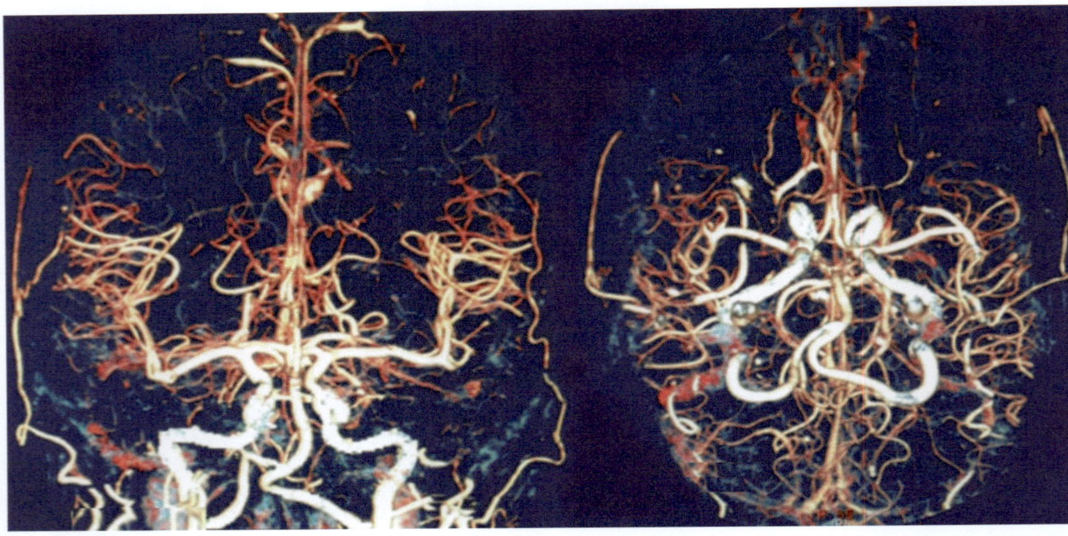

Fig. 1.5 The intense vascularity is demonstrated in the three-dimensional renderings of a brain CT angiogram in the anterior view at *left* and from superior vertex vantage point from above, as shown at *right*. © 2014 by Michael Meyer, MD

elements within the brain and play vital roles in protecting the nerve cells they envelop and also serve nutritive and supportive roles (see Fig. 1.4).

In transforming this model of this microscopic fundamental functional unit to a higher macroscopic level, the brain is an intensely vascular organ with a rich supply of capillaries that enable the efficient transfer of oxygen and nutrients to glial and neurons. The intense vascularity is demonstrated in the three-dimensional renderings of a brain CT angiogram in the anterior view at left and from superior vertex vantage point from above, as shown at right (Fig. 1.5).

Without oxygen, the brain can suffer irreversible damage if this is reduced to critically low levels over the course of only minutes; to insure this efficient supply, the great vessels leading to the brain are joined together in a fail-safe type mechanism to join vessels together within the basal structure known as the Circle of Willis. Despite these safety backup mechanisms and despite the intense vascularity of the brain as shown in

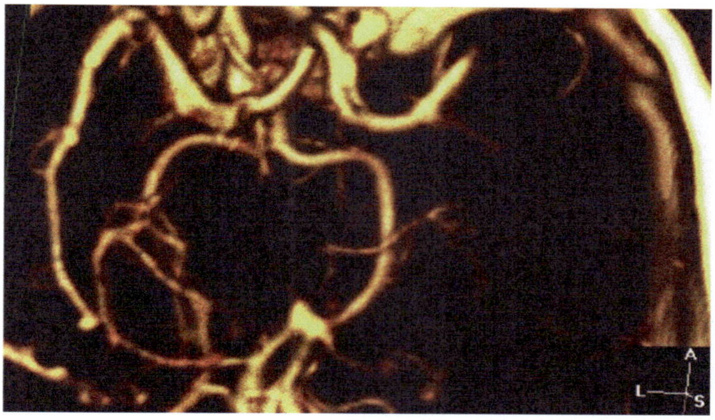

Fig. 1.6 Acute right MCA infarction. A typical CT angiogram appearance to an arterial occlusion resulting in stroke. © 2014 by Michael Meyer, MD

the above example of CT angiography, devastating brain ischemia is a surprisingly frequent event, with a stroke occurring every 40 s to someone in the United States. A typical CT angiogram appearance to an arterial occlusion resulting in stroke is shown in Fig. 1.6.

1.2.1 Neurological Diagnosis

Accurate diagnosis of neurological disease forms a fundamental part of the art and science of medicine that require skill and attention by all physicians, whether the problem develops slowly over many years as in a neurodegenerative disease process like Alzheimer's or develops abruptly in the form of a brain stem stroke. Neurological emergencies such as the brain stem stroke example often present suddenly with dire consequences for the unfortunate patient—it is therefore the responsibility of every physician to know as much as possible about this area of medicine, and to do everything possible to help the patient avoid the possibility of long-term injury once an accurate diagnosis has been rapidly made. Whether the patient is 19 years old who develops an acute brain stem stroke, or it is a 90-year-old with encephalitis, it is the job of the consulting neurologist to aggressively achieve an accurate diagnosis and rapidly institute an effective treatment plan.

The first steps towards an accurate neurological diagnosis is to conduct a neurological exam and integrate findings from tests to arrive at differential set of possibilities: A first step is to establish time frame of illness (acute versus chronic) in relation to the age of the patient and whether the problem is focal, multifocal, or diffuse—this can be gathered from the history alone. An acute focal deficit in a 90-year-old male (stroke) immediately conjures up a differential diagnosis that is distinctly different had this been a 30-year-old female with prior intermittent trouble walking and 3 days of unilateral progressive visual loss [demyelinating disease or multiple sclerosis (MS)].

An important part of modern medicine relates to disease that affects the central and peripheral nervous system, including many diseases that can affect muscle function. A comprehensive understanding of these illnesses is needed in order to understand any patient. A patient presenting with leg weakness and fever for instance could be due to one of multiple problems—arriving at the right diagnosis and treatment requires not only expertise in neurology but internal medicine as well. This text attempts to help establish a formalized logical approach to clinical problems where the ultimate diagnosis may be a primary neurologic disorder. As the reader is advised to keep an open mind about neurologic symptoms that are found as part of non-neurogenic disorders, a distinction is made here about primary versus secondary neurologic problems. This text also includes cognitive disorders such as Alzheimer's dementia, and discusses the neurologic basis for disorders that have previously been classed as psychiatric, such as schizophrenia.

Table 1.1 Acronym: vitamin D, E, and F

Vascular	Acute focal hemiparesis with aphasia, such as with acute left middle cerebral artery (MCA) occlusion
Infective	Rapid deterioration over hours as in bacterial meningitis, or over many weeks as in Creutzfeldt–Jacob disease
Traumatic	Acute stroke symptoms resulting from post-traumatic dissection, or cognitive decline over many weeks due to a subdural hygroma
Autoimmune	Severe incapacitating weakness due to autoimmune attack upon acetylcholine receptors at the neuromuscular junction (myasthenia gravis)
Metabolic	Acute to subacute confusion as in hepatic encephalopathy
Iatrogenic	Toxic medication-related neuropathy as in chemotherapy-related side effects upon peripheral nerve (e.g., vincristine neuropathy)
Neoplastic	Progressive decline with headache and possible seizure activity over weeks due to primary brain tumor, for example
Degenerative	Progressive cognitive decline over many months due to early onset Alzheimer's disease or motor neuron degeneration, for example [amyotrophic lateral sclerosis (ALS)]
Demyelinating	Acute to subacute symptoms in young adult due to optic neuritis in combination with bladder dysfunction would suggest multiple sclerosis
Deficiencies	Progressive cognitive memory decline over many months may relate to symptomatic vitamin B12 deficiency
Epileptogenic	Acute sudden cognitive change due to complex partial seizure
Familial	Familial epilepsy may be related to inherited defects in sodium and/or calcium channels, for example, with chronic time course typical for many inherited disorders

This text is organized by first presenting basic science aspects regarding the functioning of individual neurons and glia, and discusses the molecular basis of disease at the level of DNA transcription and RNA translation. By approaching neurology on a molecular basis, the clinical aspects become more apparent and provide the reader tools to understand new and different disease as they emerge and become identifiable as distinct new neurologic problems (https://www.youtube.com/watch?v=tGr9cacEKKk) [1].

1.2.1.1 Formulation of a Diagnosis

Defining *Time* (acute versus chronic) and *Space* (focal versus diffuse) to formulate Etiologic Classifications of Diagnostic Possibilities.

The basic structure to the individual nerve cell is similar to the basic structure of the nervous system, where axonal extensions from the brain are clustered in axial cylindrical arrangement (the spinal cord) with secondary effectors branching out to the periphery in the form of spinal motor neuron axons that reach out to innervate skeletal muscle. This functional unit can become dysfunctional through various mechanisms that operate in time and space as either acute, subacute or chronic, or focal, multifocal or diffuse as shown in Table 1.1.

1.3 Systematic Approach to Neurological Problems

The first aspect of care deals with obtaining and accurate history and examination. The initial visit with the patient is critical to formulating an accurate diagnosis and all collateral history needs to be obtained from family and any other witnesses to events or problems. The neurologist needs to carefully weigh all available information as to the accuracy of the information—sometimes there is very little, such as an emergency case in the ICU of a patient brought in by EMS (emergency medical services) unconscious. By sorting clinical problems in time (acute versus chronic) and space (focal versus diffuse), an accurate diagnosis can then be formulated. For example, an acute focal deficit in an 80-year-old is typical for an acute stroke event, whereas an acute focal deficit in an otherwise healthy 20-year-old would still leave stroke in the differential but other possibilities such as demyelinating disease for new onset of MS would need to be considered. The clinician needs to constantly question, "what is the worse that this could be?"—it would be devastating to miss a stroke in a 20-year-old, and therefore a prompt and comprehensive evaluation is needed.

At the turn of the century, there was little that the clinician could do other than rely upon clinical skills and correlation with pathologic findings—a master of this process with great skill in advancing the science and art of medicine at the time is exemplified by Williams Osler making rounds, trying to come to a conclusion based on history and examination (see Fig. 1.7).

Osler developed a systematic approach to the science of clinical diagnosis—the picture of him below illustrates the final step of the process as the clinician weighs all available existing evidence to form a conclusion about the nature of the illness at hand—at the turn of the twentieth century, when these photos were taken, there was little else he could rely on other his own clinical skills to formulate a diagnosis; he would be amazed with what is available today with incredible imaging technology and sophisticated lab technology.

A famous quote from Dr. Osler is also noted (Fig. 1.8):

> *"I desire no other epitaph … than the statement that I taught medical students in the wards, as I regard this as by far the most useful and important work I have been called upon to do."*

A systematic approach is needed when dealing with something as complicated as the nervous system. A fundamental first question to ask when presented with a clinical problem, is whether this actually represents a primary disease of the nervous system?

For example, consider the case of 55-year-old with a history of depression, who presents with progressive cognitive difficulty and social withdrawal; the patient not only reports short-term memory loss but also shows recall deficits on examination. Does this patient have a neurological illness, or simply pseudo-dementia due to untreated depression? It is up to the physician to explore all possibilities and understand missing

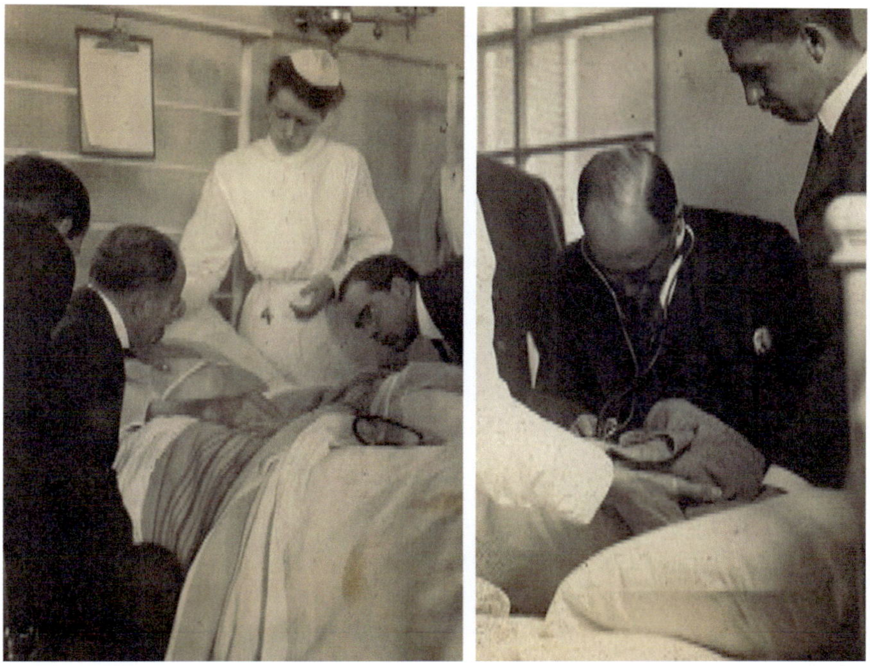

Fig. 1.7 Williams Osler making rounds, trying to come to a conclusion based on history and examination. With permission William Osler Photo Collection McGill University, Montreal, Quebec

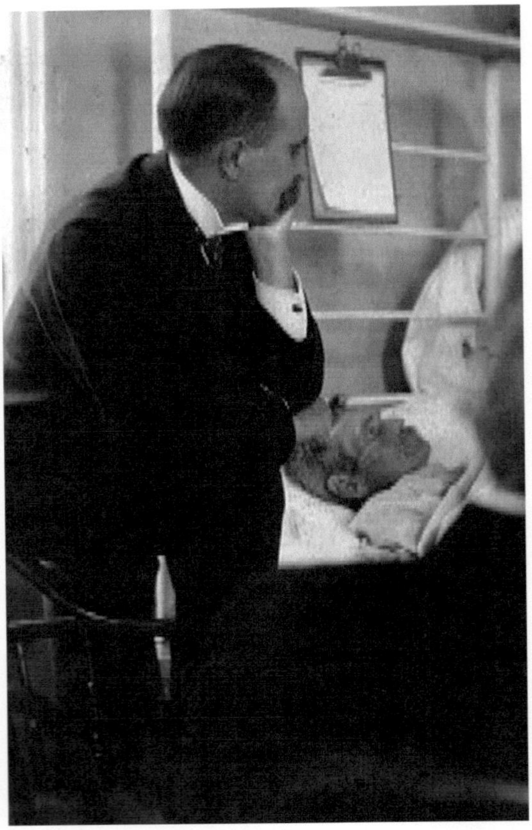

Fig. 1.8 Dr. William Osler. With permission William Osler Photo Collection McGill University, Montreal, Quebec

pieces of the puzzle that could solve the case … . a progressive cognitive decline could reflect a neurodegenerative illness in the absence of infection or neoplasm—therefore, information about the family history could be crucial in forming an accurate impression and formulation of a sensible diagnostic plan. For example, a positive history of symptoms consistent with unrecognized premature neurodegenerative illness in parents and siblings, reflective of possible familial Alzheimer's disease or Parkinson's disease (PD) could heavily influence the diagnostic impression. Lesson: take a complete and accurate history from reliable historians (this often involves interviewing unaffected family members).

Another primary question is whether the problem is clearly based in the peripheral nervous system, or does it represent a central problem? In some cases, this may be obvious when clearly referable to the brain stem upwards to the level of the cerebral cortex (for example, consider the case of an acute visual cortex infarct producing a homonymous hemianopsia). However, not infrequently, clinicians may fail to identify the importance of an acute thoracic sensory level reflective of spinal cord pathology and instead misdiagnose new sensory and motor lower extremity deficits as being attributable to Guillain Barre syndrome (GBS) rather than spinal cord compression. In the opinion of the author, this specific type of confusion leading to misdiagnosis is unacceptably high, and leads to unacceptable complications for patients. Therefore, it is important to stress that non-focal relatively diffuse impairments affecting arms and legs simultaneously with non-focal bilateral deficits which ascend and progress from distal to proximal aspect most likely suggests a peripheral nervous system problem such as GBS. Alternatively, a sharp and acute cutoff in light touch sensation circumferentially at T8, for example, in a newly ataxic patient with strong arms yet weak and numb legs clearly point to the spinal cord (emergent MRI is required in this case to evaluate cord compression at T8).

1.3.1 Diagnosis by Time and Space Factors (Table 1.2)

By defining some basic information including the age of the patient, and historical factors about the mode of onset of disease in time and space, the differential diagnosis can be ascertained fairly easily.

1.3.1.1 Clinical Examples Using the Age, Time, and Space Algorithm Approach

Sudden onset of arm weakness in 80-year-old male will have a much different set of possibilities than those of a young adult: Stroke would be more likely in the elderly, where sudden deficits in the young do not rule this out, but makes it more unlikely—the possibility of demyelinating disease needs to be considered as well. An interruption of blood flow to the motor cortex via the

Table 1.2 Neurological diagnosis by time and space characteristics

	Acute (vascular, infective, traumatic)[a]	Subacute (autoimmune, neoplastic, demyelinating)[a]	Chronic (degenerative, metabolic, toxic)[a]
Focal	Stroke	Demyelinating	Degenerative (PD)
Multifocal	Emboli	Demyelinating (MS)	Degenerative
		Metastatic disease	
Diffuse	SAH	Meningitis, GBS	Metabolic defects
			Toxins

[a]Classification by etiology; *GBS* Guillain Barre syndrome, *SAH* subarachnoid hemorrhage, *MS* multiple sclerosis, *PD* Parkinson's disease

middle cerebral artery will reliably produce ischemic dysfunction of the pyramidal neurons; these nerve cell project long fibers through the internal capsule, which decussate in the lower brain stem, and wind up on the contralateral aspect of the spinal cord as the corticospinal tract. These fibers descend upon the spinal motor neurons, which innervate skeletal muscle of limb function.

Slow progression of gait impairment in the elderly likewise will have a much different differential diagnosis than a young individual as well: normal pressure hydrocephalus and other age-related degenerative conditions affecting the spinal canal at cervical and/or thoracic levels are not problems of young individuals. The differential diagnosis for a slow cognitive decline in an elderly individual is much different than that seen in a child for instance, where leukodystrophy of childhood would be considered (examples include Krabbe and metachromatic leukodystophy).

1.3.2 Diagnosis: Signs and Symptoms

Neurologic diagnosis is based on the synthesis of historical information with observation of clinical signs coupled with specific symptoms obtained from the history. Obtaining an accurate history is of critical importance, and often needs to be obtained from multiple sources aside from the patient—in some cases it is the history which makes the entire diagnosis. A patient with marginal cognitive abilities may insist to you that in retrospect they feel that the persistent ataxia for which you are now evaluating had a sudden stroke-like onset 4 months prior, but upon interviewing family members, they may all confirm in consensus fashion that this is not true at all, but in fact represented an insidious onset with a slow and gradual progression of unsteadiness in gait and coordination. All aspects of the history often need independent confirmation; the list of current medications as relayed by the patient may in fact be different from you later find by calling the patient's pharmacy, which may confirm no filling of medications for many months. Noncompliance with seizure medication, for example, is a critically important problem to recognize, as many seizure patients will not admit to noncompliance and will avoid disclosing any responsibility for their recurrent seizure for many reasons. To enhance accuracy of diagnosis, accompanying family members and significant others should be included for the history and exam, provided the patient has no objections to this.

Family history is important for many conditions that could be explained on a hereditary basis; event for routine headache cases, all patients need to be asked about a family history for brain aneurysm, especially due to the fact the a positive family history raises the risk for the patient beyond the standard 2% prevalence rate for aneurysm.

With regard to acute stroke evaluations, the history of events over the preceding 12–24 h is of critical importance in establishing the time the patient was last known to be normal, as the window for treatment with IV tPA is only 180 min from witnessed onset or the time at which the acute stroke patient was last known to be normal [recent European trial data suggests that the window for efficacy may be out to the 4.5 h time interval; IV tPA for acute stroke treatment is

Food and Drug Administration (FDA) approved in the USA for the 180 min time window only, and not more than this].

The neurological exam can be a stressful event for the patient, and for this reason and for patient comfort it is acceptable by many practitioners to conduct the examination of the patient in their regular street clothes. It is only the occasional patient with a peripheral neuropathy or a potential amyotrophic lateral sclerosis (ALS) patient that is required to wear a hospital gown so that peripheral sensory exams can be made in detail, or that fasciculation in one or more motor groups can be more accurately assessed and visualized.

There is much mystery surrounding the neurological exam, but its essential components can be broken down in the basic elements as follows:

General appearance: older than stated age? Healthy or ill-appearing?

Mental status exam: orientation, short- and long-term recall, clock construction

Cranial nerves: look for inequalities

ENT exam: important to detail with regard to cranial nerve dysfunction

Neurovascular exam: BP (blood pressure), HR (heart rate), and auscultation for bruits and/or murmurs

Cerebellar exam: check for signs of nystagmus, ataxia, incoordination

Motor and Sensory exam of Upper extremity (*UE*)/*Lower extremity* (*LE*): look for asymmetries

Reflexes: hyper-reflexia? versus true loss of deep tendon reflexes (DTRs) as in GBS

1.3.3 Organizational Overview of the Text

The outline for the text includes key case examples that are chosen to illustrate pathophysiologic principles within clinical neuroscience:

1.3.3.1 Forming a Diagnosis: Acute Versus Chronic, Focal Versus Diffuse

- The basic unit of the nervous system: basic principles with clinical correlates
- Basic symptoms reflecting neuronal dysfunction: e.g., headache, radicular pain
- Signs of neurological disease: seizure, deficits in strength, sensation, balance

1.3.3.2 Examples of Disease Affecting Fundamental Units of Neurologic Functioning

- Neuronal degeneration: ALS, PD
- Astrocytic neoplastic proliferation: primary brain tumors
- Oligodendroglial inflammatory demyelination: MS
- Thrombotic occlusion of arterial vasculature: acute stroke
- Thrombotic occlusion of venous channels: sagittal sinus occlusion
- Spontaneous hemorrhage: ICH versus SAH (subarachnoid hemorrhage)
- Hydrocephalus: NPH (normal pressure hydrocephalus)
- Diffuse hypoxia or anoxia: brain death

1.3.3.3 An Incremental Segmental Approach to the Central Versus Peripheral Nervous System

Clinical Examples of Disease at Each Anatomic Level

- Muscle disease: myasthenia gravis, muscular dystrophy
- Peripheral nerve: GBS, chemotherapy-related neuropathy, neurofibromas
- Spinal cord: cord compression, transverse myelitis, ALS
- Brain stem: acute infarction, cavernoma, CPM (central pontine myelinolysis)
- Cerebellum: cerebellar degeneration; Chiari malformation
- Mid-brain (mesencephalon): PD
- Hypothalamus: hamartoma, VMH (ventromedial hypothalamus) versus LH (lateral hypothalamus) lesion
- Pituitary: functioning adenoma with gigantism
- Thalamus: anterior nucleus of thalamus infarct with memory impairment
- Pineal: pineal tumor, pineal cyst

- Hippocampus: memory dysfunction, complex-partial seizure activity
- Temporal lobe: epilepsy, Alzheimer's disease
- Occipital lobe: blindness, visual neglect
- Frontal lobe: Pick's disease
- Ventricles: normal pressure hydrocephalus

1.3.4 Neurologic Disease Is Very Prevalent

Neurological disease is tragic—for many of the disorders we see in neurology, there is no treatment or cure—what can be done to treat these tragic conditions? A firm foundation in understanding brain pathophysiology at the molecular level is essential as it forms the foundation for recognition of proper diagnosis and treatment of the illness. The volume of neurologic disease in the world today is staggering—in the USA alone, stroke occurs every 40 s! The incidence and prevalence numbers for other disease states are outlined below:

1.3.5 Data for USA in 2005

1.3.5.1 Prevalence

Migraine	35,461,000 m/f=0.4 (ages 12–65 years)
Cerebral palsy	207,000 for children under 21
Prevalence of epilepsy all ages	2,098,00 m/f=1 all ages
MS	266,000 m/f=0.5 all ages
ALS	12,000 m/f=1.3 all ages
Stroke	2,956,000 all ages
Alzheimer's	2,459,000 (>65 years)
PD	349,000 (>65 years)

1.3.5.2 Incidence [2]

Epilepsy	142,000
MS	12,000
Traumatic brain injury	298,000
Spinal cord injury	13,000
ALS	5000
Stroke	541,000 all ages
	401,000≥65
Alzheimer's	468,000≥65
PD	59,000≥65

1.3.6 Neurological Emergencies (Table 1.3)

Rapid yet accurate diagnostic skills are required not only for evaluating patients in the Emergency Department but also in the clinic as sometimes emergent problems present in the outpatient setting as well in the clinic. For example, GBS might present as a progression of gait instability with weakness over a few days time span; similarly, a warning leak event to an aneurismal event might present as a history of a recent severe headache, and so the clinician must be astutely aware of all possibilities (Table 1.4).

Case Example: The Complexity of Neurological Disease and Diagnosis

Neurologic disease within the central nervous system (CNS) may arise from central complications of a primary medical illness such as the relatively uncommon dilemma of sarcoidosis (see below).

In evaluating the cause of progressive cognitive decline with repeated seizures in a 34-year-old, exploring uncertain clues become important when there is limited information. The patient at first gave an unclear vague history of a skin

Table 1.3 Neurologic emergencies: cause and example

Cause	Example
Vascular	Middle cerebral artery (MCA) infarction
	Subarachnoid hemorrhage (SAH)
Infection	Meningitis
	Encephalitis
Trauma	Subdural
	Cord contusion
Metabolic	DKA
	Low Na
Neoplastic	Cord compression
Drugs	Benzodiazepines
Demyelinating	Guillain Barre syndrome (GBS)

Table 1.4 Neurologic emergencies

- Infections: bacterial meningitis, herpes encephalitis
- Compression of the brain or spinal cord by hematoma, abscess, tumor; hydrocephalus
- Massive infarction with edema, compression, and destruction of vital areas
- Uncontrolled seizures: status epilepticus

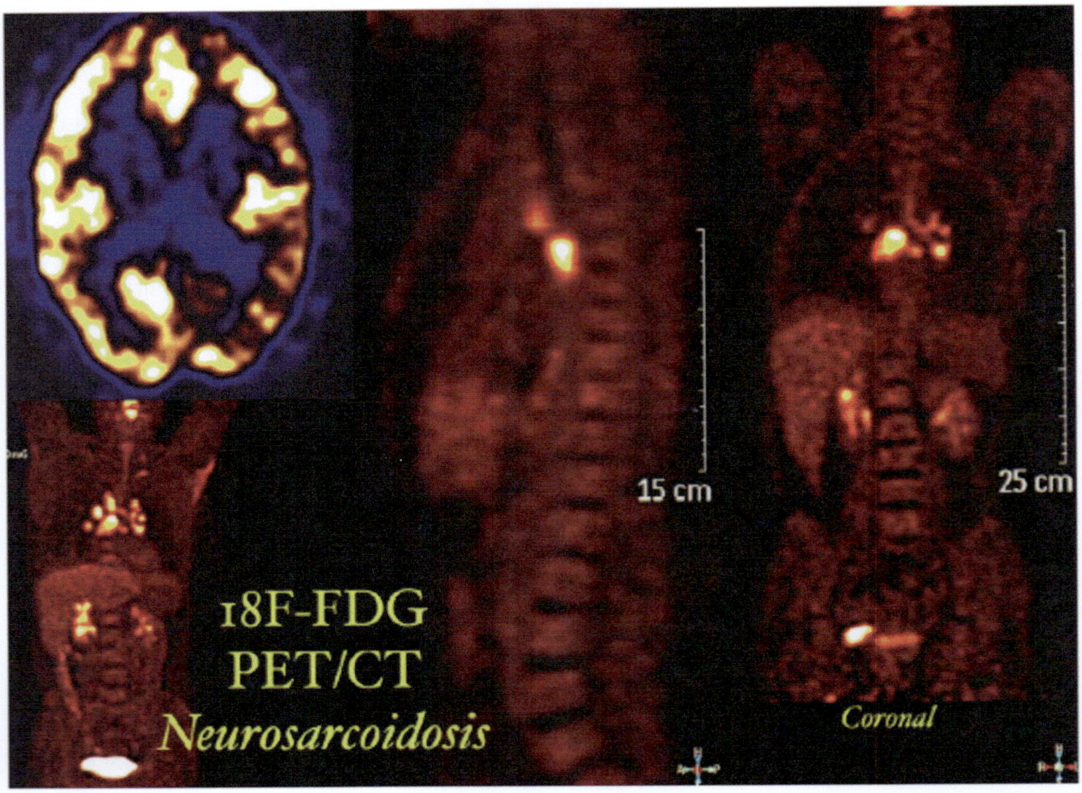

Fig. 1.9 18F-FDG imaging of CNS involvement by sarcoidosis with symptoms being acute, recurrent, and multifocal. © 2014 by Michael Meyer, MD

biopsy at age 20, which only later was found to represent a major clue to the puzzle, as it reflected the initial stages of sarcoidosis that became systemic as seen by PET at the time of presenting with intractable seizure activity. At first, the patient gave only a minimal outline of her medical history—it was only through subsequent interview of her mother that led to the understanding about the prior skin biopsy and concern for sarcoid.

Poorly understood from a pathogenesis standpoint, it is felt that sarcoidosis represents a chronic granulomatous reaction against mycobacteria; although true for selected well-studied cases, most sarcoidosis cases are idiopathic.

Case Example
18F-Fluorodeoxyglucose (FDG) imaging of CNS involvement by sarcoidosis with symptoms being acute, recurrent, and multifocal (Fig. 1.9).

MRI composite shown in Fig. 1.10 for the same case discussed above regarding neurosarcoidosis; innumerable contrast enhancing foci are revealed in panel C and windowed threshold adjusted rendering in panel D.

The case illustrates the importance of obtaining a complete history and to search for all relevant clues such as the skin biopsy at age 20; incorporation of special imaging techniques such as PET provide a more powerful insight to the burden of disease.

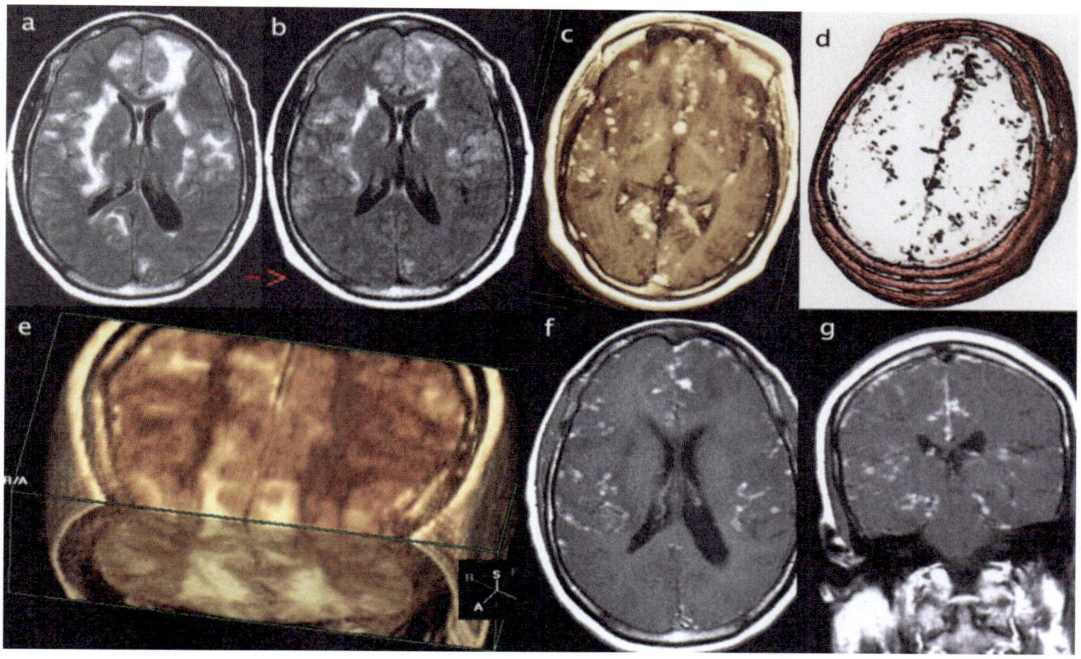

Fig. 1.10 MR imaging composite regarding neurosarcoidosis; innumerable contrast enhancing foci are revealed in panel C and windowed threshold adjusted rendering in panel D. © 2014 by Michael Meyer, MD

References

1. Neurological Diagnosis, MGMC Physician Grand Rounds 1/8/14, Selden Spencer, MD, Neurology. https://www.youtube.com/watch?v=tGr9cacEKKk. Published 8 Jan 2014.
2. Hirtz D, Thurman DJ, Gwinn-Hardy K, Mohamed M, Chaudhuri AR, Zalutsky R. How common are the "common" neurologic disorders? Neurology. 2007;68(5):326–37.

2 Cellular and Subcellular Elements of the Nervous System

A complete understanding of the structural and functional aspects to the brain at the cellular and subcellular level is needed to form links to clinical disease pathophysiology. For example, to understand the biology and pathophysiology of Parkinson's disease, it is important to understand the molecular aspects of the dopaminergic synapse. To understand Alzheimer's disease and related neurodegenerative illnesses such as ALS, an appreciation for the neuronal cytoskeleton is needed as well as to understand how disruption of axonal transport mechanisms can result in clinical disease, as shown on successive pages below. A central theme and approach is to therefore link the basic science of neuronal physiology and anatomy on a cellular level to help explain what is going on clinically.

Whereas glial cells are multipolar with diffusely radiating processes, vertebrate neurons are highly polarized into proximal dendritic trees, and distal axonal processes that give rise to synaptic contacts, as shown in Fig. 2.1 (invertebrate neurons are unipolar and lack dendrites).

Figure 2.1 emphasizes the central control aspect of genetic factors within DNA in the nucleus. This illustration as well as Fig. 2.3 also shows nuclear pores embedded within the dual membrane nuclear envelope and mediate the import and export of key signaling compounds as well as RNA and ribosomal proteins that shuttle across the nuclear pore complex. The average vertebrate cell has about 2000 nuclear pore complexes and can accomplish up to 1000 translocations every second. Cargo tagged by special nuclear localization signal (NLS) amino acid sequences have particularly efficient and selective transport into the nucleus (NLS example: PKKKRKV).

The most fundamental and central aspect that determines cellular functioning is DNA coiled within the nucleus. Minor defects in the sequence of DNA base pairs can give rise to tragic illnesses such as Duchenne muscular dystrophy or Huntington's disease (HD), as shown in the example summary (Fig. 2.2) with other genetically defined nervous system diseases listed including ALS (in certain cases only—most sporadic cases of ALS have no gene defect identified) and the very rare DRPLA.

Maintaining circulation is vital to neuronal health and involves not only circulation of oxygenated blood on a cellular capillary level, but also involves circulation of key proteins and organelles up and down the axon via the processes of slow and fast axonal transport. Exchange of glutamate versus glutamine occurs between neuron and glia as well, with neurons shuttling information in the form of neurotransmitter release mediated chemical activation at the synapse. A major form of circulation is in the form of cerebrospinal fluid that literally keeps the brain afloat within the cranial vault and is buoyant in a suspended form; this vital fluid is produced inside the ventricular cavities within choroid plexus and flows from one chamber into

M.A. Meyer, *Neurologic Disease*, DOI 10.1007/978-3-319-39581-4_2

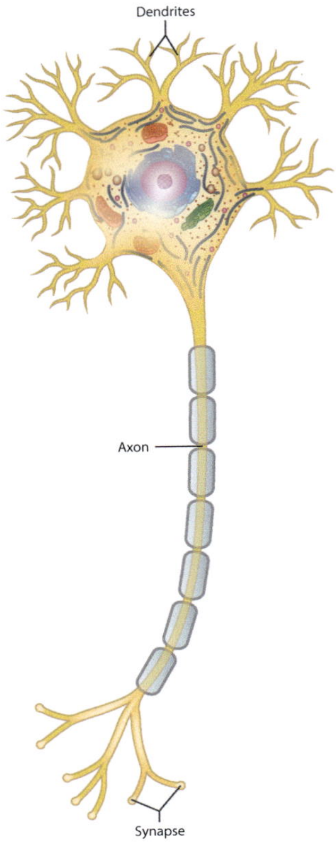

Fig. 2.1 The vertebrate neuron is highly polarized into proximal dendrites, with singular distal axonal processes that arborizes and give rise to synaptic contacts

the other (lateral ventricles into the central third ventricle and then into the midline central fourth ventricle).

With regard to this concept of intracellular circulation, a fundamental principle of neuronal function relates to the neuronal cytoskeleton shown in Fig. 2.3, which provides the framework for delivery of key proteins and organelles that shuttle back and forth along the microtubule system within the cell; disruption at any point can be deadly, with disruption of axonal transport being especially problematic as it isolates the cell body from its synaptic terminals.

Neurofilaments (NFs) are intermediate filaments within nerve cells that provide structural support for the neuronal cytoskeleton and can contain three types of subunits: neurofilament light chain (NF-L), medium chain (NF-M), and heavy chain (NF-H).

Neurofilaments assemble with neuronal cell bodies and then are shipped out down the axon via slow transport mechanisms along microtubules, at rates as fast as 2 cm per week. In actuality, this represents the net effect of an erratic stop and go pattern that at times is actually bidirectional, and sometimes rapid interspersed with periods of long pauses [1].

Fig. 2.2 Defects in the sequence of DNA base pairs can give rise to tragic neurologic illnesses such as Duchenne muscular dystrophy or Huntington's disease (HD). DNA encoding of neurological diseases: dystrophin gene deletions: Duchenne muscular dystrophy; SMN_1 gene deletion: spinal muscular atrophy; SOD_1 mutation: Familial ALS; Heavy neurofilament gene mutation: ALS; Huntington CAG expansion: HD; Atrophin CAG expansion: DRPLA

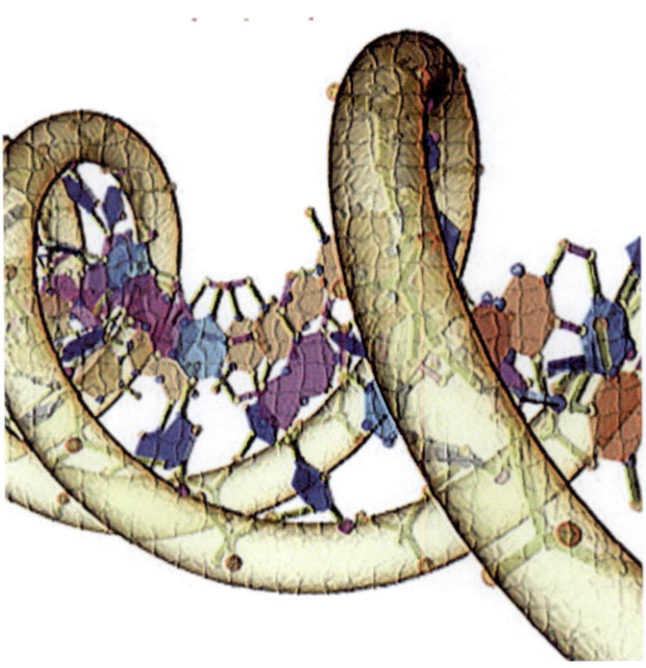

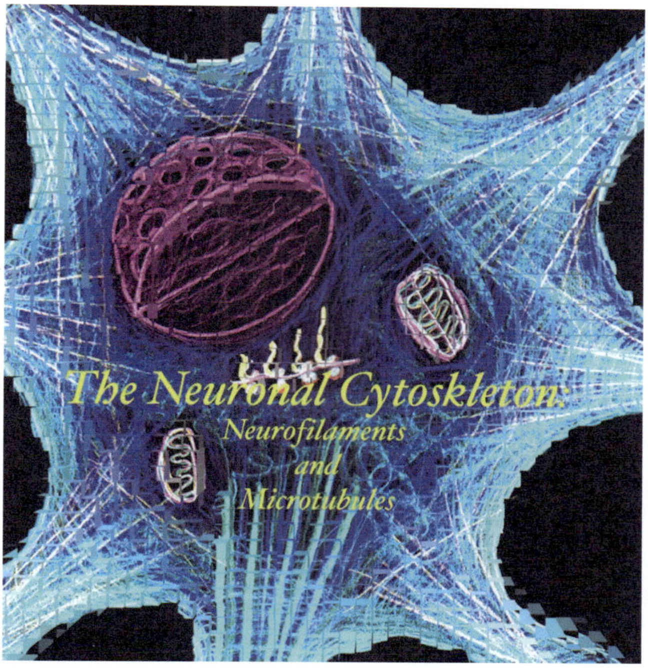

Fig. 2.3 The neuronal cytoskeleton provides the framework for delivery of key proteins and organelles that shuttle back and forth along the microtubule system within the cell

Defects in the transport mechanism and/or the genetic encoding of the neurofilament subunits may lead to pathologic neurofilament aggregations and induce neurodegenerative diseases, including ALS, where genetic defects in NF-H have been found.

Many illnesses have cytoskeletal disruptions at the microtubule level as a key aspect, including Alzheimer's disease where the microtubule framework falls apart due to alterations in the microtubule-associated protein Tau (see Fig. 2.4).

In general, one type of microtubule-associated protein is found only within the dendrites (MAP2) whereas the other type, associated with Alzheimer disease when phosphorylated (tau) is found only in the axon in healthy brain tissue (abnormally phosphorylated pathologic types of tau protein may be found in degenerative conditions within dendrites as well).

The microtubule motor proteins kinesin and dynein have polarity with respect to providing anterograde transport of kinesin bound proteins, filaments, and organelles from the cell body down the axon to the synapse, and up the reverse retrograde direction towards the cell body for dynein (see Fig. 2.5).

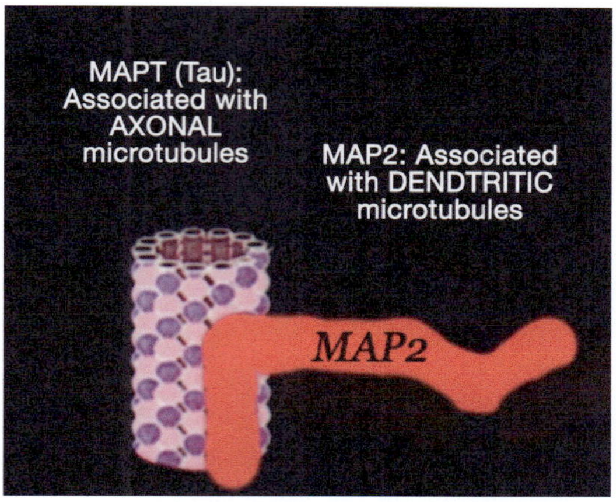

Fig. 2.4 In general, one type of microtubule-associated protein is found only within the dendrites (MAP2) whereas the other type, Tau, is found only in the axon in healthy brain tissue

Integrity of the microtubule system is critical for these transport processes to take place; the differences between slow and fast transport is summarized in Table 2.1.

In diseases such as Alzheimer's where the microtubule system has fallen apart due to mutations in the microtubule-associated protein Tau,

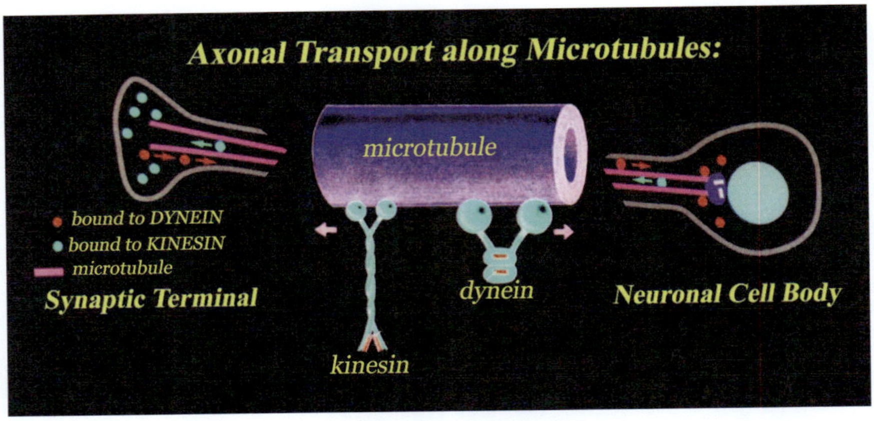

Fig. 2.5 Anterograde transport of kinesin bound proteins, filaments, and organelles travel from the cell body down the axon to the synapse

Table 2.1 Summary showing the differences between fast versus slow anterograde axonal transport

Fast transport rates are measured as high as 400 mm per day in sciatic nerve	Slow transport rates are usually found to be 1–5 mm per day
Fast transport is mainly for elements related to synaptic transmission and neurotransmitter vesicles	Slow transport is not significantly affected by colchicine
Microtubules mediate fast transport	Microtubule protein, enzymes, and mitochondria can travel slow route

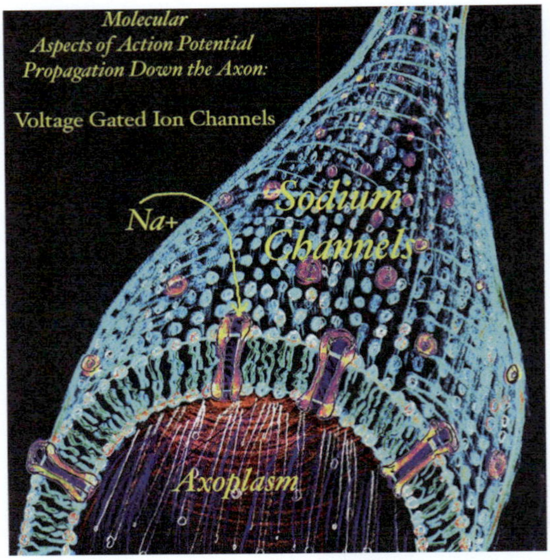

Fig. 2.6 Influx of extracellular sodium across voltage-gated channels is a key first step in propagating an electrical nerve impulse

the vital transport link between the nerve cell body and synaptic targets is lost.

With regard to the circulation of electrical impulses and flow of ions across channels embedded within axonal membranes, it is important to examine the key role played in this process by sodium channels in health and disease (see Fig. 2.6).

Using the squid giant axon for research on the basis of neural action potentials, it has been established since the 1950s that influx of extracellular sodium across voltage-gated channels is a key first step in propagating an electrical nerve impulse, followed by conductance changes for the efflux of intracellular potassium across separate and distinct channel protein complexes that are voltage sensitive; the process completes itself with local repolarization after sodium channel inactivation takes place. Much of the knowledge about sodium currents across nerve membranes can be attributed to the use of selective channel blockers in squid axon studies, such as the puffer fish poison tetrodotoxin that binds to the extracellular portions of the sodium channel, and thereby cause fatal blockade of neural impulse conduction.

Recent research has disclosed a key link between sodium channel defects and neurologic diseases with special reference to epilepsy [2].

Although 40 % of seizure disorders have no obvious cause, most of these are likely due to genetic mutations, possibly within transmitter receptors or within axonal conductance channels.

Voltage-gated sodium channel gene mutations are now known to cause multiple types of seizure disorders including GEFS+ (genetic generalized epilepsy with febrile seizures Plus) and the Dravet syndrome (severe myoclonic epilepsy of infancy).

Whereas GEFS+ is linked to a missense mutation that alters sodium channel properties, the catastrophic Dravet syndrome is due to a loss of function, with status epilepticus occurring by about 6 months.

Most of these epileptic sodium channel gene mutations occur in the *SCN1A* gene, with patterns of dominant inheritance.

A key point of communication between one nerve cell and the other is the synaptic juncture, where the axonal impulse terminates to induce an influx of calcium on the presynaptic side, causing synaptic vesicles to fuse with presynaptic membrane leading to transmitter release across the synaptic cleft with activation of postsynaptic receptors. The drawing in Fig. 2.7 and electron micrograph in Fig. 2.8, both by the author, illustrate the structure of a chemical synapse with synaptic vesicles containing quanta of neurotransmitter chemical, to be distinguished by the less common but more immediate contact known as the electrical synapse (gap junction structure to permit further spread of a depolarizing impulse to the next cell).

The structure of the synaptic juncture is basically the same, whether it is sampled from a human patient as part of a diagnostic brain biopsy for encephalitis (Fig. 2.9) or from a mouse (Fig. 2.10); what is unique to humans is the vast

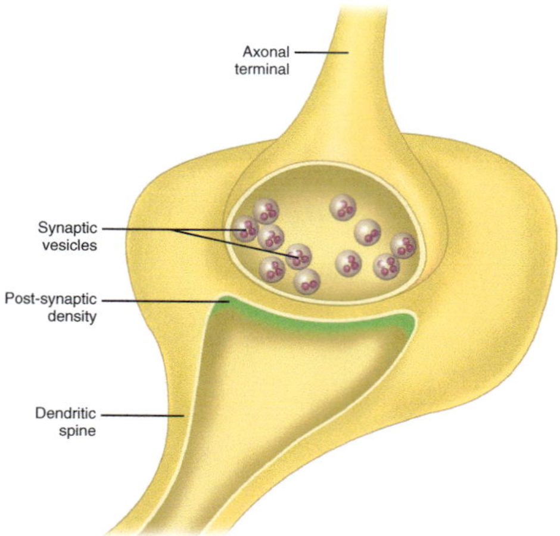

Fig. 2.7 The synaptic juncture, where the axonal impulse terminates to induce an influx of calcium on the presynaptic side, causing synaptic vesicles to fuse with presynaptic membrane

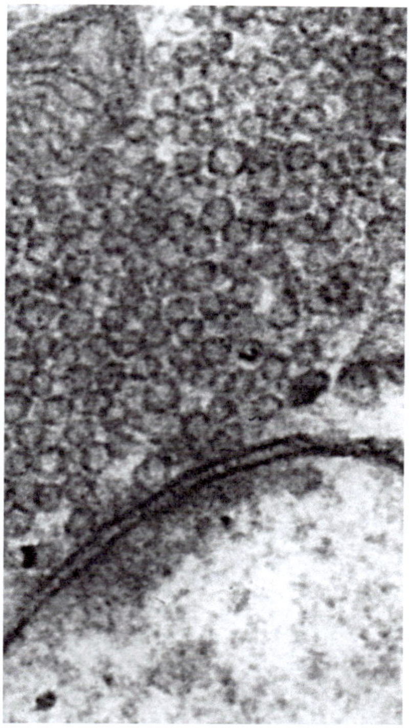

Fig. 2.8 Electron micrograph of a synapse within the mouse brain

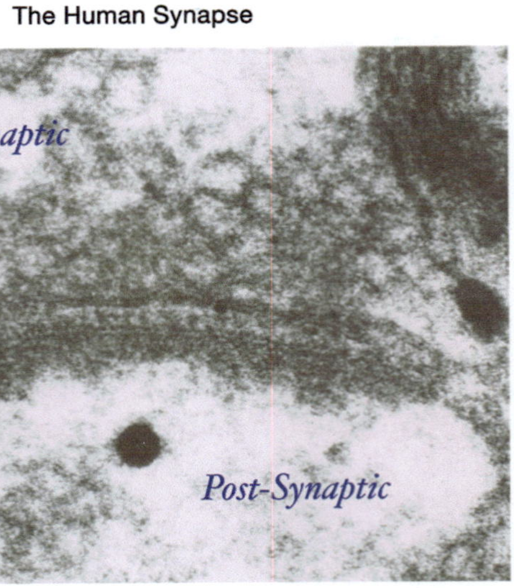

Fig. 2.9 Electron micrograph of a synaptic juncture sampled from a human patient as part of a diagnostic brain biopsy for encephalitis

number of synapses (150 trillion for the human neocortex alone) as well as the greater capability to form dendritic spines that may be linked to learning and memory through enhanced synaptic contacts. Interestingly, the density of synaptic contacts in the brains of rodents and humans is more or less constant at around 1100–1300 million/mm^3 [3].

Studies with animals show that stimulating environments and memory tasks produce greater densities of deep invaginating presynaptic contacts surrounded and encircled by the postsynaptic membrane in the form of well-developed dendritic spines (see Fig. 2.10, for example).

The electron micrograph by the author in Fig. 2.10 reveals the structure of a dendritic spine that forms a more direct contact with presynaptic structures that surround the invaginating postsynaptic finger-like projection. It is believed that neuronal plasticity of the synapse is linked to the growth of dendritic spines; spine formation and morphology are linked to the process of learning and memory.

Although multiple types of chemical synapses exist within the brain, and include transmitter

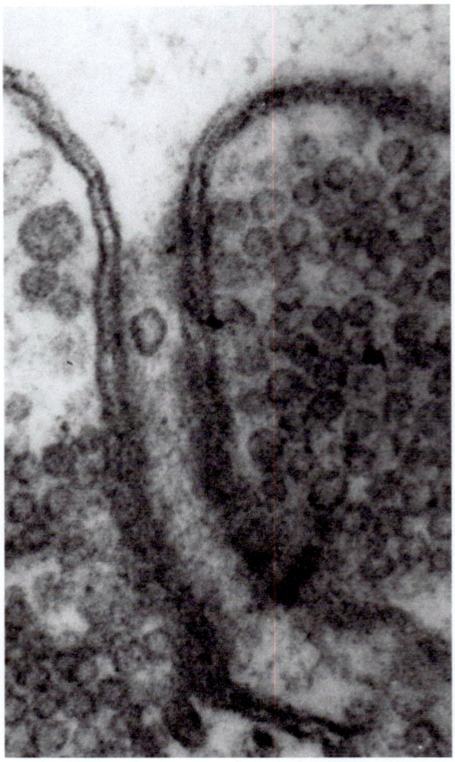

Fig. 2.10 Electron micrograph of a dendritic spine synapse

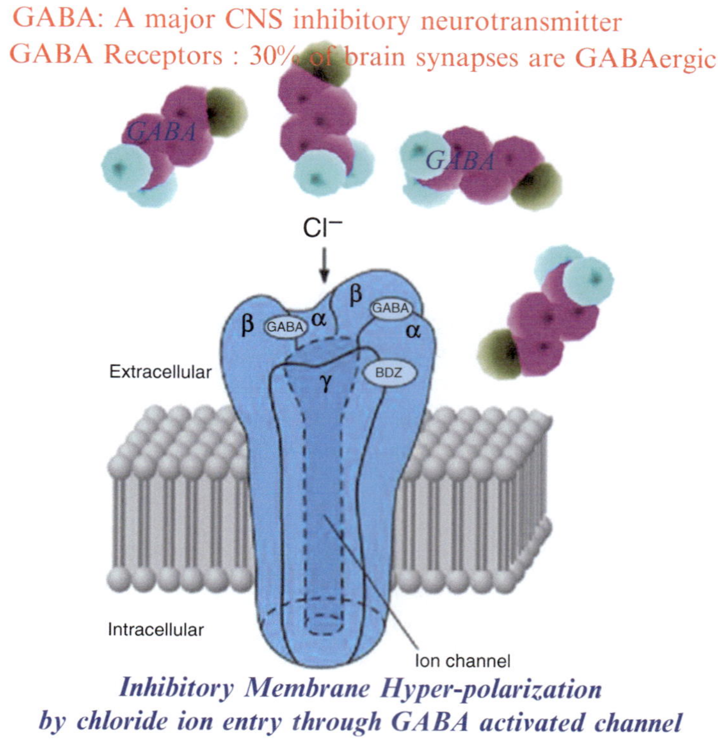

Fig. 2.11 Synapse for GABA (gamma amino butyric acid), which generates hyperpolarization of the postsynaptic terminal, thereby inducing inhibition

release specific for dopamine, or serotonin, or acetylcholine, for example, a particularly important synapse is for GABA (gamma amino butyric acid), which generates hyperpolarization of the postsynaptic terminal, thereby inducing inhibition (see Fig. 2.11).

About one-third of all synapses within the brain rely on GABA as the neurotransmitter, which mediates inhibition through the intracellular influx of chloride ions. Focal lack of synaptic inhibition from loss of GABAergic nerve terminals can predispose the region to become epileptogenic, as seen in postinfarction seizures that arise at the borderzone rim of tissue that straddles healthy fully innervated brain tissue and chronic encephalomalacia comprising dead scar tissue from an old infarct. By emergent administration of benzodiazepines to such a patient experiencing a seizure, the excessive electrical firing can be reduced through this inhibitory mechanism, as the GABA channel is a multimeric complex with multiple subunits, one of which has a specific binding affinity for benzodiazepine compounds.

GABAergic synapses can be visualized in health and disease by PET imaging of 11C labeled flumazenil; whereas diminished receptor density has been found by PET imaging of epileptogenic foci, normal GABA receptor density has been found in Alzheimer's disease [4].

Glial cells play important nutritive and supportive roles for neuronal function, which is entirely dependent on intact perfusion at the capillary level as shown below in Fig. 2.12.

As illustrated in Fig. 2.12, Glial cells are anatomically interposed between capillaries and neurons, and play important supportive roles for neuronal functioning.

From an evolutionary perspective, glial cells are more highly developed within the human brain than other mammals. For example, with regard to brain weights and glia–neuron ratios for layer II/III of prefrontal cortical area 9 L, the cotton-top tamarin (*Saguinus oedipus*) is a small New World monkey with a brain weight of only 10 g with a glia-to-neuron ratio of 0.446 versus 1.21 for the gorilla's 509 g brain; the 1373 g human brain is at the top of the evolutionary ladder with the highest glia-to-neuron ratio of 1.65 [5].

Human protoplasmic astrocytes have volumes that are 27 times greater than those found in the mouse brain, which enables the human protoplasmic astrocyte to contact and surround two million synapses versus only 100,000 synapses being contacted and covered by the same type of glial cell in mice [6].

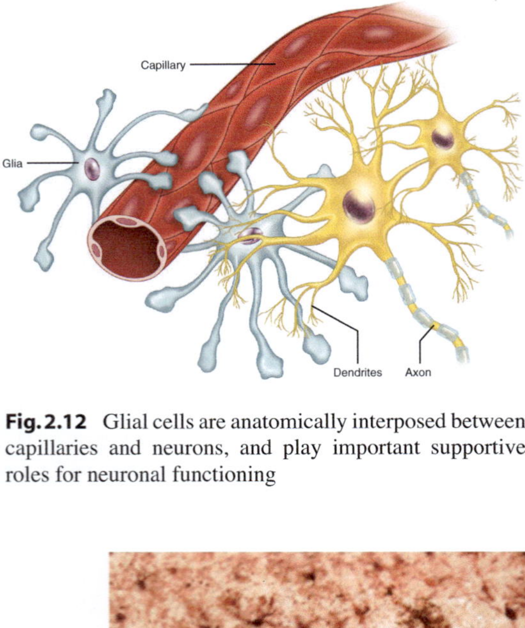

Fig. 2.12 Glial cells are anatomically interposed between capillaries and neurons, and play important supportive roles for neuronal functioning

One study on the cytologic aspects of the brain of Albert Einstein revealed higher glia-to-neuron ratios for cerebral cortex area 39 [7].

Recently, a unique type of astroglia has been found only in humans and certain primates known as the interlaminar astrocytes and polarized astrocytes; these specialized glia are absent from the brains of other species; intralaminar astrocytes are thought to be linked to information transfer between cortical layers [8].

With regard to information transfer between glia, it is important to note that glia show widespread expression for connexin proteins, which comprise gap junctions; 11 different connexin proteins have been found within the brain. Connexins have also been linked to the propagating waves of astrocytic intercellular calcium waves underlying the phenomenon of spreading depression, which moves across the cortex in both epileptiform and migrainous events [9].

Interconnection of glia via gap junctions allows for rapid and widespread sharing of information about the metabolic and ionic aspects of the extracellular environment.

Glia have specific biochemical specializations; for example, as shown in Fig. 2.13, the natural angiogenesis inhibitor thrombospondin 2 is selectively expressed within protoplasmic astrocytes; recent studies show that thrombos-

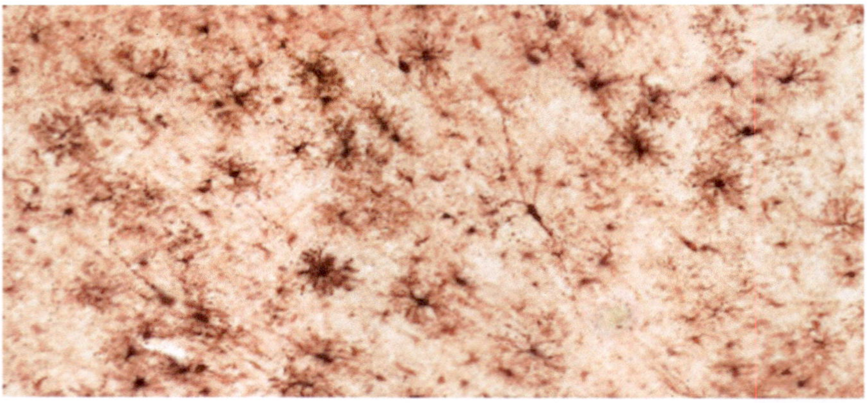

Fig. 2.13 Normal astrocyte morphology: Thrombospondin 2. Thrombospondin 2 is selectively expressed within protoplasmic astrocytes. Human gene map locus 6q27. THBS2 is a potent endogenous inhibitor of tumor growth and angiogenesis

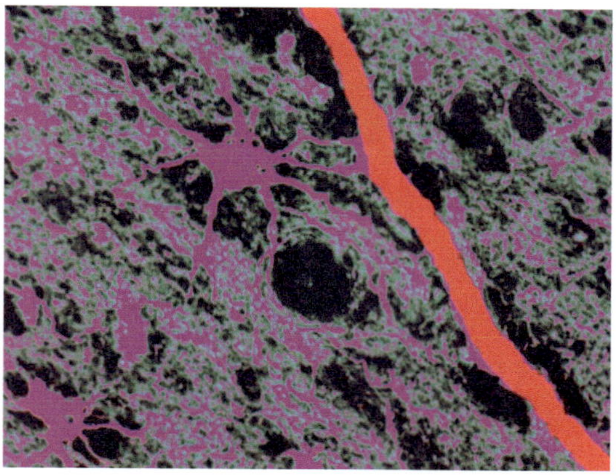

Fig. 2.14 The key nutrient role played protoplasmic astrocytes (*purple*) is illustrated in relation to end-feet processes that adhere to the walls of local capillaries (*red*)

pondins promote the formation of new synapses during development and in general act as key regulators of synaptogenesis in the central nervous system [10].

In Fig. 2.14, the key nutrient role played protoplasmic astrocytes (purple) is illustrated in relation to end-feet processes that adhere to the walls of local capillaries (red); initial absorption of nutrients needed the neuron takes place at the glia level initially, which passes this on to nearby neurons as needed; glucose is thought to shuttle across in this manner, with glia building limited supplies of glycogen in reserve as needed.

Whereas the cytoarchitecture of glial cell types remains constant throughout different regions of the brain, the shape and appearance of the neuron itself is characteristically and uniquely different for each region of the brain, as shown in the Fig. 2.15 composite.

Not only does the neuronal cytoarchitecture vary, the 18 F-FDG PET scan also illustrates significant metabolic heterogeneity for gray matter structures, with the cerebral cortex being far more active in utilizing glucose to support the activities of densely arborizing large pyramidal neurons, versus the relatively inactive globus pallidus that contains simpler, spindly neurons that have less rich arborizations.

Artistic renderings of the cytoarchitecture unique to cerebral cortex pyramidal neurons versus those found within the hippocampus is portrayed in Figs. 2.16 and 2.17, respectively.

Out of the 130 billion neurons present in the normal human brain, about 31 million are lost annually as part of normal aging, representing a small fraction of 0.024 % annually [11].

However, consider the extreme situation if they were all lost overnight, as shown in the tragic case example within Fig. 2.18 where major head trauma led to fatal surges in intracranial pressure leading to cessation of intracranial circulation with herniation and brain death; the dynamic PET scan revealed no flow and metabolism within the brain.

The normal whole body appearance on 18F-FDG PET scan studies at extreme left highlights the marked dependence the brain has on glucose metabolism relative to the rest of the body; any transient interruption as in the case of cardiac arrest can also lead to brain death despite successful resuscitation and restoration of circulation.

Successful efforts to minimize the damage is shown in Fig. 2.19 through the use of mild therapeutic hypothermia; by maintaining core temperature at 33 °C for 24 h after resuscitation from cardiac arrest, postanoxic brain injury can be minimized with many patients showing excellent outcomes when the loss of circulation is brief; the mechanism presumably relates to hypothermic inhibition of the endogenous unfolding of programmed cell death, otherwise known as apoptosis, where caspase 9 is a key factor in the cascade.

Programmed cell death, otherwise known as apoptosis, is an event common to both the birth and development of the nervous system as well as brain death after global hypoxia with prolonged interruption of cerebral blood flow. Figure 2.20 outlines the final steps of apoptosis, where the final executioner pathway driven by caspase 3 arises through astrocytic generation of caspase 8 through TNF alpha, versus neuronal mitochondrial release of cytochromes to generate caspase 9.

As shown in Fig. 2.21, development of the brain and spinal cord is a complex event.

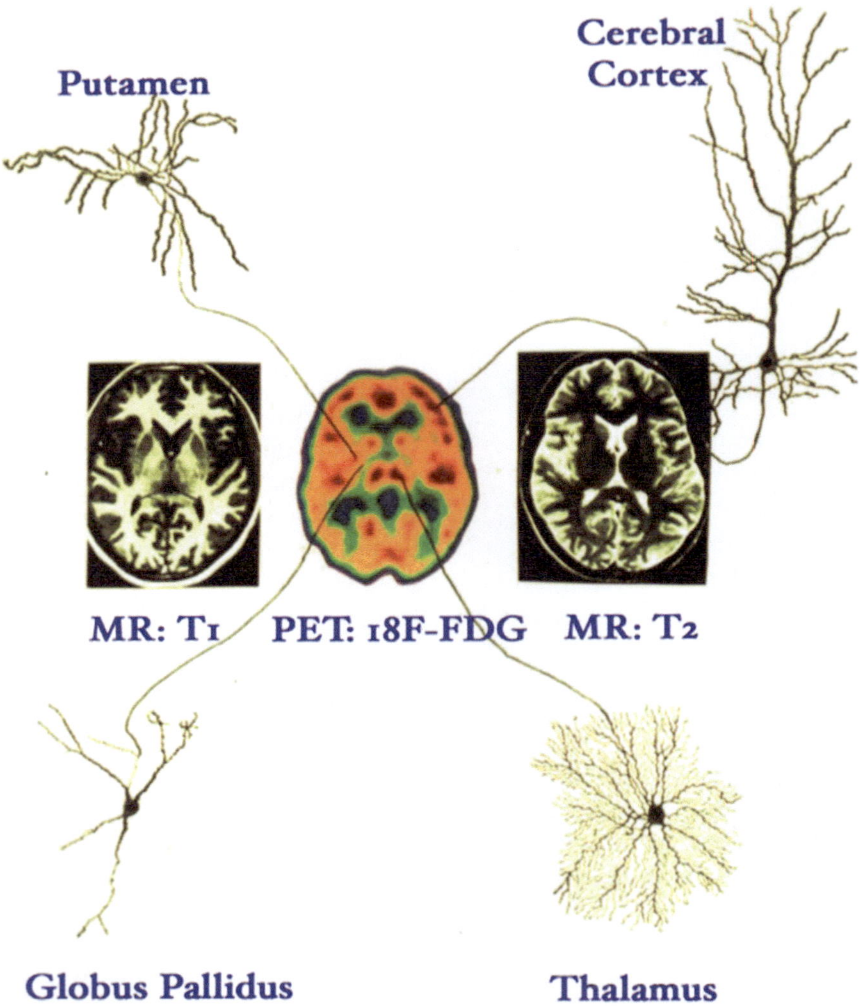

Fig. 2.15 The shape and appearance of the neuron itself is characteristically and uniquely different for each region of the brain

Fig. 2.16 Cerebral cortex neurons. Artistic rendering of the cytoarchitecture unique to cerebral cortex pyramidal neurons

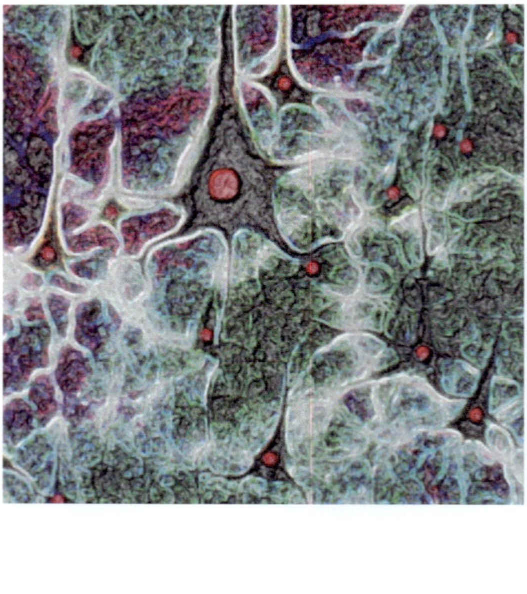

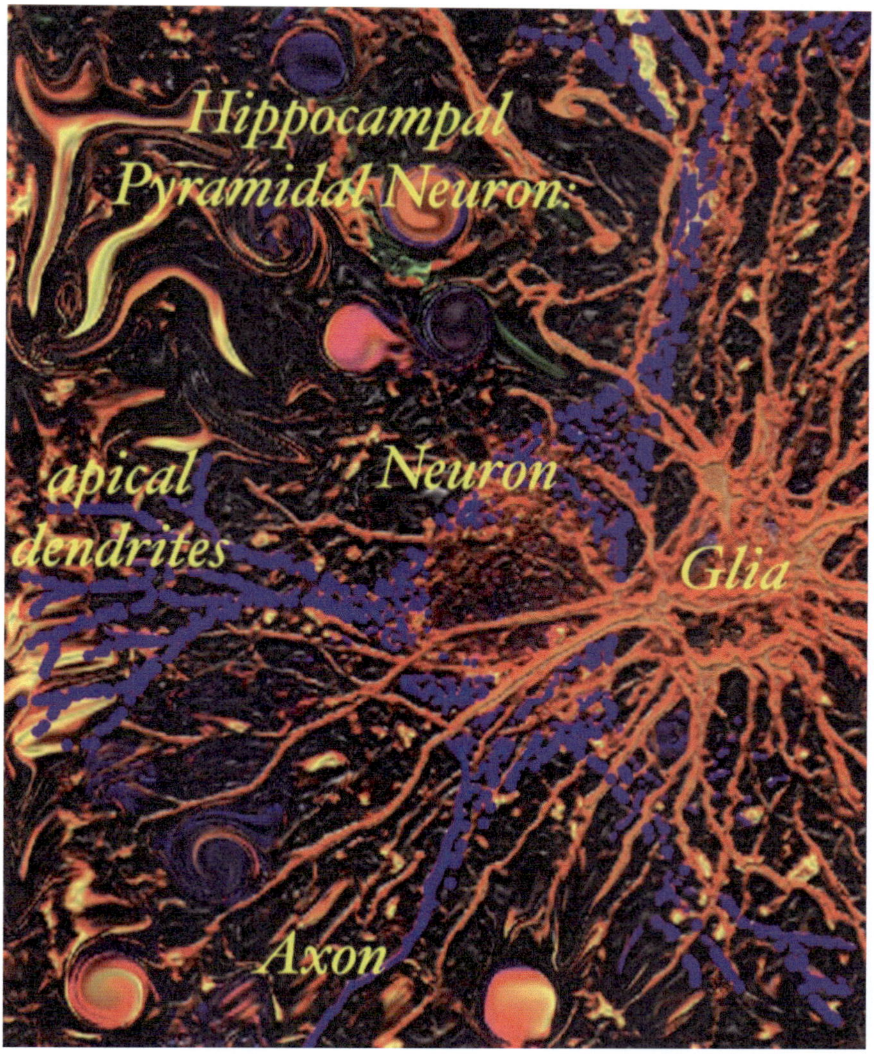

Fig. 2.17 Artistic rendering of the cytoarchitecture unique to hippocampal pyramidal neurons

Starting out as the primordial neural plate that fold upward to form a tubular structure, with central remnants persisting as the central canal of the spinal cord in adults which communicates with the ventricular system. Molecular analysis of neural crest migration indicates that a gradient of bone morphogenic protein (BMP) activity initially demarcates the neural plate borders, followed later by a transformation of this border of the neural plate into neural crest cells by a combination of Wnt signaling factors, fibroblast growth factors (FGFs), and retinoic acid (RA); connexin proteins also become upregulated during neural crest migration. The subsequent anterior–posterior patterning of cellular migration is controlled by semaphorins/neuropilins and Eph/ephrins [12].

Although there is great cellular proliferation during development, programmed cell death (Apoptosis) also takes place to refine and reduce the cell populations to the appropriate levels. Programmed cell death is actually an important

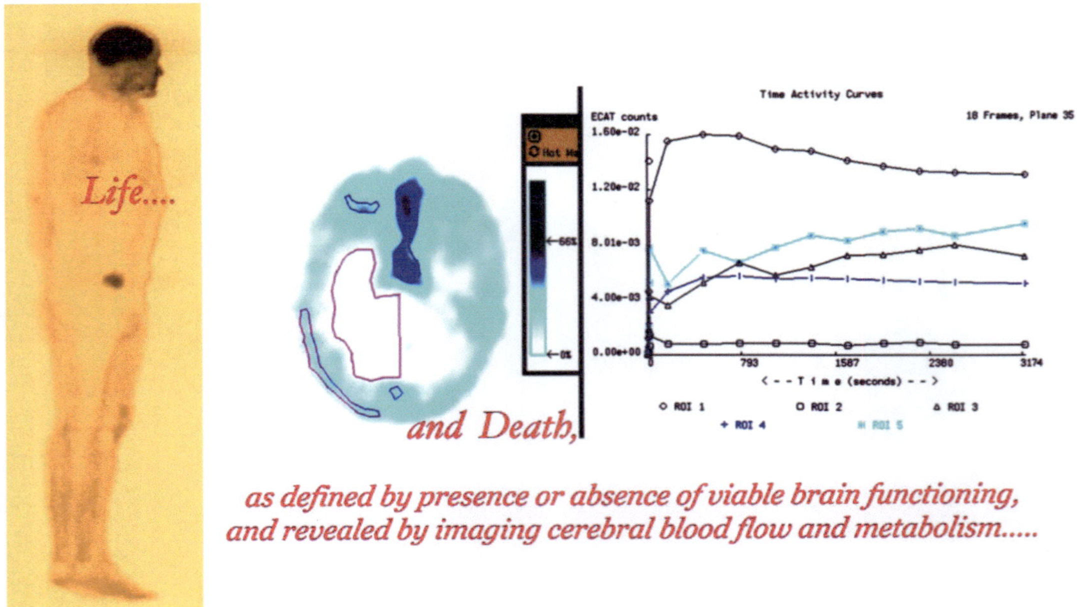

Fig. 2.18 The dynamic PET scan study at right revealed no flow and metabolism within the brain, making the diagnosis of brain death certain

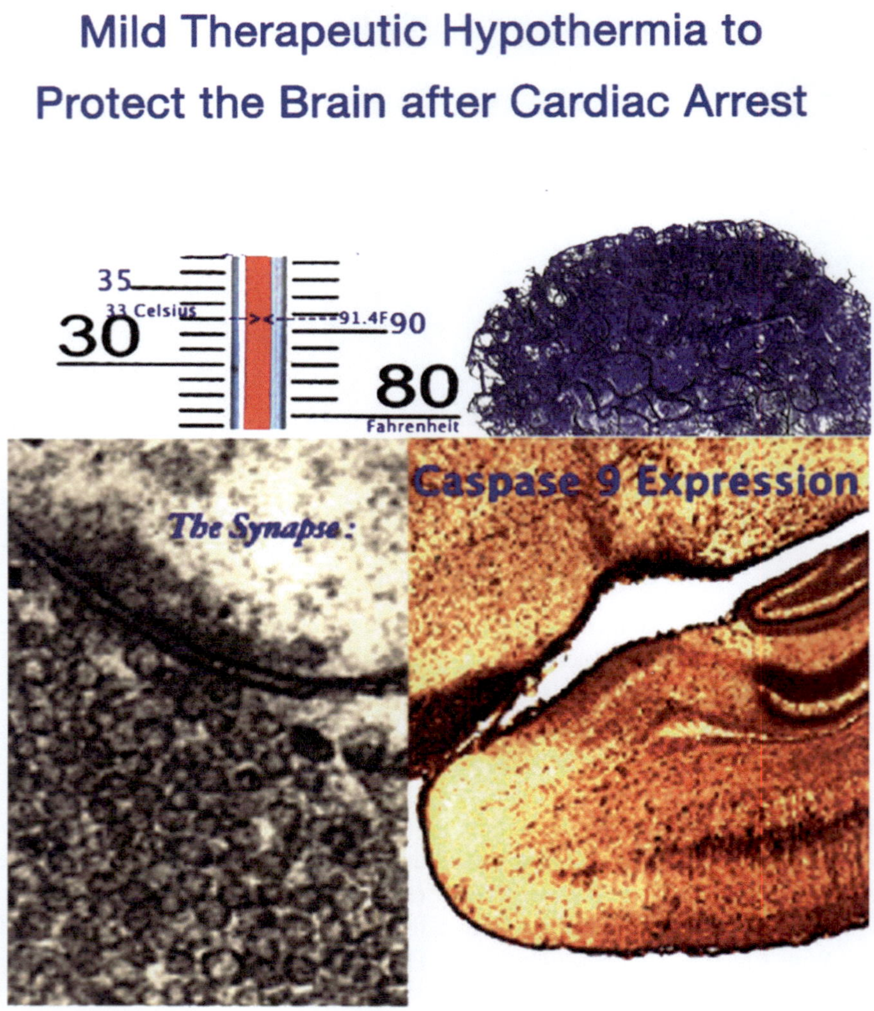

Fig. 2.19 Successful efforts to minimize postanoxic damage through the use of mild therapeutic hypothermia

Fig. 2.20 The final steps of apoptosis

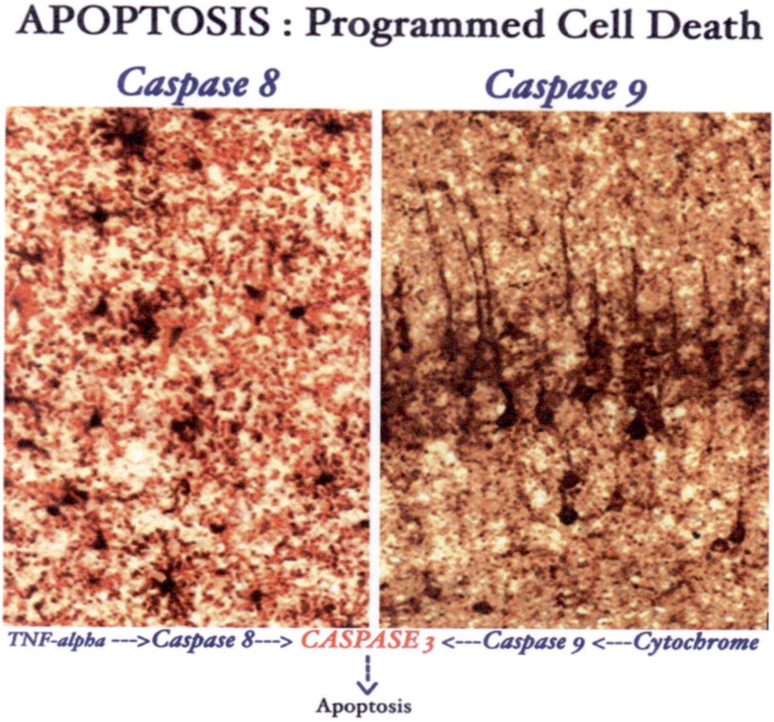

process in neuronal development that acts to eliminate certain areas and remove excess neurons that had proliferated. As suggested by Fig. 2.21, pyramidal neurons within the cerebral cortex proliferate during development—through the process of programmed cell death, not all of these neurons and associated glial cells survive. Recent research indicates that ephrin molecules play a role in this brain region-specific apoptosis process in regions where erythropoietin-producing hepatocellular (Eph) receptor tyrosine kinases (RTKs) cluster with their ephrin (Eph receptor interacting proteins) through direct cell to cell contact [13].

The final product is a masterpiece of the developmental process: containing 130 billion neurons and 150 trillion synapses in the human neocortex alone, each brain is uniquely different with regard to fine details of interconnections and patterns of cortical gyration. As shown in Fig. 2.22, the MRI study by the author showed a surprising variability to the patterns of cortical infoldings for the primary central fissure and neighboring cortical sulci.

The effects of age on these infoldings producing mild global cortical atrophy is shown in Fig. 2.23 for the case example of a 68-year-old male with new onset of mild to moderate cognitive impairment, who also displayed mild prominence to the ventricular system thought to be less likely of a congenital nature.

The development of the ventricular system of the brain is influenced by many genes and proteins; recent research indicates that one of these influencing factors is SOCS7, which is a member of the suppressor of cytokine signaling (SOCS) family of proteins. Lack of this protein in the developing mouse brain was found to be linked to hydrocephalus [14].

Whereas the intrasulcal cerebrospinal fluid spaces are readily visible on 3D surface renderings of MR brain images, the 3D morphology of the

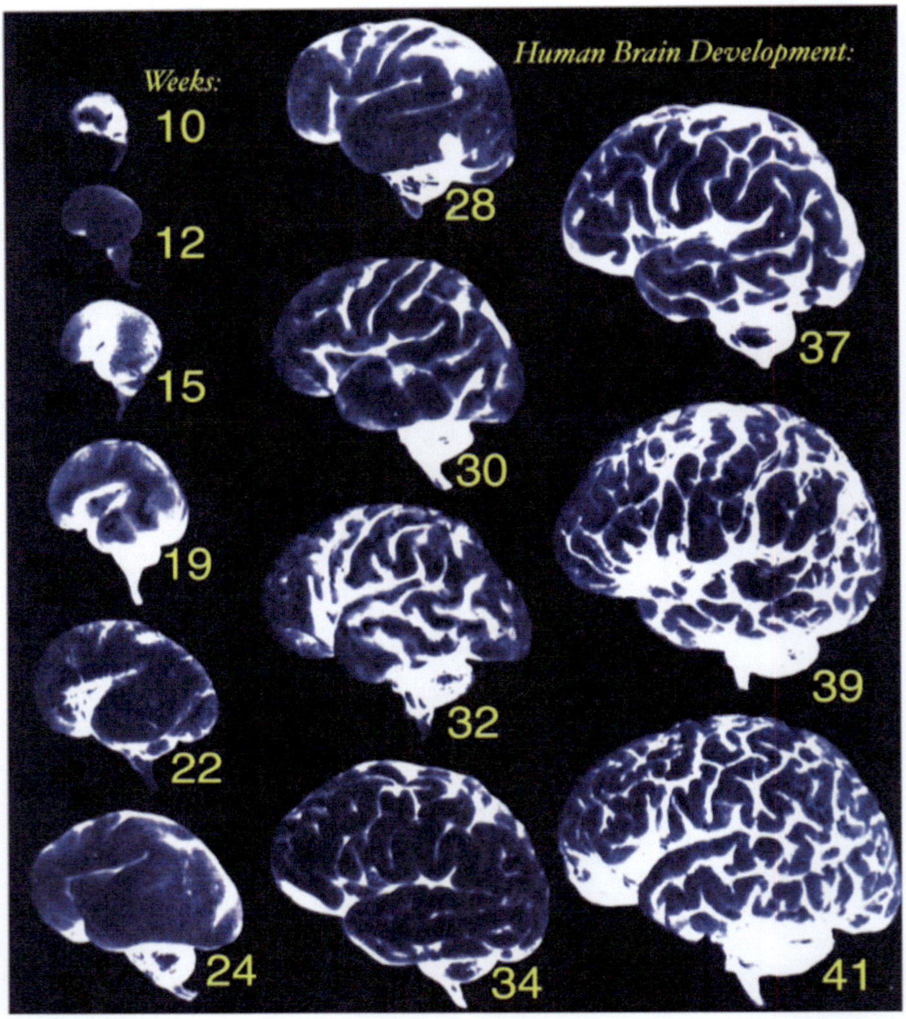

Fig. 2.21 In utero development of the brain

internal ventricular spaces are not readily apparent. As shown in Fig. 2.24, the drawings by Leonardo da Vinci on his studies of the ventricular system were reasonably accurate and also included making a wax corrosion cast of the ventricular system post-mortem using molten hot liquid wax.

Lower panels reveal a MRI-derived 3D computer reconstruction dating to 1991 that selectively outlined the morphology of the ventricles at various viewing angles (overlying cerebellar and cortical structures are shown at right).

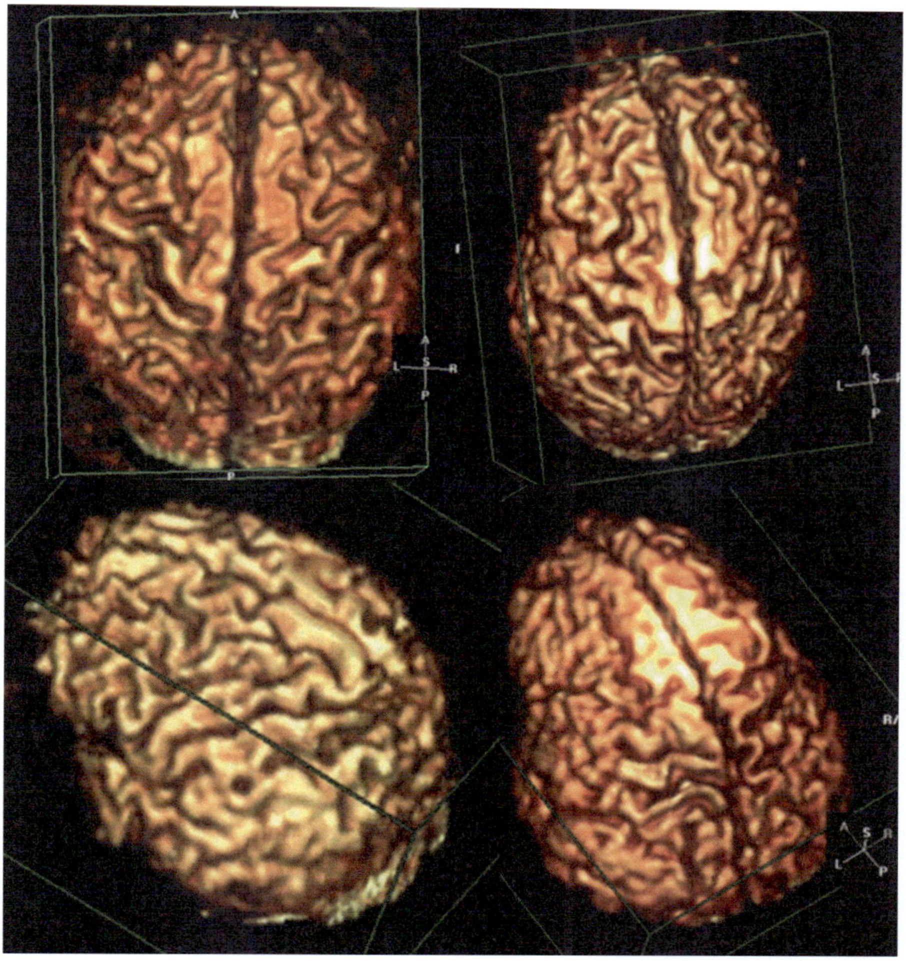

Fig. 2.22 3D reconstructions of brain MR data for four patients show a surprising variability to the patterns of cortical infoldings for the primary central fissure and neighboring cortical sulci

Fig. 2.23 Mild global cortical atrophy for the case example of a 68-year-old male

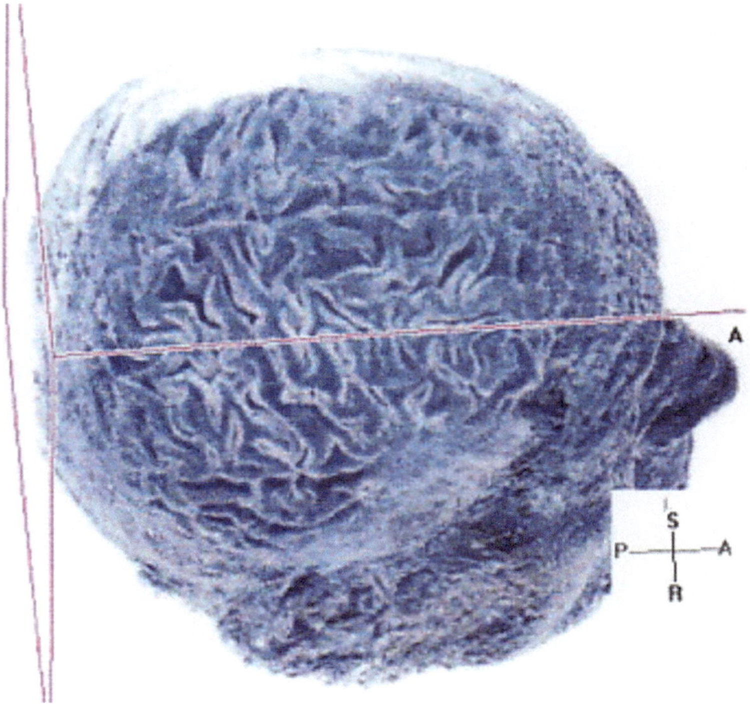

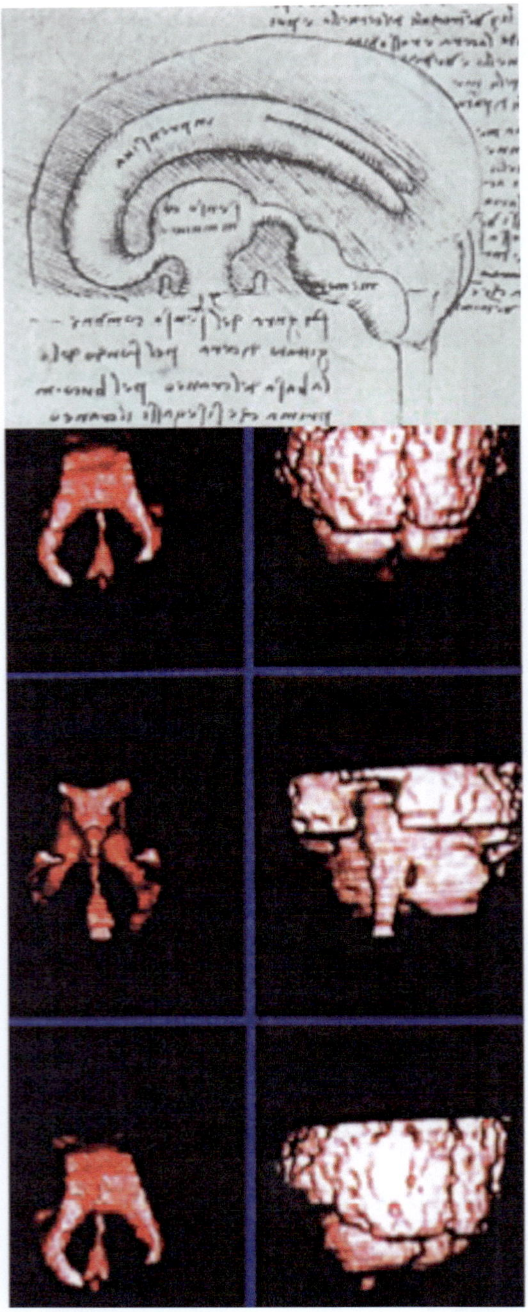

Fig. 2.24 Drawings by Leonardo da Vinci (*above*) on his studies of the ventricular system were reasonably accurate; compare with a MRI-derived 3D computer reconstruction (*below*) that selectively outlined the morphology of the ventricles at various viewing angles

References

1. Wagner OI, Ascano J, Tokito M. The interaction of neurofilaments with the microtubule motor cytoplasmic dynein. Mol Biol Cell. 2004;15(11):5092–100.
2. Escayg A, Goldin AL. Sodium channel SCN1A and epilepsy: mutations and mechanisms. Epilepsia. 2010;51:1650–8.
3. DeFelipe J, Alonso-Nanclares L, Arellano JI. Microstructure of the neocortex: comparative aspects. J Neurocytol. 2002;31:299–316.
4. Meyer M, Koeppe RA, Frey KA, et al. Positron emission tomography measures of benzodiazepine binding in Alzheimer's disease. Arch Neurol. 1995;52:314–7.
5. Sherwood CC, Stimpson CD, Raghanti MA, et al. Evolution of increased glia–neuron ratios in the human frontal cortex. Proc Natl Acad Sci U S A. 2006;103(37):13606–11.
6. Oberheim NA, Wang X, Goldman S, Nedergaard M. Astrocytic complexity distinguishes the human brain. Trends Neurosci. 2006;29:547–53.
7. Diamond MC, et al. On the brain of a scientist: Albert Einstein. Exp Neurol. 1985;88:198–204.
8. Giaume C, Kirchhoff F, Matute C, et al. Glia: the fulcrum of brain diseases. Cell Death Differ. 2007; 14:1324–35.
9. Theis M, Zho JR, Speidel D, et al. Accelerated hippocampal spreading depression and enhanced locomotory activity in mice with astrocyte-directed inactivation of connexin43. J Neurosci. 2003; 23:766–76.
10. Risher WC, Eroglu C. Thrombospondins as key regulators of synaptogenesis in the central nervous system. Matrix Biol. 2012;31:170–7.
11. Saver JL. Time is brain—quantified. Stroke. 2006; 37:263–6.
12. Kuriyama S, Mayor R. Molecular analysis of neural crest migration. Philos Trans R Soc Lond B Biol Sci. 2008;363(1495):1349–62.
13. Park E, Kim Y, Noh H, et al. EphA/ephrin-A signaling is critically involved in region-specific apoptosis during early brain development. Cell Death Differ. 2013;20:169–80.
14. Krebs DL, et al. Development of hydrocephalus in mice lacking SOCS7. Proc Natl Acad Sci U S A. 2004;101(43):15446–51.

3 Stroke

3.1 Introduction

In terms of morbidity and mortality implications, stroke is one the most common as well as one of the most important areas of neurology to be familiar with as it is the cause of six million deaths annually around the world. Accurate recognition that a patient may have had a true stroke warning sign (transient ischemic attack: TIA) could lead to an 80 % reduction in risk for stroke if proper measures are taken to start prophylactic measures (i.e., antiplatelet medications such as clopidogrel). Once a stroke has occurred, urgent action by the physician can effectively improve the likelihood in reversing the ischemic deficit and result in little to no long-term disability if tPA is promptly started according to protocol within 180 min of symptom onset.

Despite great access to imaging technology that can help assess stroke risk, and despite the availability of stroke prevention medications, factors such as smoking and uncontrolled hypertension lead to surprisingly high rates of stroke in the USA, where a new stroke occurs every 40 seconds.

3.2 General Facts About Stroke

As noted (Fig. 3.1), the stroke mortality rate has strong regional characteristics with most of the stroke deaths occurring in the Southeastern USA ("Stroke belt") and follows a pattern related to lung cancer mortality as well as heart disease mortality [1].

This chapter reviews the major causes of stroke with ischemic factors representing 85 % or more of all stroke cases versus hemorrhagic explanations being 15 % or less. The diagnostic approach is again emphasized as reasoning through clinical cases: the symptoms for stroke most often present acutely in terms of time with spatial factors within the nervous system as being focal for most events or multifocal for those which are cardio-embolic in origin, for example. The chapter reviews hemorrhagic etiologies first [2] and then discusses TIA and acute stroke along with treatment options in detail with the aid of multiple case examples.

The challenge to the neurologist is to determine the etiologic cause of the stroke, as this will lead to the proper treatment (Fig. 3.2). CT imaging readily identifies the 15 % presenting with acute stroke-like symptoms secondary to hemorrhage. For the remaining 85 % that present as ischemic stroke events, modern imaging techniques such as diffusion-weighted MRI have greatly improved accuracy of diagnosis and subsequently treatment decisions and patient outcome (Fig. 3.3).

3.3 Establishing a Stroke Diagnosis

By applying the principles of establishing factors of time (chronic vs. acute) and space (focal vs. diffuse vs. multifocal) the clinician can arrive at

M.A. Meyer, *Neurologic Disease*, DOI 10.1007/978-3-319-39581-4_3

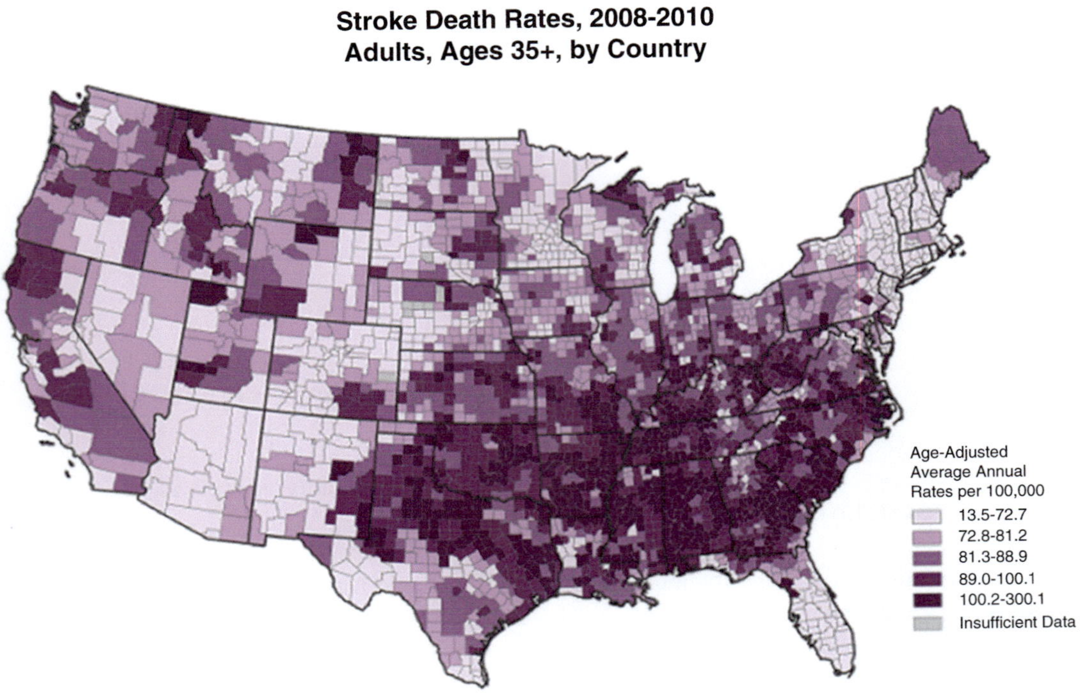

Fig. 3.1 Stroke mortality across the USA; note the high incidence in the Southeastern USA

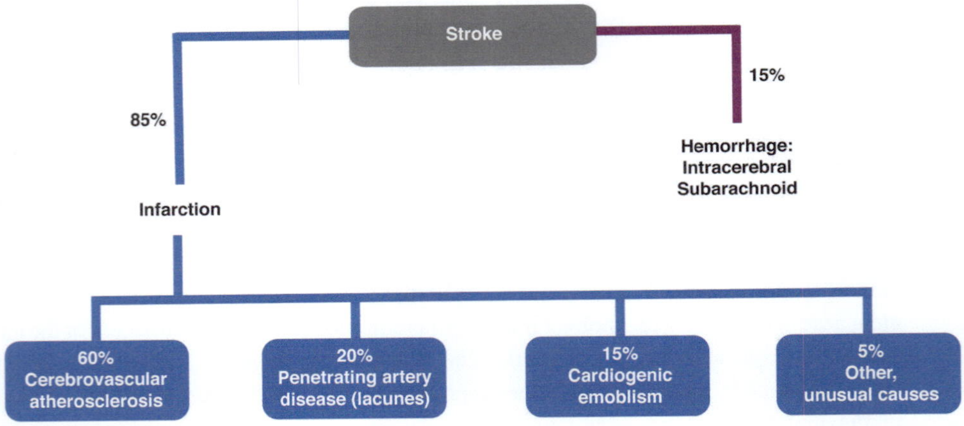

Fig. 3.2 Majority of stroke-like presentations in the ER are ischemic in nature

a tentative diagnosis that can then be supported or refuted by correlative neuroimaging data. For example, in the case shown above (Fig. 3.3), a 60-year-old male with hypertension and diabetes developed sudden and abrupt weakness in the left hand, suggesting acute focal stroke. The time factor is key to the diagnosis—any abrupt and sustained focal deficit should suggest stroke in the differential diagnosis list, especially for an individual with stroke risk factors being noted. Had the patient been in his early 20s and had a history for unilateral vision loss, the differential would be different and instead suggest demyelinating disease.

Neuroimaging helps narrow the list of possibilities down further for this case example of a

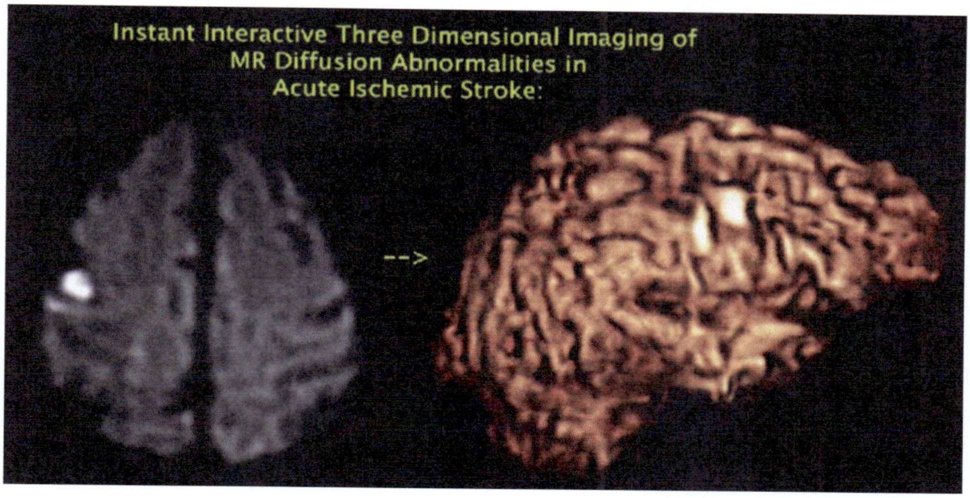

Fig. 3.3 Diffusion-weighted MRI is a very sensitive tool in identifying acutely ischemic brain tissue

60-year-old hypertensive diabetic, as CT typically shows no significant hypodensity within the first few hours after infarction—the absence of hemorrhage on CT is critical in the assessment for the event as being representative of ischemia due to an obstruction of flow (of additional note, CT can be very helpful in establishing a time line when no details are available or the patient is aphasic—acute ischemic events within the first 3 h generate little to no significant CT hypodensity in general). MR angiography would then be important to carry out to understand the mechanism of the event as being due to intracranial disease such as embolic occlusion of a distal middle cerebral artery (MCA) branch from ipsilateral proximal M1 segment atherosclerotic disease of the MCA; alternatively, another possibility might be embolic material from atherosclerotic disease from the ipsilateral internal carotid artery. Other sources of emboli include the aortic arch as well from the heart (cardiac emboli, as in atrial fibrillation, result more often in multifocal defects with multifocal diffusion-weighted signal changes).

3.4 Historical Aspects of Cerebrovascular Disease

One of the earliest but most important concepts in cerebrovascular disease is illustrated in Fig. 3.4. A key safety mechanism and feature about large vessel interconnections is the Circle of Willis that can lead to alternate paths of perfusion in the event of a stroke-like large vessel occlusion, as shown in the original 1664 drawing below by Thomas Willis with highlighting in red of major trunks of arterial supply (Fig. 3.4).

3.5 Modern Concepts in Cerebrovascular Anatomy and Disease

Modern concepts in cerebrovascular anatomy and disease have advanced greatly over the past decade to understand the molecular basis for vital functions, such as the blood brain barrier (Fig. 3.5). From the ultrastructural perspective, the blood–brain barrier is now known to be formed by tight junctions that adhere one endothelial cell to the other within the cerebral vasculature, as reveled by light microscopy of claudin staining (Fig. 3.5) as well as electron micrographs of tight junction contacts between endothelial cells.

From the Gross Anatomy Perspective, it is amazing that ischemic stroke occurs at all, given the extreme vascularity of the brain. Despite the rich vascularity and mechanism to open up collateral circulation, stroke remains prevalent with advancing age; a natural question that subsequently arises with respect to age relates to other

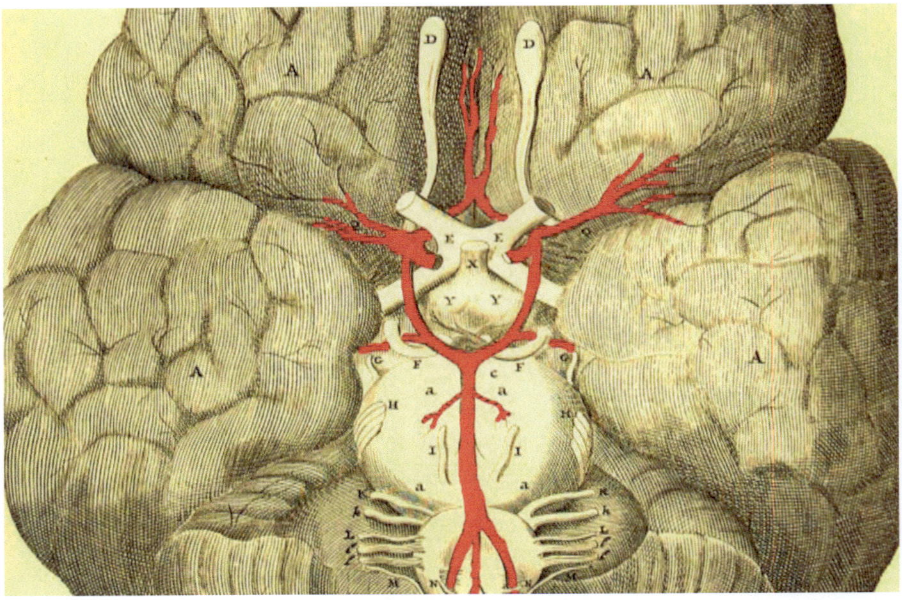

Fig. 3.4 Historical aspects: 1664 drawing by Thomas Willis portraying the important conjoining of vessels now named for him as the Circle of Willis [48]

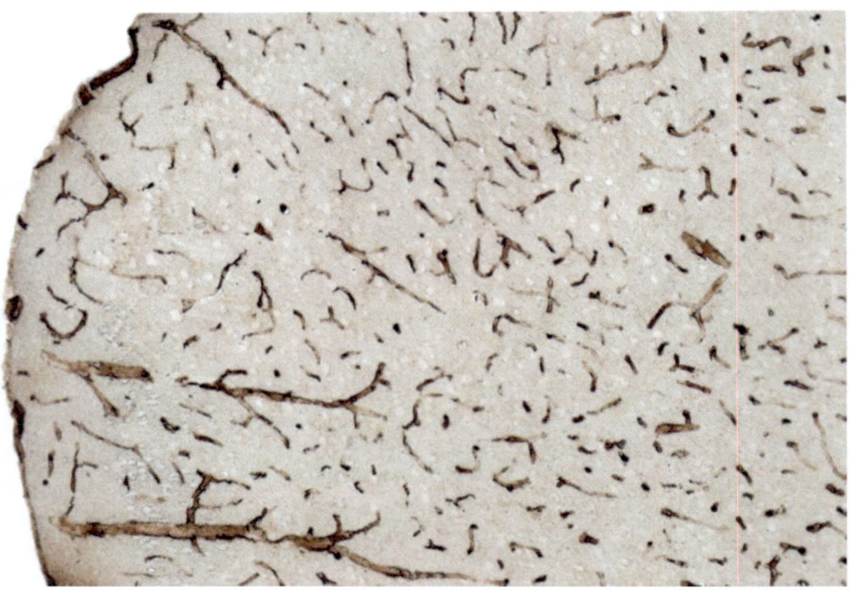

Fig. 3.5 Histochemical localization of Claudin to the cerebral vasculature

personal risk factors that may predispose an individual to stroke (Table 3.1).

Case Example

Acute infarction (left panel, Fig. 3.6) in a 64-year-old female with extreme hypertension and acute speech deficit; long-term outcome was relatively good as shown in the right hand panels, with only a mild disruption in the rhythm and pattern to speech (focal ischemic deficit seen at right for left peri-sylvian cortex). In other cases, a small well placed infarction can have devastating

Table 3.1 Risk calculator

Are you at risk for stroke?
Understand your risk factors with the Stroke Risk Calculator [3]
Abstract result summary:
The following regression parameters were used to produce 10-year stroke-risk estimates and assign risk points:
Age (one point/year after age 20 years), Male sex (three points), Low education (four points), Renal disease (eight points), Diabetes (seven points), CHF (congestive heart failure) (five points)
PAD (peripheral arterial disease) (two points), High BP (blood pressure) (two points)
CAD (ischemic heart disease) (one point), Smoking (eight points), Alcohol (>7 alcoholic drinks per week) (three points), Low physical activity (two points), Indicators of anger (four points), Depression (four points), Anxiety (three points)

According to MyRiskStroke Calculator, a person with <50, 75, and 90 risk points has a 10-year stroke risk of <3%, 28%, and >75%, respectively

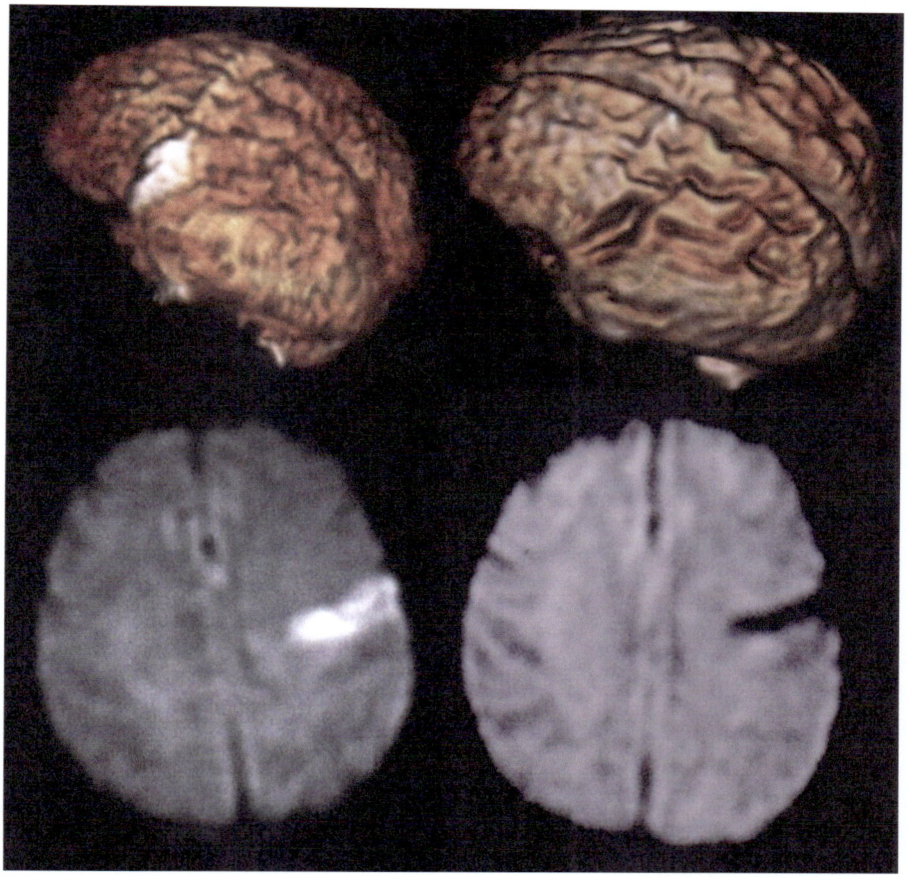

Fig. 3.6 Case example showing typical classic representation of speech within the left hemisphere: *left hand panel* shows acute disruption of speech as a bright DWI positive peri-sylvian area of cortical ischemia (*right hand panel* shows this as cortical defect with focal encephalomalacia at follow-up when some speech alteration still persisted)

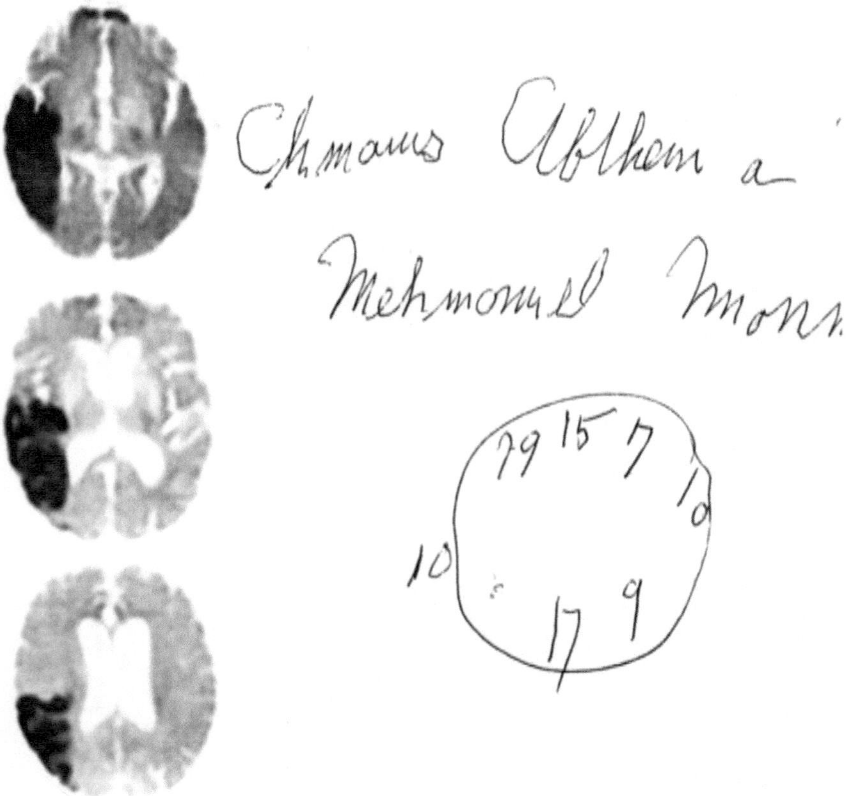

Fig. 3.7 Rare case of right hemisphere dominance for speech and language; acute right MCA infarct appearing as DWI positive regions in a patient with sudden expressive aphasia with alexia and agraphia

consequences, particularly if it occurs within the brain stem; in other individuals with strict unilateral language dominance and less compensatory abilities, a dominant hemisphere cortical infarct similar to what is shown above not infrequently can cause permanent and significant language deficits.

Case Example

Acute Focal Deficit with speech in the form of expressive aphasia in an 81-year-old male; clinical exam and history suggested the likelihood of a dominant left hemisphere infarct, as even the majority of left hand dominant individuals will still show a left hemisphere speech dominance. Surprisingly, the MR diffusion images at left confirmed that instead, the infarct was in the right hemisphere.

In summary, this case displays a right-sided MCA infarction with acute and persistent aphasia in a rare case of right hemisphere dominance for speech; this case emphasizes the need to make radiographic correlation with clinical signs and symptoms as the clinical exam would predict a left hemispheric ischemic insult being most likely (Fig. 3.7).

Other technologies used for stroke evaluations include CT angiography, which can readily portray brain perfusion in the normal state (Fig. 3.8) or in the setting of acute stroke.

This 3D view in the sagittal projection of a patient undergoing CT angiography in a noninvasive manner (Fig. 3.8) provide surprisingly fine details that compare in quality to postmortem radiographs of sagittal sections after dye injection to the major arterial vessels.

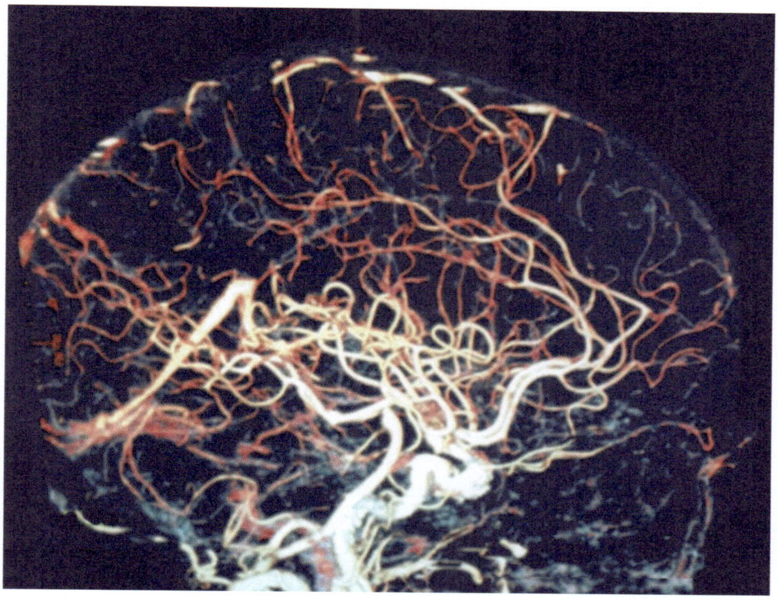

Fig. 3.8 Normal CNS vasculature revealed by CT angiography

When viewing acquired disability on a global basis, stroke is the leading cause worldwide and is the second most common cause of death. A great majority of these fatal stroke events occur in low- and middle-income countries across the globe [3, 4].

A TIA event marks the risk for a subsequent stroke within the next 1 week to be as high as 13 %; however, prompt and comprehensive evaluation and treatment of the TIA patient can prevent about 80 % of recurrent events. Large studies have clearly demonstrated the dramatic reduction in stroke by immediate evaluation of the cause of the TIA and promptly starting treatment with appropriate medications, including antiplatelet agents.

Stroke or TIA occurrence is very significant and reflects an elevated risk for not only recurrent stroke but also other potentially fatal vascular events such as myocardial infarction. Immediate evaluation is needed after a TIA or stroke event to reduce disability and overall stroke risk. Simple measures such as starting antiplatelet agents, anti-hypertension medications, and statins as needed can make a great difference in addition to simple lifestyle modifications such as discontinuation of smoking, better diet, exercise, and loss of excess weight.

Other measures may be required that include surgery for those with symptomatic severe carotid stenosis, or may need anticoagulation for stroke and/or TIA due to atrial fibrillation.

The task of the physician evaluating an acute stroke patient is to categorize it according to etiologies, with ischemic stroke being the most common (at least 80 % or more of cases) versus intracerebral hemorrhage (15 %) versus other causes including subarachnoid hemorrhage (5 %).

In contrast, a TIA event represents a transient acute deficit usually lasting minutes to hours that fully resolves without residual clinical signs or symptoms or changes seen on CT or MR imaging. For those events that do not fall into this category of TIA, and represent ischemic stroke, the major categories for causation include:

Cardioembolism (e.g., atrial fibrillation):

Large-artery disease

Small-vessel occlusion (lacunar stroke)

Stroke of other determined cause (e.g., dissection, drug-related, hypercoagulable state)

Stroke of undetermined cause ("cryptogenic stroke")

Note: this useful classification is adopted from the Trial of Org 10172 in Acute Stroke Treatment (TOAST) categorization for ischemic stroke causation.

In the landmark Introstoke study on stroke risk factors amongst 3000 stroke patients from 22 countries compared to 3000 controls [5], high blood pressure was found to be the strongest risk factor with an odds ratio of 2.64 with nine other risk factors noted as follows: smoking, elevated waist-to-hip ratio, diet, inactivity, diabetes mellitus, alcohol, stress/depression, cardiac factors such as myocardial infarction or atrial fibrillation, apolipoprotein B to apolipoprotein A ratio. Collectively, these ten risk factors accounted for 90 % of the risk for stroke with five of these ten being more important for hemorrhagic stroke (hypertension, smoking, waist-to-hip ratio, diet, and alcohol).

Clearly, blood pressure is the single most important modifiable risk factor to treat in an effort to reduce stroke; this is supported by many large studies that have demonstrated the value of blood pressure reduction in reducing recurrent stroke risk. One placebo controlled randomized trial study involved 6105 patients with a history of stroke or TIA and showed a 28 % lower risk of stroke over 4 years in the ACE-inhibitor treatment group, blood pressure dropped by an average of 9/4 mmHg [6].

Lipid profiles are important in the evaluation of stroke as current guidelines advocate that LDL cholesterol levels of 100 mg per deciliter should be treated with statin medications. Despite their benefits, the risks of disabling statin myopathy need to be weighed as well as the controversial opinions that statins may slightly increase the risk for intracerebral hemorrhage (ICH); the latter point is debatable as there are other studies that refute the risk and remain an area of relative uncertainty for those with ICH.

Antiplatelet agents are widely accepted cornerstones of treatment for stroke or TIA, with meta-analysis of trial data showing definite risk reductions with aspirin. One meta-analysis of eight trials involving 41,483 patients found that for every 1000 people treated with aspirin, 13 will avoid death or dependency [7].

Common treatment regimens also include clopidogrel (an adenosine diphosphate-receptor inhibitor) as well as the combination of low dose aspirin plus dipyridamole (a phosphodiesterase inhibitor) as ways to enhance protection beyond aspirin monotherapy. Although the latter approach with dipyridamole may be limited in some patients due to the not infrequent problem of headache, the use of clopidogrel is generally well tolerated with recent data showing significant risk reduction when combined with aspirin for limited time spans after an initial event. As shown in a recent randomized study involving 5170 patients with minor stroke or high risk TIA, the combination of clopidogrel and aspirin started within 24 h of symptom onset is superior to aspirin alone for reducing the risk of stroke in the first 12 weeks without any increased risk for bleeding; clopidogrel had been started with a 300 mg loading dose and continued at 75 mg per day for 12 weeks, while daily aspirin continued for only 3 weeks [8].

Carotid endarterectomy is indicated for those patients with symptomatic stenosis of exceeding mild to moderate ranges of narrowing—although 70–80 % may be a gray zone in terms of measurement precision, clearly defined stenosis of 80 % or more is of great significance when the TIA event or stroke episode is referable to the ipsilateral highly stenosed carotid artery and serves as a justified need for surgical intervention. As determined by the randomized North American Symptomatic Carotid Endarterectomy Trial (NASCET), a 17 % reduction in stroke risk was found over a one and a half year time period for those undergoing carotid endarterectomy for high-grade narrowing. No benefit was found for NASCET trial participants who underwent surgery for mild stenosis (under 50 %) with some reduction of risk amounting to only 6.5 % over 5 years for those undergoing endarterectomy for moderate narrowing. For those who have not incurred infarction and had a TIA directly referable to a high-grade carotid stenosis, early surgical intervention within the first 2 weeks may be preferable. The CREST and European stenting trials found better outcomes for those symptomatic patients older than 70 years of age who underwent carotid endarterectomy as opposed to carotid artery stenting.

Atrial fibrillation accounts for about one out of every seven ischemic stroke cases with anticoagulation being the key therapeutic intervention where risks of bleeding do not exceed potential benefits; a full investigation to other potential stroke etiologies still is warranted despite the readily obvious evidence for paroxysmal or persistent atrial fibrillation.

New alternatives to traditional forms of anticoagulation with warfarin exist now with published evidence for safety and efficacy. For example, dabigatran is a direct thrombin inhibitor that was found to more effective than warfarin for preventing ischemic stroke with lower risks for intracranial bleeding and comparable overall risk for major systemic bleeding episodes.

Overall, patent foramen ovale (PFO) can be an incidental finding for many young stroke patients with an overall incidence of 22 % for the general population, but it is found at somewhat higher rates among those with cryptogenic stroke and becomes very significant when the PFO size is large and a large excursion off the midline septum is noted for an inter-atrial septal aneurysm demonstrated by ECHO, and may therefore require closure of the PFO to prevent recurrent stroke events. However, a recent trial showed no benefit to PFO closure in those with cryptogenic stroke of unknown cause; specifically, they noted no significant effect whether an atrial septal aneurysm was present or absent; likewise, the degree of shunting also made no difference in the findings [9].

Likewise, a major trial known as SAMMPRIS determined that aggressive medical management was superior to percutaneous transluminal angioplasty and stenting (PTAS) to prevent recurrent stroke in patients with high-grade intracranial stenosis; the randomized trial had to be stopped early after 451 patients had been enrolled, because the 30-day rate of stroke or death was 14.7 % in the PTAS group versus 5.8 % in the medical-management group [10]. However, with regard to the utility of endovascular techniques in stroke care, a recent large randomized trial from the Netherlands known as MR CLEAN involving 500 anterior circulation acute stroke patients (90 % of whom already had been given IV tPA) found better outcomes with emergent endovascular intervention within 6 h of onset by a microcatheter delivery of a thrombolytic agent, mechanical thrombectomy, or both [11].

Carotid atherosclerotic disease accounts for about one-fifth of all strokes, with the degree of stenosis correlating to the degree of risk. Plaque within the walls of the carotid can lead to thrombus formation that can dislodge and produce distal embolization to the brain. Specifically, an unstable irregular ulcerated carotid plaque can present high risk for a combination of platelets with thrombotic fragments containing calcific material to break free and produce acute stroke symptoms; to prevent stroke, such cases may require urgent intervention by surgery when antiplatelet therapy with clopidogrel and aspirin may be insufficient [12].

Clinical recognition of the problem is critical, with an important presenting symptom of carotid atherosclerotic disease may be unilateral transient visual loss, termed amaurosis fugax and involves direct retinal artery ischemia from emboli migrating from an ulcerated carotid plaque lesion; immediate evaluation is needed by carotid Doppler and/or CT or MR angiography techniques. Should the stenosis be less than 70 %, medical therapy is preferable to surgical intervention.

Of additional note, one-fourth of all individuals have a fetal origin to the posterior cerebral artery (PCA) where the vessel originates off the internal carotid; this is important to know in consideration of whether a carotid lesion is truly symptomatic or not as unilateral carotid emboli may lodge within the ipsilateral PCA territory.

Carotid stenting is an alternate procedure to endarterectomy, especially for those under age 70 who are considered to be a high surgical risk. Stenting may be an option for those with carotid dissection, which can result from trauma of various types including impingement by the styloid process.

Dissection is an important consideration for stroke in young adults, and can occur spontaneously in the absence of trauma, especially in those with genetically determined collagen defects such as Ehlers–Danlos syndrome. With carotid dissection, the patient often complains of linear pain radiating up the neck (more than 60 % of dissections have significant ipsilateral face and/or neck pain). Relevant signs on exam include Horner's syndrome (ptosis, miosis, enophthalmos) as a result of traumatized sympathetic nerves that ascend around the arterial wall. In these circumstances, embolic stroke can result from hematoma formation within the tunica media that ruptures through the intimal layer, creating a false lumen and limits flow through the true lumen. Fibromuscular dysplasia, which is more often found in women, can be a predisposing causative factor for dissection as well as aneurysm formation.

Exam findings for carotid disease include the detection of a bruit by auscultation, but are not specific for stenosis as 5 % of the population between ages 45 and 80 have incidental bruits in the absence of carotid stenosis.

The first major trial to define risk versus benefits to medical versus surgical therapy for carotid disease management depending on the level of stenosis was the NASCET trial, which found clear benefit to endarterectomy for those with 70 % stenosis or more. Subsequent meta-analysis of this data with other trials representing an aggregate total of 6092 patients showed that for patients with carotid near-occlusion, benefit to endarterectomy is marginal in the short-term. However, for those with 70–99 % symptomatic stenosis without near-occlusion, endarterectomy provided a significant absolute risk reduction of 16 % for incurring ipsilateral ischemic stroke [13].

The Carotid Revascularization Endarterectomy versus Stenting Trial (CREST) concluded in 2011 that there were no significant differences in the primary endpoint outcomes between carotid endarterectomy (CEA) and stenting but periprocedural stroke and death rates were significantly lower for symptomatic patients undergoing CEA which may reflect the early stages of technical development for stenting that remain to be improved upon; furthermore, those over age 70 did better with surgery [14].

Intracerebral hemorrhage, or ICH, is a highly serious problem affecting over 50,000 people in the USA annually. ICH occurs in more than one million people annually across the globe; unfortunately, it remains a devastating form of stroke where the median 1 month case fatality rate is 40 % with only one in five survivors having made full functional recovery by the half year mark [15].

Half of the mortality due to ICH occurs within the very first 24 h, emphasizing the critical need to aggressively control hypertension in the early stages to reduce hematoma expansion [16].

Risk factors for ICH include male sex, advanced age, and Asian ethnicity; it is also twice as frequent in low- to middle-income countries compared to high-income countries. Within the United States, ICH is known to be more common amongst African Americans and Hispanics.

A major risk factor for ICH is hypertension, with end-vessel vascular territories being especially predisposed such as the deep penetrating vessels from the lenticulostriate and thalamostriate arteries that supply the basal ganglia and thalamus respectively. Without anastomosing vessels, the fairly linear terminal branches of these deep penetrating vessels bear the brunt of injury from the pounding effects of excessively high blood pressures leading to lipohyalinosis around the tips of these vulnerable fragile branches; another similar terminal end-vessel terminus is within the fine deep penetrating vessels within the brain stem. With regard to peripheral lobar hemorrhages that is centered within the cortex, this is characteristically due to the age-related change known as amyloid angiopathy. Other factors that could promote the risks for hypertension-related ICH within the deep basal ganglia and thalamus or the less common lobar cortical hemorrhage from amyloid angiopathy include the following:

(a) Alcohol intake: dose-dependent risk
(b) Cholesterol: paradoxically, and opposite to risks for ischemic stroke, low levels of total serum cholesterol are risk factors for ICH
(c) Genetics: apolipoprotein E (APOE) ε2 and ε4 alleles are ICH risk factors
(d) Anticoagulation: ICH annual risk for those on warfarin ranges from 0.3 to 1.0 % per patient-year with much higher risk when the INR is >3.5.
(e) Drug abuse: sympathomimetic drugs (i.e., cocaine)

3.6 Acute Management Issues with ICH

Airway protection is a key and vital priority and, therefore, those with massive ICH and/or depressed level of consciousness need rapid sequence intubation with propofol sedation preferable thereafter with transfer into ICU setting to aggressively control blood pressure. Recent AHA guidelines [17] published from 2010 include the following recommendations:

(a) Patients with ICH whose INR is elevated due to oral anticoagulants should have their warfarin withheld, receive therapy to replace vitamin K-dependent factors and correct the INR, and receive intravenous vitamin K.
(b) In patients presenting with a systolic BP of 150–220 mmHg, acute lowering of systolic blood pressure to 140 mmHg is probably safe.
(c) Glucose should be monitored and normoglycemia is recommended.
(d) Patients with a Glasgow Coma Scale score of ≤8, those with clinical evidence of transtentorial herniation, or those with significant IVH or hydrocephalus might be considered for ICP monitoring and treatment. A cerebral perfusion pressure of 50–70 mmHg may be reasonable to maintain depending on the status of cerebral autoregulation.
(e) Ventricular drainage as treatment for hydrocephalus is reasonable in patients with decreased level of consciousness.
(f) Patients with cerebellar hemorrhage who are deteriorating neurologically or who have brainstem compression and/or hydrocephalus from ventricular obstruction should undergo surgical removal of the hemorrhage as soon as possible.

New data on the use of Prothrombin complex concentrate shows promise in the setting of warfarin-associated ICH; one small study from Hong Kong showed encouraging clinical outcomes when compared to fresh frozen plasma with mean INR reduced from 2.81 to 1.21 within 24 h [18]. For ICH due to warfarin use, where warfarin has inhibited vitamin K-dependent carboxylation of coagulation factors 2, 7, 9, and 10, vitamin K infusion should be given slowly but promptly at a dose of 5–10 mg. Despite the potential for allergic reactions, Fresh Frozen Plasma (FFP) infusion can provide all the necessary coagulation factors to correct the prolonged INR effect of warfarin and is a frequently elected option for use in acute ICH management.

A relatively uncommon yet very important cause of ICH in young adults is an intracerebral arteriovenous malformation. Found in only 0.01 % of the general population, 12 % of these vascular lesions become symptomatic during a patient's lifetime. Congenital in origin, some are linked with other disorders such as Osler–Weber–Rendu disease and the Sturge–Weber syndrome [19].

Arteriovenous malformations carry an annual bleeding rate 2–4 % per year, with each event linked to a 5–10 % chance of death with one-third to one-half of affected patients being left with permanent or disabling neurologic deficits. The risk for a second subsequent bleed is estimated to be 6 % for the first year after the initial hemorrhage.

Due to the vascular steal effects within high flow shunts within unruptured arteriovenous malformations often present with new onset seizures; one study found that seizures were the initial clinical manifestations of AVMs in about one-third of cases [20].

AVMs may not be detectable on a noncontrast head CT but be strikingly obvious as a web of serpiginous flow voids on T2-weighted noncontrast brain MR exams. When examined by PET metabolic imaging, the area surrounding the vascular malformation may appear as a metabolic defect due to the vascular steal effect from high flow arterial to venous shunting.

With regard to management, the ARUBA trial showed that better outcomes are afforded in patients with unruptured brain arteriovenous malformations by medical management as opposed to interventional therapy (i.e., neurosurgery, embolization, or stereotactic radiotherapy, alone or in combination). The trial had to be stopped early after a mean follow-up time of 33 months as the primary endpoint of death or symptomatic stroke had been reached by 10.1 % in the medical management group compared versus 30.7 % in the interventional therapy group [21].

Despite the fact that intracranial aneurysms are surprisingly common with a prevalence of 1–5 % of the adult population, most aneurysms are small, and never rupture. Despite the fact that 5–15 million Americans may harbor an aneurysm, only 1 in 10,000 rupture, correlating annually to about 30,000 new cases of aneurysmal subarachnoid hemorrhage [22].

Other factors that predispose patients to aneurysm formation include autosomal dominant polycystic kidney disease where 5–40 % of cases have an intracranial aneurysm with 10–30 % of these positive individuals harboring multiple aneurysms. Other predisposing factors include fibromuscular dysplasia, as well as Marfan's syndrome, Ehlers–Danlos syndrome type IV, and intracerebral arteriovenous malformations. Amongst family members of those with an identified aneurysm, the prevalence rate for incidental aneurysms may be as high as 21 %.

Insight into the natural history of aneurysms is gained from a recent study from Finland where a group of unruptured aneurysm cases identified between 1956 and 1978 were followed for 21 years on average in the absence of intervention. As noted by the investigators, "Cigarette smoking, location of the aneurysm in the anterior communicating artery, patient age inversely and aneurysm diameter ≥7 mm independently predicted subsequent aneurysm rupture, as did alcohol consumption" [23]. Other studies have documented the importance of hypertension for aneurysm growth and rupture.

Family history of intracranial aneurysm is critically important in management decisions when an aneurysm is detected as the annual rupture rate for 6 mm or less is approximately 17 times higher than the rupture rate for subjects without a family history. This elevated risk can markedly influence the management of small aneurysms that may otherwise be delegated a conservative role of observation; furthermore, familial aneurysm patients who smoke and/or have hypertension are at an especially high risk [24].

As aneurysms are surprisingly common, and headache is one of the most common problems patients face in daily life, it is critically important the educated physician be keenly aware of the fact that the first signs of aneurysm rupture may be the sentinel warning headache that occurs in about one-fourth of subarachnoid bleeds and timed on average 11 days in advance of the potentially fatal event [25].

Clinical factors such as "worst headache of my life" descriptions coupled with family history of cerebral aneurysms should signal the need for immediate evaluation by brain MR angiography whenever possible as a more sensitive test than CT angiography. Should an aneurysm rupture, about 10 % are immediately fatal before reaching the emergency department; for the remaining group, 2–4 % experience a repeat bleed within the first day and 15–20 % chance of the same within 14 days.

For those who survive the initial bleed, complications that can ensue include hydrocephalus in 15–20 % as well as vasospasm in the 3–12 day time frame; this is a major feared complication that can lead to fatal or disabling stroke. Nimodipine over 3 weeks can help prevent this unfortunate complication of vasospasm, as well as a combination regimen of hypertension, hypervolemia, and hemodilution ("triple H" therapy). To assess likelihood of developing vasospasm as well determine responses to therapy, transcranial Doppler measurement of middle cerebral artery flow velocities can be very helpful (a trend towards increasing velocities may signal the development of vasospasm).

Alternative treatment options to craniotomy with clipping include endovascular occlusion with the use of detachable coils. Recent studies now show excellent long-term outcomes with coiling, as shown by long-term follow-up data extending out to 18.5 years on patients enrolled in the randomized International Subarachnoid Aneurysm Trial (ISAT): "… . the probability of death or dependency was significantly greater in the neurosurgical group than in the endovascular group. Rebleeding was more likely after endovascular coiling than after neurosurgical clipping, but the risk was small and the probability of disability-free survival was significantly greater in the endovascular group than in the neurosurgical group at 10 years" [26].

3.7 Cerebral Aneurysms

Case Example

Time and Space Factors in the Diagnostic Approach to Sub-arachnoid Hemorrhage.

Typically, the symptom of overwhelmingly severe headache of a global nature is abrupt, sudden, and described by the patient in dramatic terms (explosive, or worst headache in the life) with associated nausea, vomiting (Fig. 3.9). In essence, an acute, sudden, and severe headache should include SAH in the differential diagnosis; other factors, such as a family history of polycystic kidneys (known to associate with aneurysms) should immediately raise the level of suspicion. CT can help confirm SAH; however, if the CT is negative, but the history is still suggestive of true SAH, further testing is required and may include lumbar puncture, and/or going directly to MRA or CTA.

The pathophysiology of a unilateral third nerve-related ptosis has been reviewed by Fukushima et al. [27] in relation to a case report of a rare case of a symptomatic infundibulum, which is a funnel-shaped outpouching that is not truly aneurysmal but found in 7–25 % of cases. Regarding pathophysiology of aneurysmal third nerve compression, it is important to note that the oculomotor nerve supplies motor innervation to the levator palpebrae superioris, superior rectus, middle rectus, inferior rectus, and inferior oblique muscles, and parasympathetic innervation to the sphincter muscles of the iris and to the ciliary body. Oculomotor nerve palsy has a wide range of causes that include diabetes mellitus, hypertension, multiple sclerosis, trauma, and compressive lesions such as tumors and aneurysms; compression of the oculomotor nerve in the subarachnoid space usually manifests as partial isolated nerve palsy including pupillary dysfunction.

Case Examples

3D renderings of MRA (Fig. 3.10) or CTA (Fig. 3.11) provides powerful insight to aneurysm morphology.

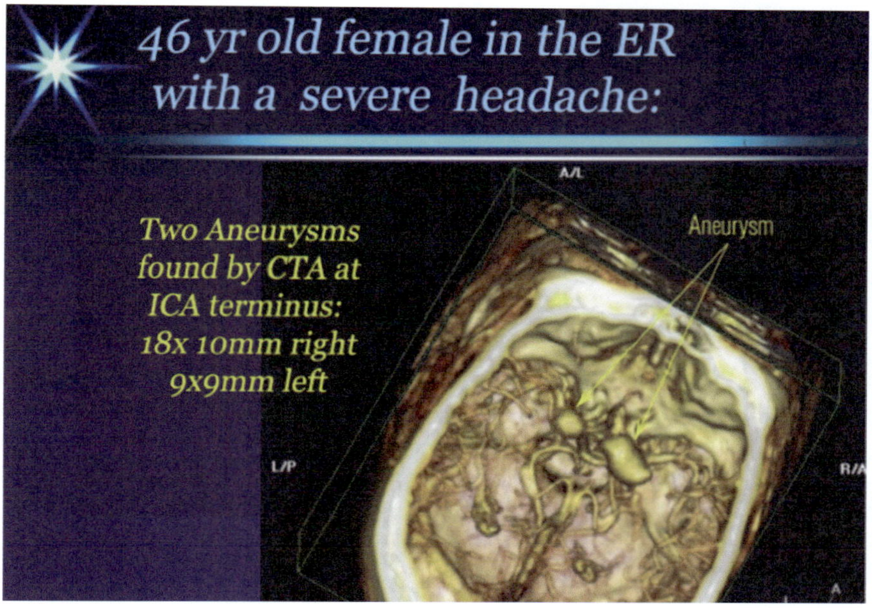

Fig. 3.9 CT angiography aids in ER evaluations in revealing cerebral aneurysms

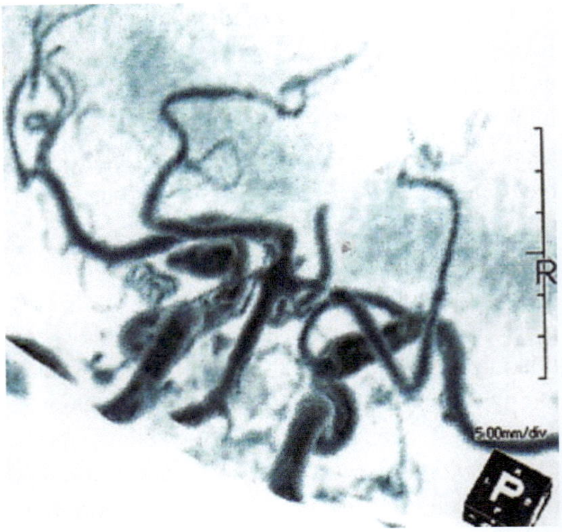

Fig. 3.10 Large intracavernous aneurysm revealed by 3D reconstruction of a brain MRA

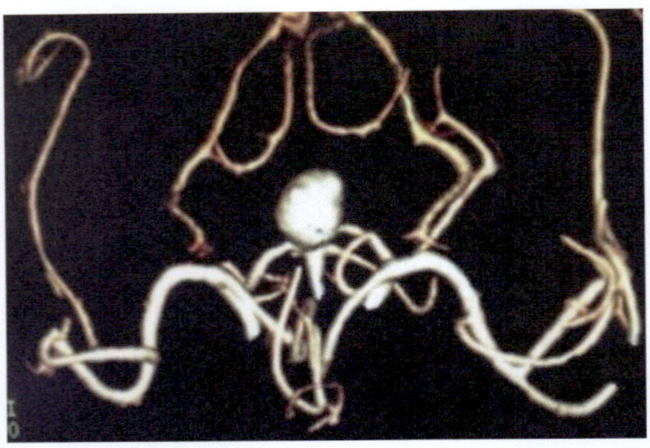

Fig. 3.11 Basilar tip aneurysm seen by CT angiography

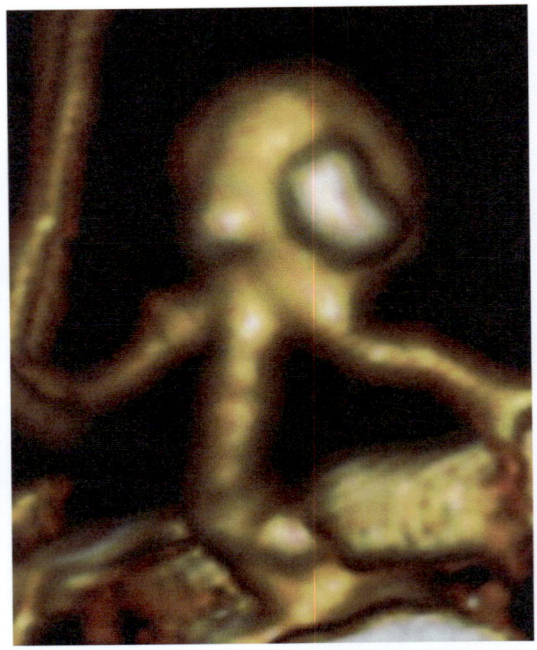

Fig. 3.12 Chronic calcific changes to the wall of an aneurysm discovered by CT angiography

Case Example
Calcific change to walls of a chronic aneurysm discovered incidentally by CT angiography (Figs. 3.12).

Case Example
This MRA was originally read by radiology as negative; however, it reveals an obvious bilobed left ICA terminus aneurysm that was coiled shortly thereafter with good resolution to the pattern of sudden severe headaches in this 62-year-old female (Figs. 3.13 and 3.14).

Case Example
Unusual morphology to left ICA terminus aneurysm well outlined by the 3D reconstruction of the MRA data (Fig. 3.15). Most aneurysms lie in the anterior aspects of Circle of Willis (Fig. 3.16).

Case Example of SAH Mimic
Acute baro-trauma from rapid descent in flight producing acute severe headache in patient with chronic right frontal sinus obstruction due to sinusitis (negative MRA). The patient was brought directly from the airport to the local hospital complaining of the worst headache ever with MRA found to be negative for aneurysm. Sequence of images from top left panel downward include CT, T2, Diffusion, FLAIR for MRI (Fig. 3.17).

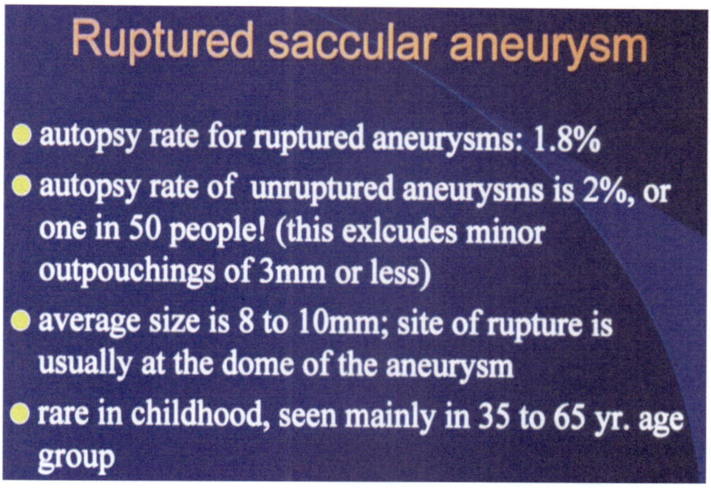

Fig. 3.13 Unruptured aneurysms are found in 2 % of the population

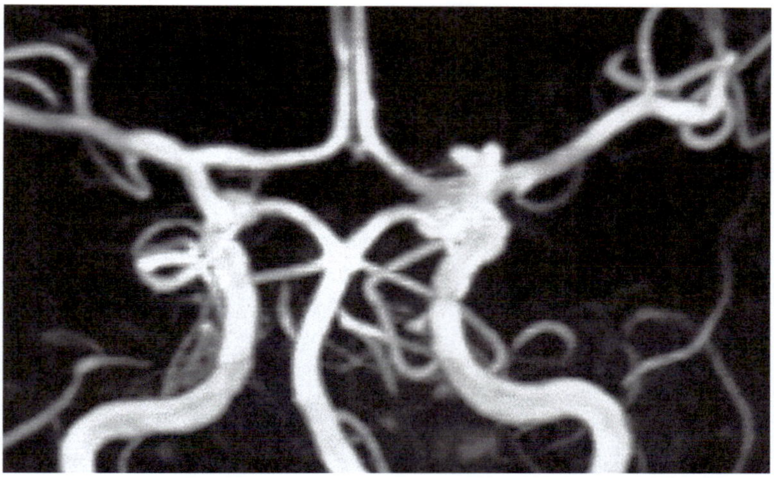

Fig. 3.14 Unusual bilobed appearance to a symptomatic aneurysm that was later successfully coiled

Case Example
Massive sudden fatal ICH. An 82-year-old female who was at home having an afternoon meal with her husband who suddenly became completely unresponsive and was rushed to the local ER where CT imaging was performed immediately—as shown, a massive ICH is revealed with midline shift already apparent within 30 min of the bleed (Fig. 3.18).

3.7.1 Hypertension-Related Intracranial Hemorrhage

Case Example
Shows a typical location for hypertension-related ICH being the lenticulostriate artery distribution—the hemorrhage shown above was in a recurrent form and in the setting of uncontrolled hypertension (Fig. 3.19).

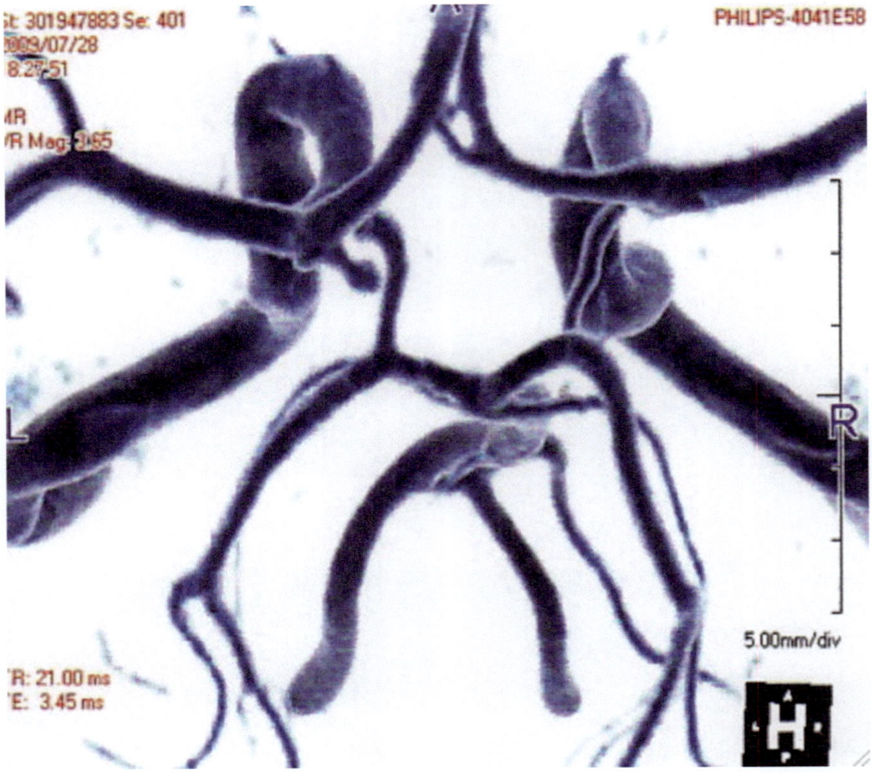

Fig. 3.15 3D rendering of 3 T brain MRA showing a left ICA terminus aneurysm

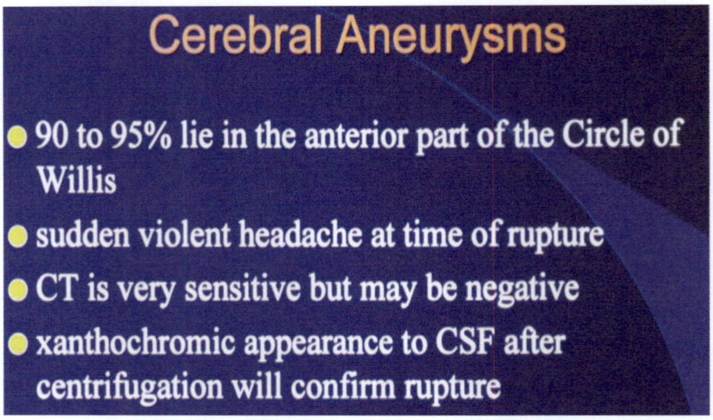

Fig. 3.16 Most aneurysms lie in the anterior aspects of Circle of Willis

3.7.2 Intracranial Hemorrhage: Relation to Thrombocytopenia

Case Example

ITP-related ICH in a 57-year-female with severe headache, new onset (Fig. 3.20).

Case Example

In an investigation regarding the incidentally reported spells of unexplained syncope, an underlying AVM of the left parietal region was uncovered as shown above in an otherwise healthy 74-year-old male; conservative management was elected. Metabolic effects of

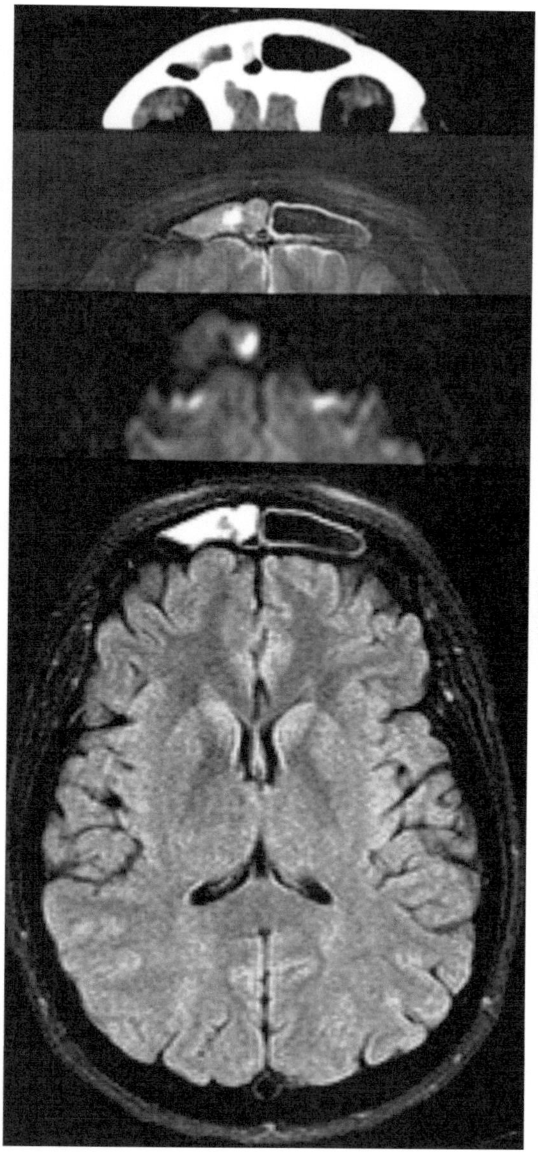

Fig. 3.17 Frontal sinusitis mimicking subarachnoid hemorrhage with "worst headache ever" event with barotrauma while descending in an airplane about to land. *Top* to *bottom*: CT, T2, diffusion, FLAIR

Vascular "Steal" Phenomenon from Arterio-Venous Malformations (AVMs) are illustrated in Figs. 3.21, 3.22, 3.23, and 3.24).

The dynamic study above shows the metabolic effects of the presumed vascular "steal" effect from the high flow AVM shown above within the

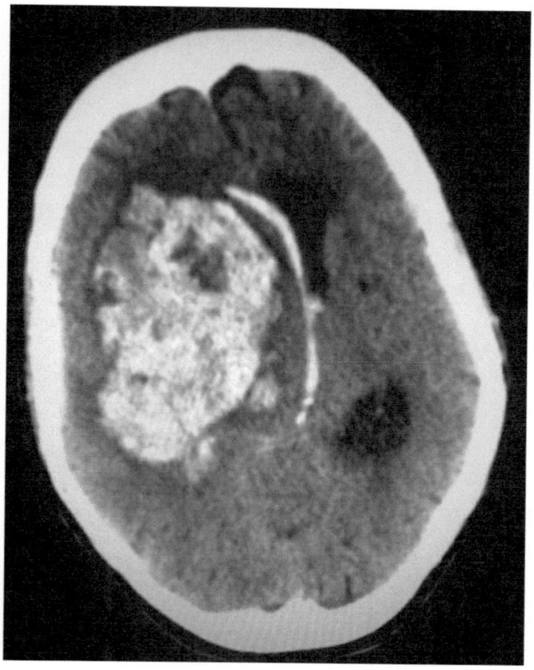

Fig. 3.18 Sudden fatal hypertension-related right lenticulostriate artery area intracerebral hemorrhage

left parietal cortex; this steal effect renders areas of cortex in a marginally perfused state, thereby forming a predisposition to seizure activity (Figs. 3.23 and 3.24).

Case Example

De novo evolution of a highly symptomatic lower pontine cavernoma that was successfully treated by surgery (Figs. 3.25 and 3.26).

The Cerebral Venous Circulation: A neglected yet important aspect to stroke in the cerebral venous system (Fig. 3.27).

As shown in the examples set forth below, stroke symptoms and changes suggesting hemorrhage can arise with major sagittal sinus occlusions; in other cases, it may be partial as in the case of the straight sinus shown below, or may be a cortical branch vein occlusion, also shown here in this section. Anatomy of the cerebral venous system shown in Figs. 3.28, 3.29, and 3.30 depicts Chiari-related venous hypertensive change to the straight sinus.

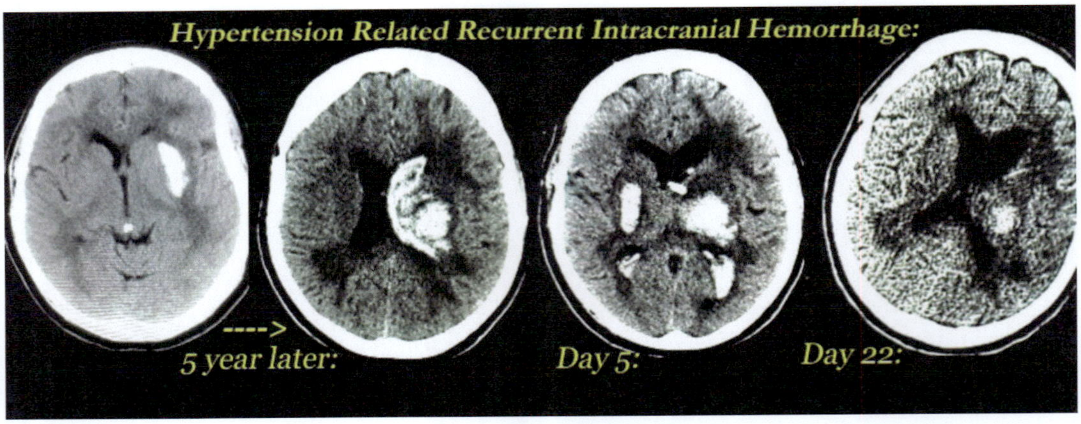

Fig. 3.19 Recurrent left lenticulostriate area bleed secondary to hypertension

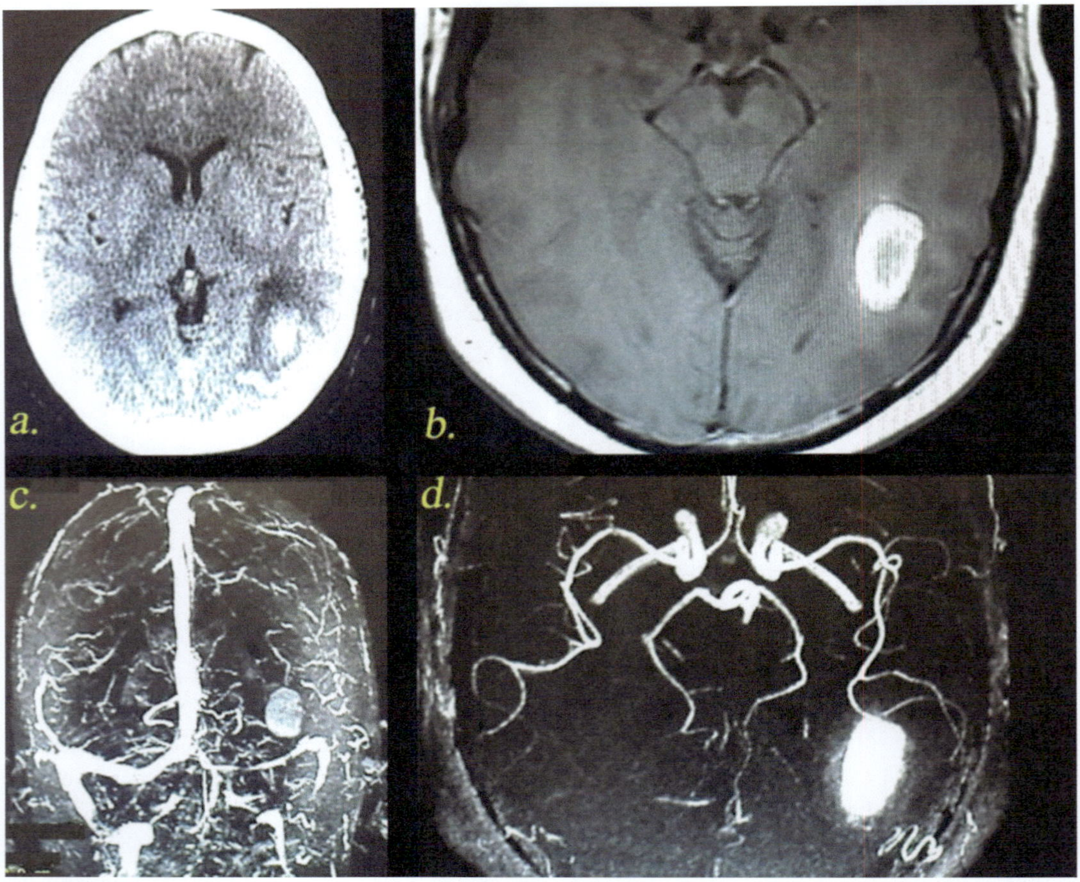

Fig. 3.20 ITP-related spontaneous bleed within the posterior left temporal area that resorbed and resolved with conservative management within 10 weeks

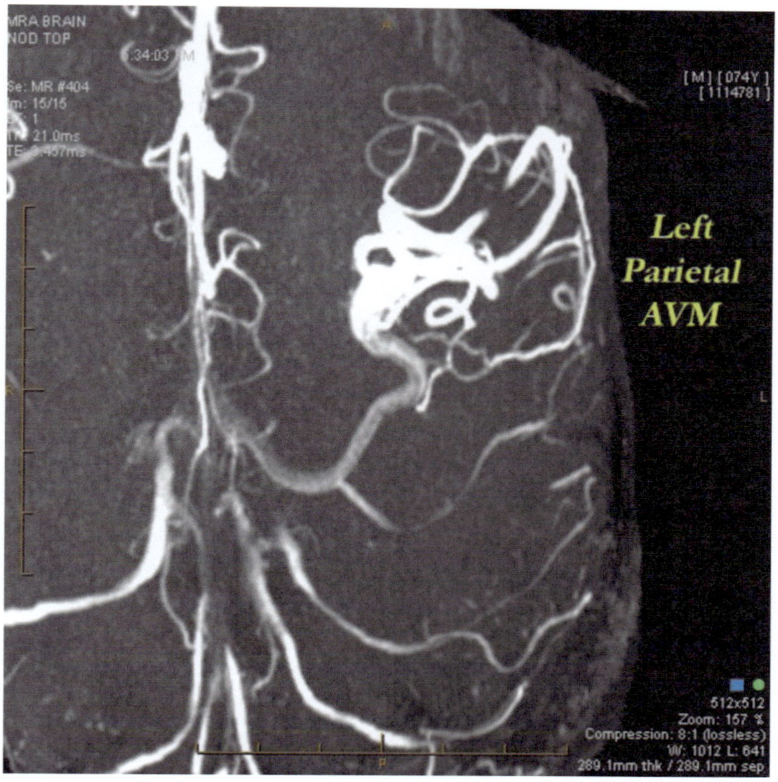

Fig. 3.21 Left parietal AVM revealed by MRA; conservative management elected

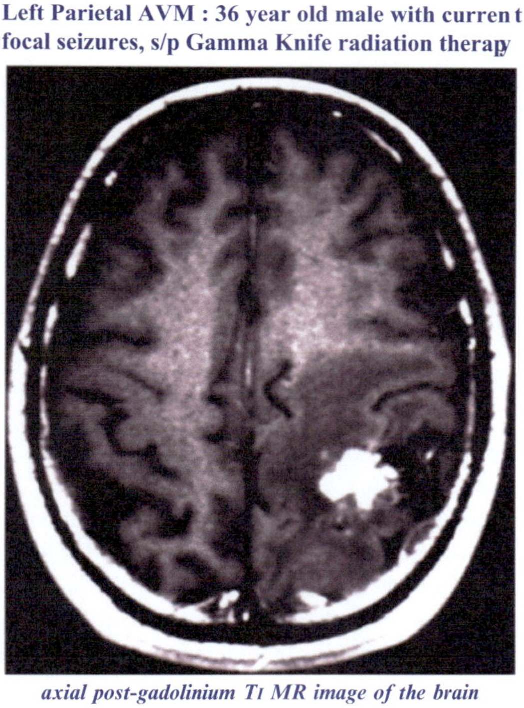

Fig. 3.22 Persistent AVM despite gamma knife radiotherapy in 36-year-old male with seizures

Case Example Sagittal Sinus Thrombosis

A 24-year-old female presented to the ER with the worst headache of her life that was becoming progressively severe and extreme, leading to generalized seizure activity within the MR scanner, where MR venography could eventually be performed after giving anticonvulsant medication with sedation (Fig. 3.31a). As shown in Fig. 3.31b, complete superior sagittal sinus thrombosis was evident, and found to be related to not only ongoing irregular oral contraceptive use, but also homozygosity for the Factor V Leiden gene mutation but also being pregnant with twins, which she was unaware of. Angiography clearly revealed the morphology of the occlusive thrombi (Fig. 3.31c)—after 30 h of Urokinase infusion, this occlusion was resolved with good restoration of flow (Fig. 3.31d) and great clinical outcome with the patient leaving in a fully intact state.

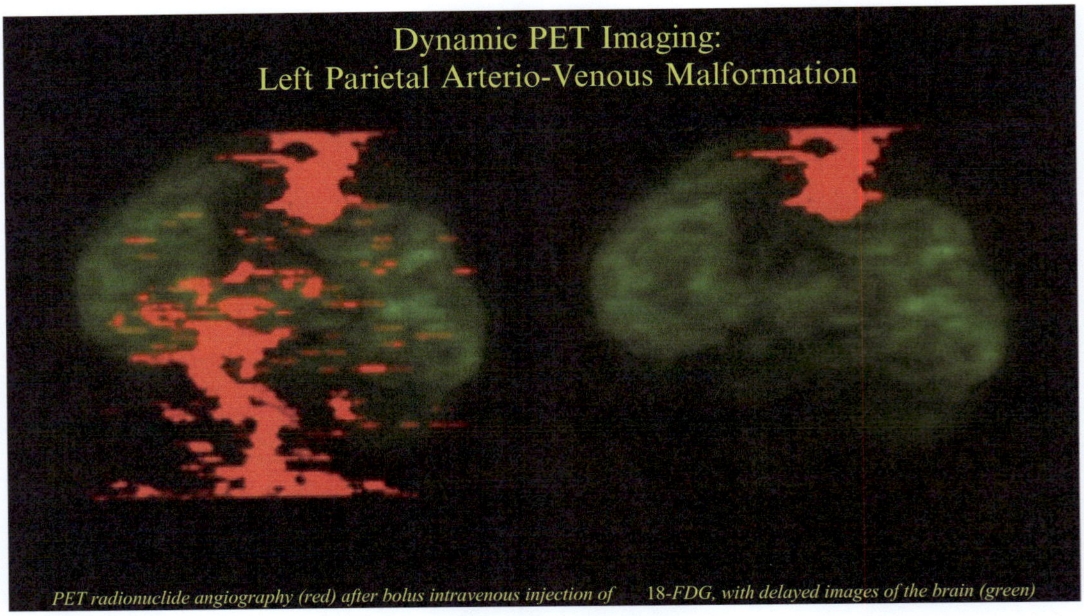

Fig. 3.23 Metabolic depression within AVM area as revealed by dynamic PET imaging with 18F-FDG

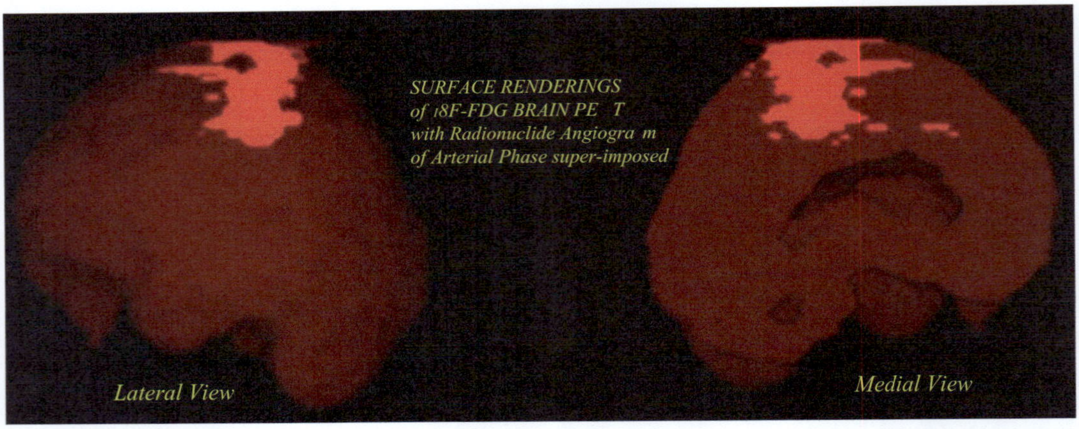

Fig. 3.24 Arterial phase after 18F-FDG bolus injection outlining extent of the AVM shown in Fig. 3.28

Case Example
Straight Sinus Thrombosis (Fig. 3.32). A 46-year-old female with progressively severe headaches and hyper-dense CT changes within the straight sinus, corresponding to a filling defect on the CT Venogram shown at right. Clopidogrel on a daily basis was given with good resolution of symptoms as well CT changes.

Case Example
Focal Right Vein of Labbe Thrombosis (Fig. 3.33). A 50-year-old male with sudden focal right parietal headache consistent with a focal right vein of Labbe thrombosis; conservative management in this particular case with anti-platelet agents led to a successful outcome without deficit.

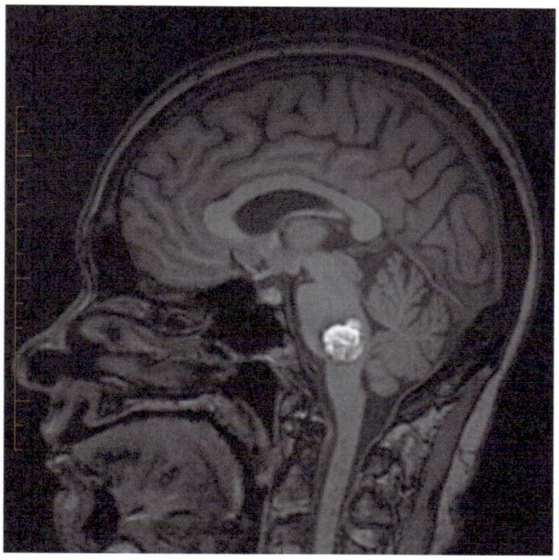

Fig. 3.25 Brain stem cavernoma that arose de novo as assessed by serial MR brain exams with successful resection at surgery

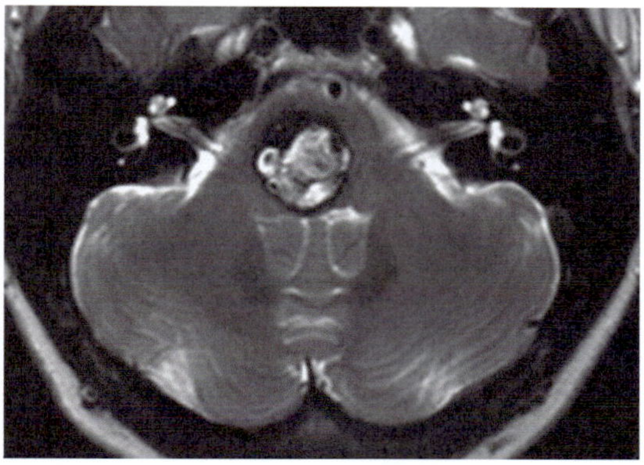

Fig. 3.26 Axial T2 image of same cavernoma lesion; patient was highly symptomatic preoperatively with leg weakness and ataxia that improved after surgery

Case Example (Fig. 3.34)

Forty-six-year-old with multiple TIA episodes due to multiple rare vascular anomalies with areas of critical stenosis at the origins of both middle cerebral arteries, reflecting a highly unusual pattern (likely of developmental origin) where fortunately no infarction had yet occurred. This case is presented to highlight and contrast the transiently symptomatic patient versus those presenting with major acute and sustained deficits

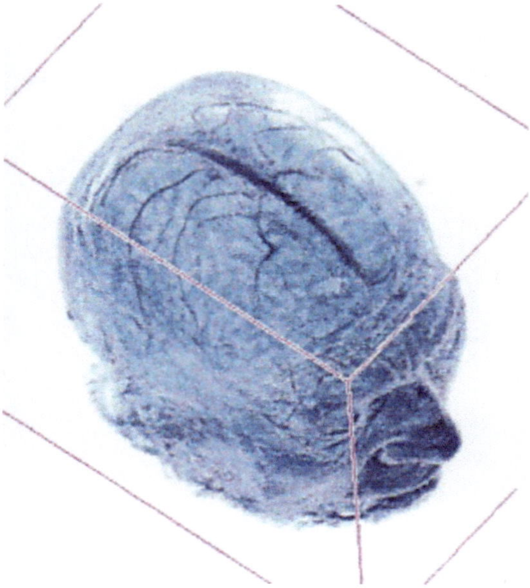

Fig. 3.27 Normal appearance to superior sagittal sinus as seen by MR venography

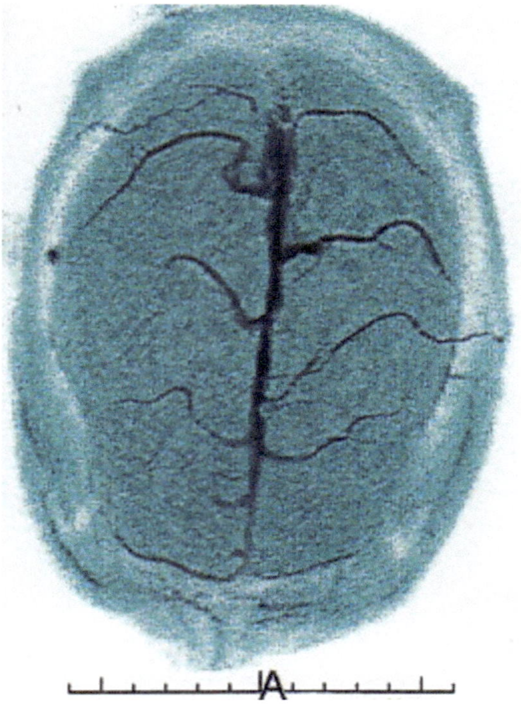

Fig. 3.28 Normal superficial venous anatomy shown by MR venography

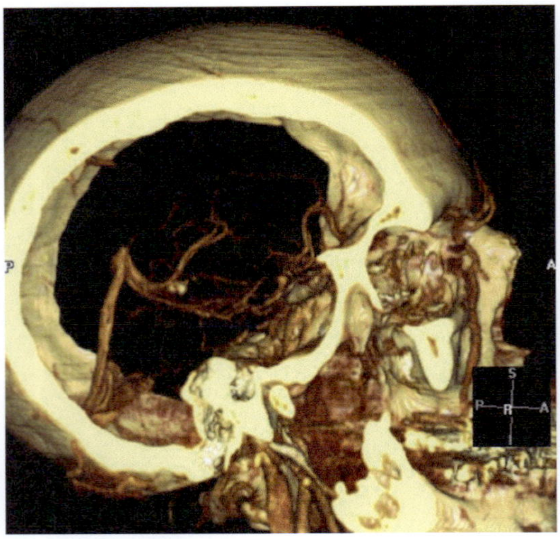

Fig. 3.29 Deep venous anatomy as shown by CT angiography

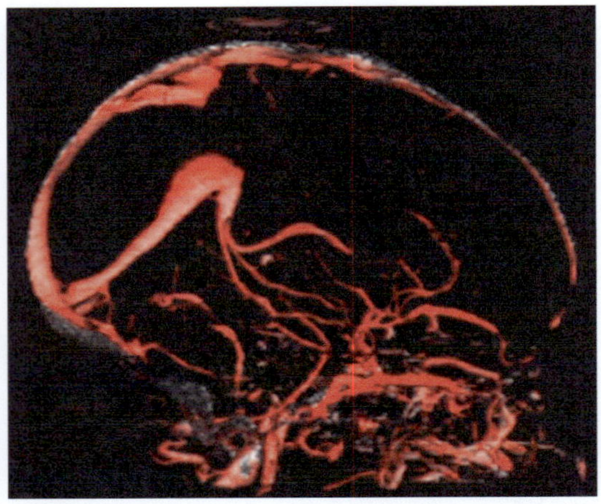

Fig. 3.30 Extreme venous hypertension in 32-year-old female with headaches, papilledema, and high intracranial pressure due to Chiari-related tonsilar herniation that improved dramatically after emergent decompressive surgery; note the dilated plump appearance to the straight sinus on this preoperative CT venogram study

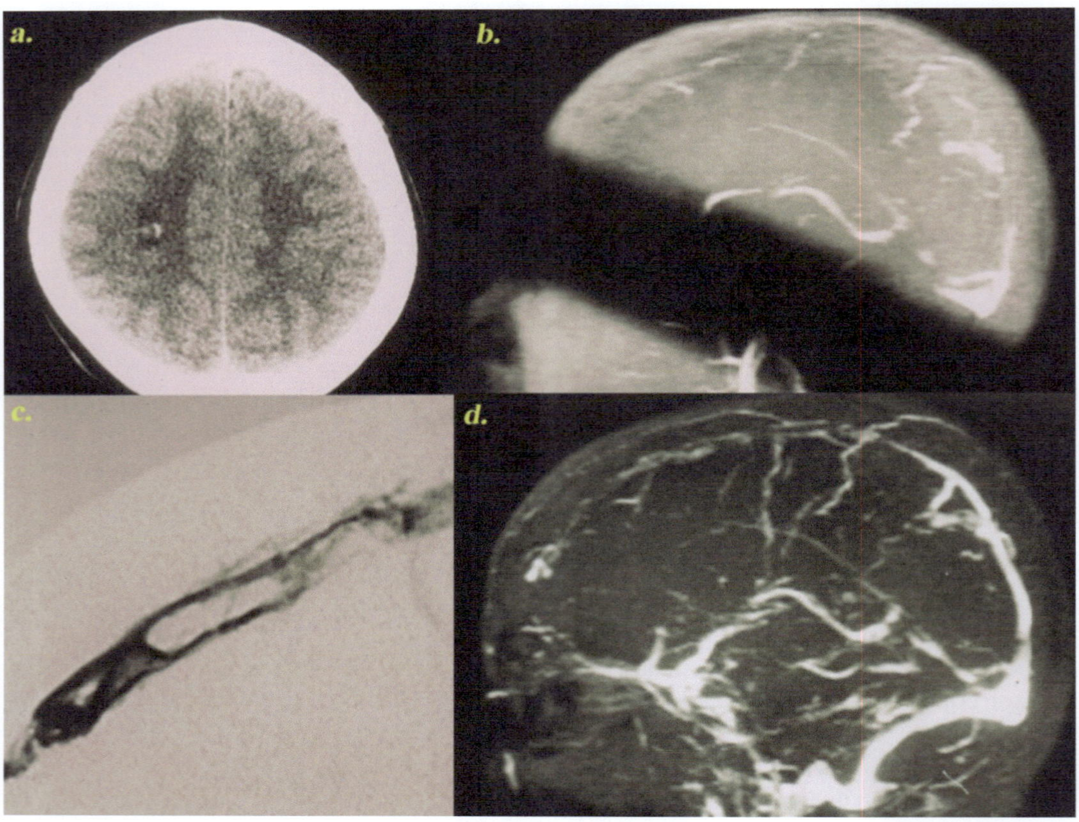

Fig. 3.31 (**a**) Extreme venous hypertension in young woman due to complete sagittal sinus occlusion (**b**) secondary to oral contraceptive use without awareness of being pregnant with twins while being homozygous for the factor V Leiden gene mutation; intraluminal thrombus (**c**) was successfully lysed by catheter directed urokinase infusion (**d**); 10 days later, patient walked out of the hospital, free of deficit

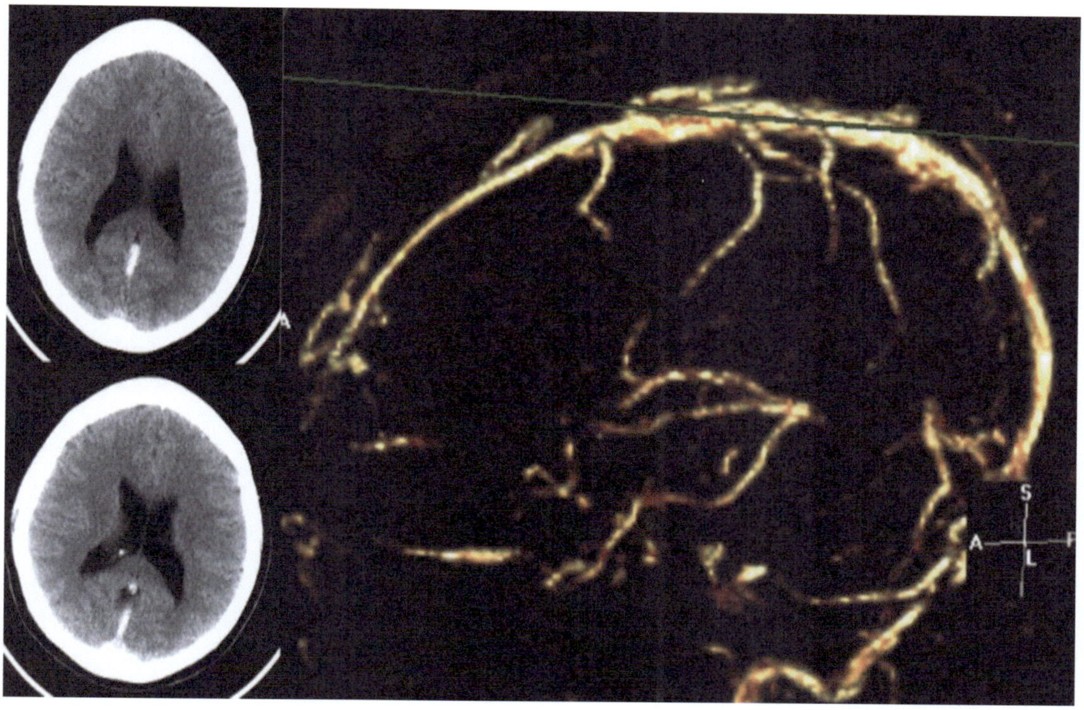

Fig. 3.32 Thrombotic deep straight sinus occlusion successfully managed by conservative treatment with clopidogrel

from acute ischemic stroke, requiring thrombolytic therapy with IV tPA if meeting criteria within 180 min after onset. Figure 3.35 shows a case well outside the thrombolytic time window.

3.7.3 Facts on TIA

Transient ischemic attack (TIA) is a serious problem that occurs in at least one-quarter of a million Americans annually and signals a sharply elevated risk for a damaging stroke event that may be imminent. Half of all strokes that do ensue within the first 1-month after a TIA do so within the first 1 day after the onset of TIA, which is why TIA is regarded as a true medical emergency that requires immediate attention; one Canadian study showed the 1 year stroke risk was almost 15 %. As shown by the EXPRESS study [28], immediate attention makes a huge difference in outcome as it can reduce the 3-month risk for stroke by 80 %!

Although technically defined as a fully resolved transient neurologic deficit lasting no more than 24 h, 60 % of all TIAs are completed within 1 h (actually two-thirds of these brief events last no more than 10 min). As the risk for stroke can be as high as 10 % over the next 1 week, it is important to immediately identify the mechanism for the TIA event through comprehensive evaluation by CT or better yet MR vascular imaging techniques along with cardiac monitoring and ECHO so that the most appropriate treatment plan can be formulated and instituted right away.

Unlike the urgent pain involved with myocardial ischemia that readily brings patients to their local hospital emergency department, a TIA is painless and often neglected and/or not appreciated by many individuals as significant; about one-third of those interviewed about their TIA do not recall seeing a doctor in the first day after the event.

As shown by the landmark British study known as EXPRESS, involving 1278 patients presenting with TIA or minor stroke, an aggressive approach to the problem with immediate evaluation and treatment gave superior outcomes when compared to a slower, non-emergent process. The 90-day risk for stroke for the latter slow

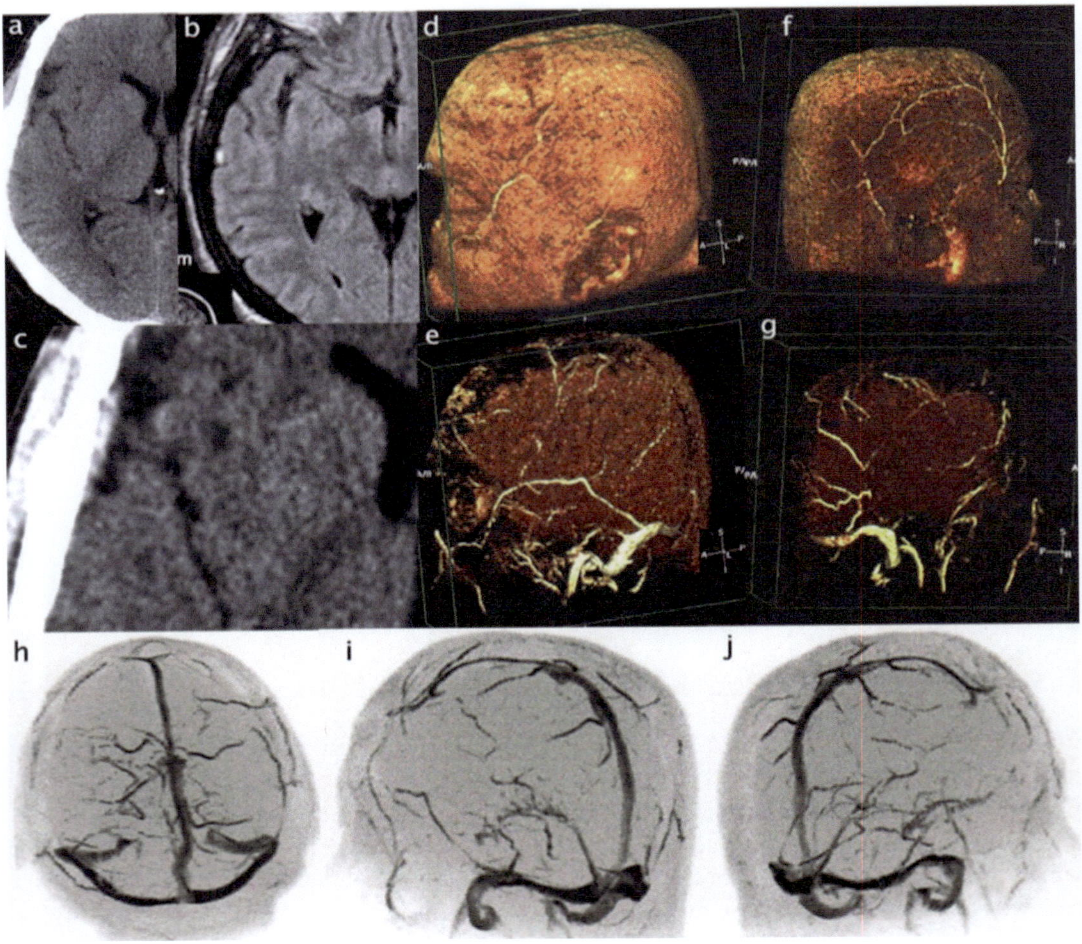

Fig. 3.33 Thrombotic occlusion of the right vein of Labbe (**g**) with associated headaches; normal vein of Labbe is seen on the left (**e**); the patient was successfully managed by conservative treatment with clopidogrel

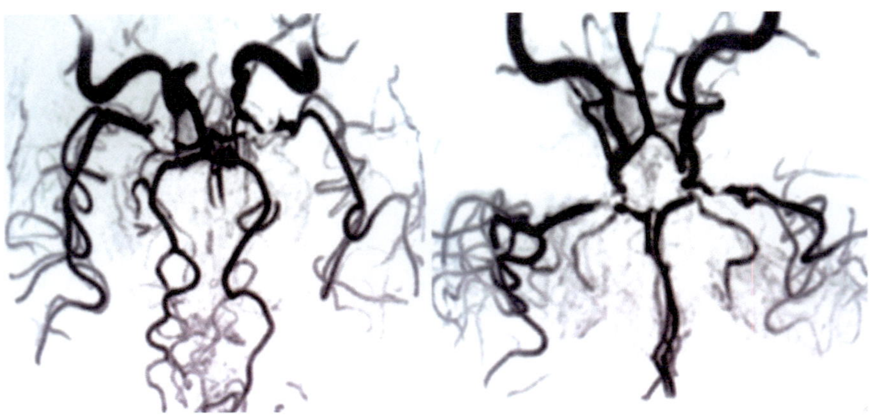

Fig. 3.34 Multiple TIA events in 46-year-old female led to the discovery of multiple congenital vascular anomalies with hypoplasia to origins of both middle cerebral arteries

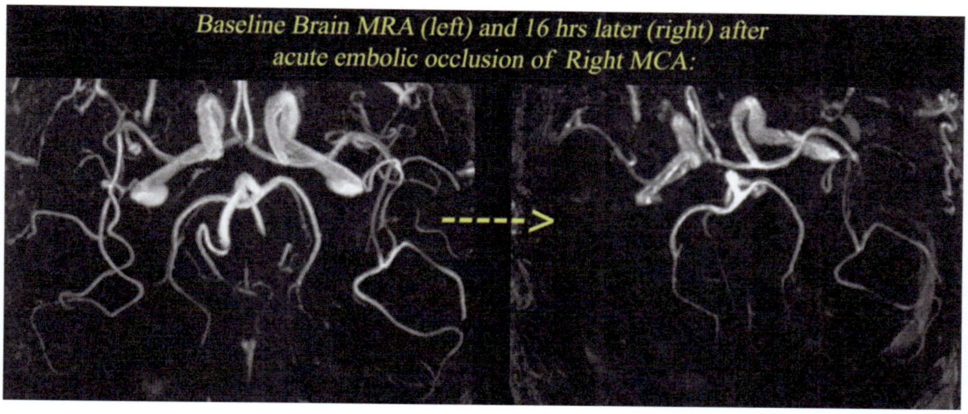

Fig. 3.35 Embolic occlusion to right middle cerebral artery as shown by sequential MRA exams

approach was 10.3 % versus 2.1 % for the urgent evaluation method, equating to an 80 % reduction in the risk of early recurrent stroke [29].

3.8 Thrombolytic Therapy

A major advance in stroke care has been the introduction of thrombolytic therapy with intravenous recombinant tissue plasminogen activator (r-tPA). First approved in 1996 by the FDA after publication of the landmark trial sponsored by the NINDS [29], it has become the standard of care for acute significant ischemic stroke occurring within the 180-min time window. The mechanism of action for this naturally occurring serine protease is that its enzymatic activity is selectively limited to the site of thrombus and does not generate a systemic fibrinolysis. The tPA molecule binds to lysine side chains that cross-link fibrin monomers within an occluding thrombus; this binding of lysine to tPA activates plasminogen only locally around the clot, inducing plasminogen to convert to active plasmin which can then enzymatically reduce the thrombus into fibrin degradation products.

Although not FDA approved for use beyond 180 min, there is European data from the ECASS III study that shows comparable safety and efficacy for tPA to be used in the 180–270 min time window (3–4.5 h). As noted by the investigators, higher favorable outcomes were seen with tPA than for placebo (52.4 % vs. 45.2 %; odds ratio, 1.34; $p=0.04$). Although higher rates of symptomatic intracranial hemorrhage was found (2.4 % vs. 0.2 %), mortality did not differ significantly between the two groups [30].

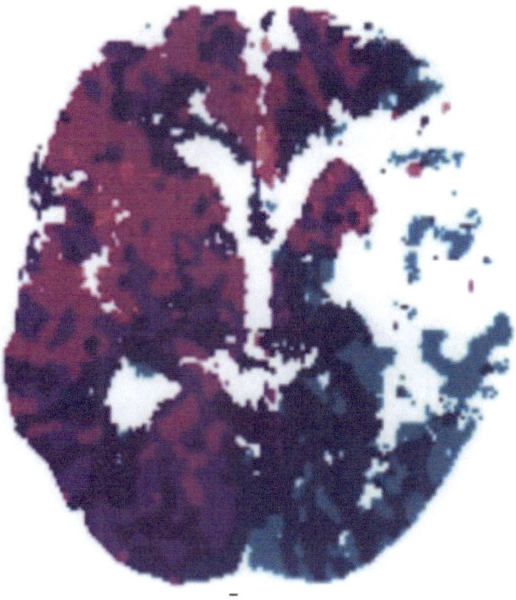

Fig. 3.36 Major acute left MCA occlusion revealed by CT perfusion techniques

Perfusion CT exam mapping time to peak on a voxel by voxel basis, revealing a massive acute left MCA ischemic event in a 92-year-old; as the changes extended into the left PCA area as well, this may represent a fetal origin of the left PCA from the left ICA, which may be occluded in this case. Normal perfusion is seen for the right hemisphere (Fig. 3.36).

Case Example
Acute stroke effectively treated with IV tPA (Fig. 3.37).

Clinical Case Example
Use of tPA in acute stroke (Fig. 3.38).

3.9 Clinical Analysis by Time and Space Methodology

The history described above reflects an acute focal deficit, most likely consistent with stroke, especially in conjunction with obvious risk factors being

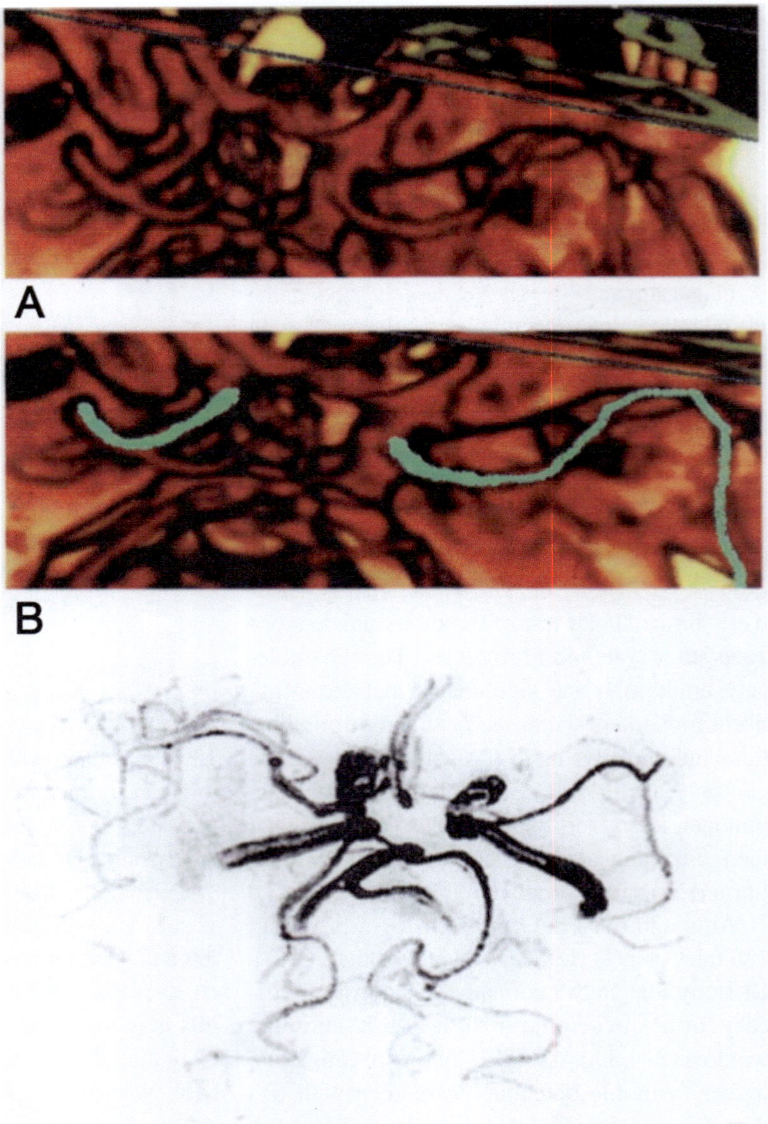

Fig. 3.37 Successful thrombolysis of an acute left MCA occlusion using IV tPA. (**a**) Acute left MCA occlusion (CT angiogram prior to i.v. tPA). (**b**) MRA obtained 1 week later after successful treatment with i.v. tPA with good functional improvement in acute right hemiparesis and recanalization of flow into the previously occluded left middle cerebral artery (MCA)

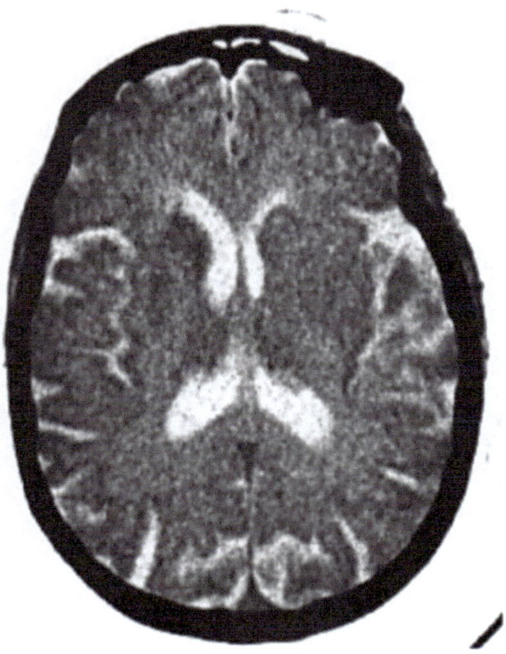

Fig. 3.38 Case example: acute stroke management in the elderly with use of tPA. An 88-year-old female who becomes aphasic and falls into the arms of her husband in her kitchen with a sudden right-sided paralysis; CT head exam obtained later in ED was negative for hemorrhage (Fig. 3.38)

advanced age of 88 years. If this had been a hemiparetic event in a 22-year-old, the breadth of possibilities would be greater and include etiologies such as demyelinating disease, and if there was associated headache, hemiplegic migraine; however, given the markedly severe deficit of not only language but motor strength being affected in an abrupt manner, hemorrhage or infarction remain at the top of the differential diagnosis list, regardless of age and constitutes a true Neurological Emergency.

Acute Stroke Protocol: Every regional medical center needs to formulate its own decision tree that is practical for its hospital facility. Although IV tPA is a requisite core responsibility, the details may vary depending on the availability of Point of Care (POC) for near instant lab test result determination; other details include the possible need to transfer to a tertiary care center if endovascular therapy is needed; MR/MRA is not required for tPA use but may be helpful if readily available for patients who can be effectively and safely screened. For those presenting late, the 3–4.5 h window represents a special use that is reserved for individual consideration, as tPA has FDA approval only for 0–180 min. Contraindications for tPA use is shown in Fig. 3.39.

tPA ContraIndication Summary

CONTRAINDICATIONS:

- ▲ Evidence of intracranial hemorrhage on pretreament evaluation
- ▲ Suspicion of subarachnoid hemorrhage
- ▲ Recent intracranial surgery or serious head trauma or recent previous stroke
- ▲ History of intracranial hemorrhage
- ▲ Uncontrolled hypertension at time of treatment (e.g., >185 mm Hg systolic or >110 mm Hg diastolic)
- ▲ Seizure at the onset of stroke
- ▲ Active internal bleeding
- ▲ Intracranial neoplasm, arteriovenous malformation, or aneurysm
- ▲ Known bleeding diathesis, including but not limited to:
  - — Current use of oral anticoagulants (e.g., warfarin sodium) with prothrombin time (PT)>15 seconds
  - — Administration of heparin within 48 hours preceding the onset of stroke and an elevated activated partial thromboplastin time (aPTT) at presentation
  - — Platelet count < 100,000/mm^3

tPA Dose **EXACT BODY WEIGHT NEEDED:**

DOSING INFORMATION FOR ACUTE ISCHEMIC STROKE:

0.9 mg/kg; maximum dose 90 mg

10% of the total dose administered as an IV bolus over 1 minute
Remaining 90% infused over 60 minutes

Fig. 3.39 IV tPA protocol: list of contraindications with dosing instructions

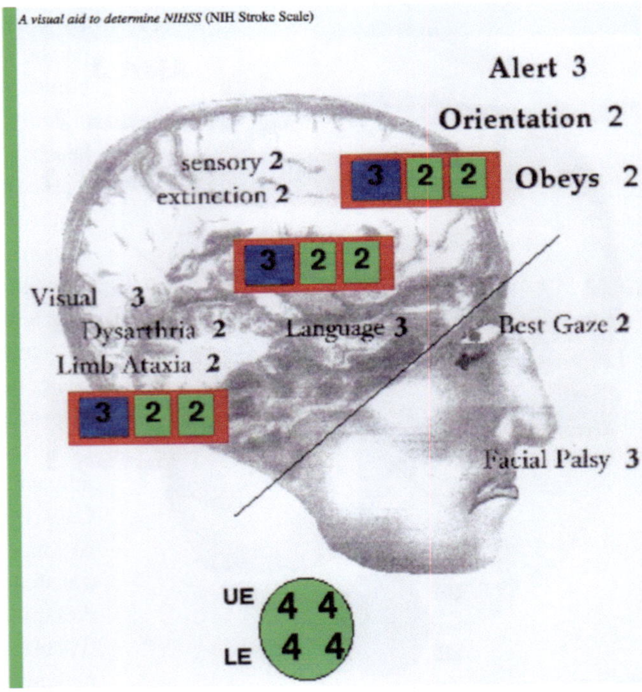

Fig. 3.40 Rapid method to determine level of stroke deficit using the NIHSS system

The NIH Stroke Scale (NIHSS) score is an accepted standard part of all acute stroke evaluations and represents a semiquantitative summation of clinically observable deficits that reflect the overall severity to the stroke-like event. As many feel this can be a cumbersome effort that consumes limited time available when tPA may be an option, a quick estimation is proposed above using the Stroke Quick Score (Fig. 3.40) [31].

3.9.1 Details of the Ninds Stroke Protocol (Fig. 3.41)

Actual Acute Stroke Case Example: CT angiography with 3D reconstruction software produced the following interactive windowed reconstructions generated by the attending Stroke Neurologist over the span of 90 s from start to finish, as illustrated in the sequence of 10 images shown below that finally localized the site of occlusion to the left MCA M1 segment as shown at the lower right panel (Fig. 3.41).

The sequence of windowed images not only revealed the site of occlusion, but also revealed extensive calcific changes to the left carotid bifurcation (Fig. 3.42).

With regard to Fig. 3.43, the baseline CT head was negative for hemorrhage (a), clearing patient for IV tPA use, with the immediate post tPA infusion MRA still revealing the left MCA M1 occlusion (b), which resolved with recanalization evident on the MRA at 1 week (e and f). At 219 min after onset, and within 40 min of tPA infusion completion, the DWI image (c) confirms that damage was limited to the left lenticulostriate artery distribution which was later evident on the CT 1 week later (d) that showed spotty hemorrhagic transformation within the basal ganglia infarct; these hemosiderin changes become magnified with MRA where the associated left basal ganglia signal changes are readily seen in (e) and (f). Reasonably good clinical outcome was achieved for this 88-year-old stroke patient, who had incurred a major left MCA M1 occlusion that cleared with the use of IV tPA as shown in the above follow-up MRA at 1 week where the left MCA was wide open (Fig. 3.43).

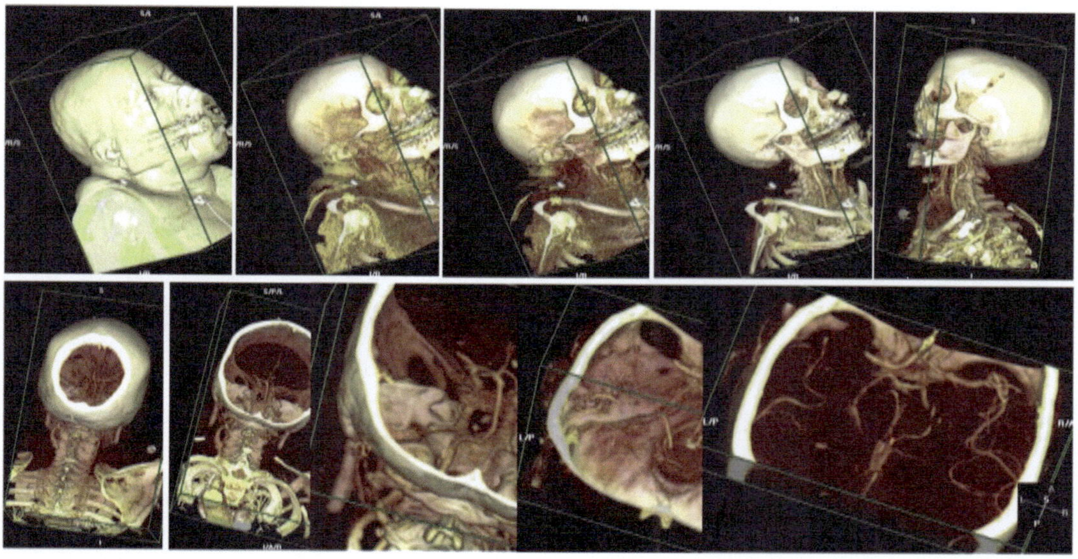

Fig. 3.41 Rapid determination of the site and severity of obstruction using CT angiography

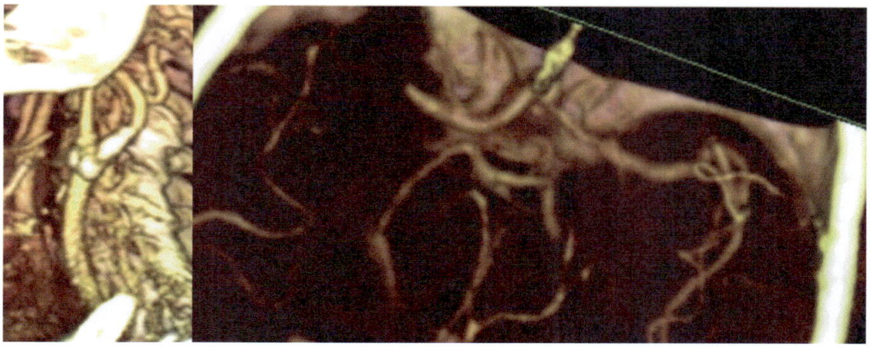

Fig. 3.42 Left MCA occlusion as seen by CT angio prior to IV tPA

Case Example

A 78-year-old with major left MCA ischemic deficits of an acute nature treated with IV tPA failed recanalize immediately after treatment (MRA at left) but later improved within 3 h after tPA as confirmed by CT perfusion (middle) and repeat MRA (right); final NIHSS was zero with full reversal of initial speech and motor deficits (Fig. 3.44).

Case Example

Small infarct producing major clinical deficits (Fig. 3.45).

Acute right leg weakness in an elderly patient with hypertension—emergent MR diffusion scan defines this as small vessel related and after weighing risk versus benefits, the patient was taken out of consideration for thrombolytic therapy and deferred to medical therapy due to elevations in her blood pressure (Fig. 3.45).

3.10 Stroke in Young Adults

Case Example

Cryptogenic Stroke in 32-year-old male, fully reversed by IV tPA.

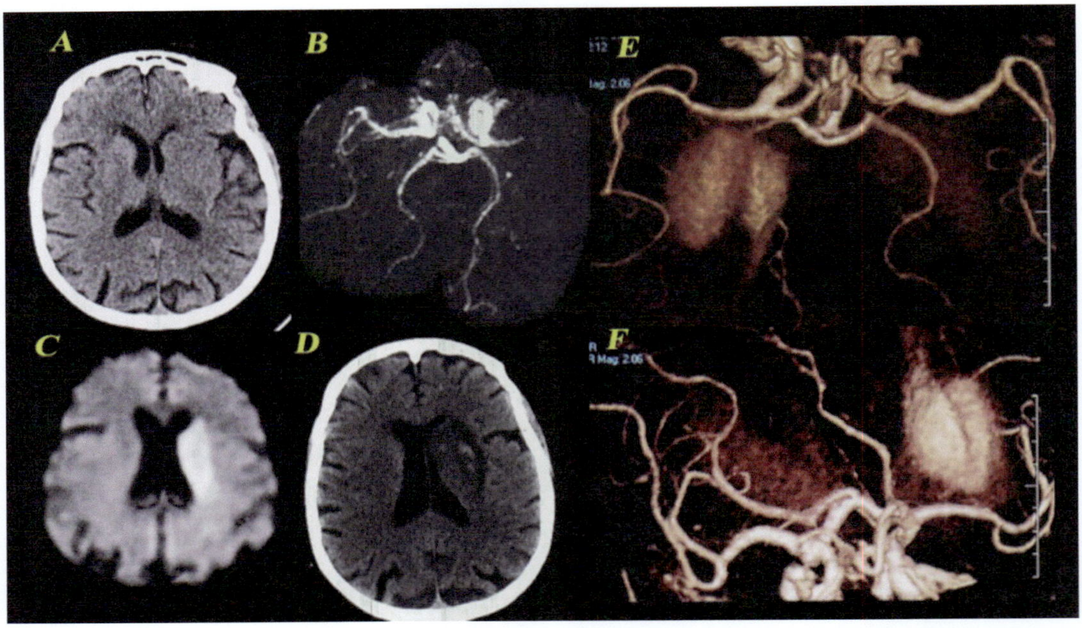

Fig. 3.43 Successful outcome using tPA to restore flow into left MCA (**e, f**) with good clinical outcome

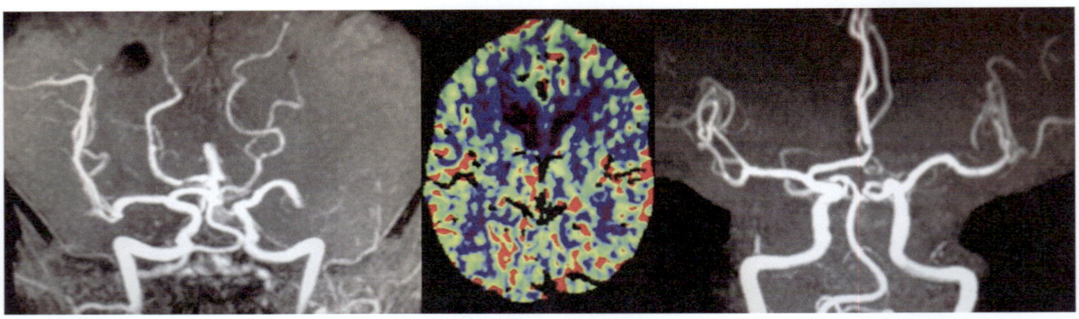

Fig. 3.44 Acute left MCA occlusion (*left*) successfully treated with IV tPA as shown by CT perfusion (*middle*) and the MRA (*right*) obtained within 3 h of treatment with tPA

".....Within a few weeks of successfully treating a young woman with a very unusual cause for hemorrhagic stroke, my beeper went off in the middle of the afternoon while I was at clinic. I rushed over to the ER to find out what the STAT page for the stroke team was all about. The ER was fully of its usual daily activity, with a nurse brushing aside my question not to worry as our Senior Chief of Neurology had already been by and said that it turned out to be "psyche case"—she told me that he thought that "he must be crazy." Bed 14 revealed a frantic young man with his wife by his side; he appeared to be somewhat hysterical yet unable to fully express himself in any clear manner. I tried to calm him a little bit, and carefully examine him—he had asymmetric strength in his arms and legs. Someone approached the bed who looked familiar to me and identified himself as a coworker of the man, who turned out be a young physician at the hospital in residency. The details now became clear, as the young man was too frantic and seemingly

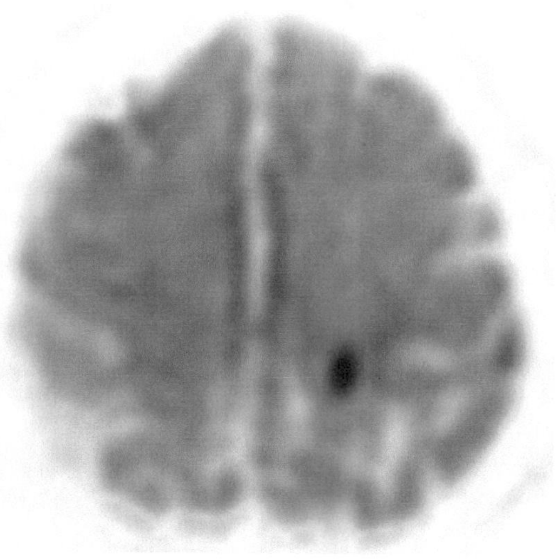

Fig. 3.45 Acute right leg weakness due to a solitary focal DWI positive ischemic zone affecting exiting motor fibers from midline left motor cortex representation of the right leg

incapacitated to explain what had happened: while peering into a microscope at 1:30 PM, this young physician was witnessed to fall to the floor with unilateral weakness and trouble with his speech. This young doctor knew exactly what was happening to him—at the young age of 32, this father of two young children was suddenly fearful that he was about to leave his wife a widow… he knew that he was having a major stroke, and did not know why, and was extraordinarily panicked and frightened.

Having been part of the major NIH sponsored trial for the use of tPA as a clot busting agent for acute stroke, I knew as well what was going on, and tried to reassure him and his wife that we might be able to use this new clot busting medicine that had been approved for clinical use only within the past 2 years at that time. I knew that he was not crazy, but need to get him into MRI as soon as possible to determine the site and size of his ischemic change invisible to us on his CT, while not delaying our team from working through the checklist of inclusion and exclusion criteria for tPA. The lab was busy working on his blood counts and chemistries, while we were getting him into MRI and calling pharmacy to deliver tPA to the MR imaging suite STAT. Just as he emerged from the scanner, and his major acute diffusion-weighted scan abnormality flashed across the computer screen, the pharmacist rushed in with the tPA and the infusion equipment. Within the 180-min time limit, we assembled everything we needed right there in the middle of the MR prep room and began the infusion. I will never forget, nor will the patient or his wife who was present, the sudden melting away of his major deficit, right before our eyes. This was not immediate, but very clearly starting to take place within 15 min of the 10 % bolus followed by the infusion, and by the end of the 1-h of the infusion, I had a very happy patient who was smiling and fully able to move all his arms and legs normally.

Ten years later, I still get Christmas cards of thanks from this physician and his family, who was left without any visible or obvious deficit. We never figured out what happened despite an exhaustive set of tests that also included a transesophageal echocardiogram. My departmental chairman had initially thought "he must be crazy"—he had heard the hoof-beats of something that led him to think incorrectly as this being a psychotic reaction in a young adult to something unknown—the zebra in this case was that young adults (and even children) can develop acute stroke. Common knowledge about stroke in the elderly is easy to apply, but by neglecting uncommon modes of presentation in young adults could have led to devastating consequences if others were not more aware."

Case Example

The above example illustrates the value of tPA in reperfusing acute occlusions in young adults. The case shown above illustrates an oral contraceptive use related stroke event in a 30-year-old female who presented with an acute right homonymous hemianopsia with headache, clinically simulating a migrainous event—however, the recent start of oral contraception use in conjunction with abrupt onset of symptoms that remained

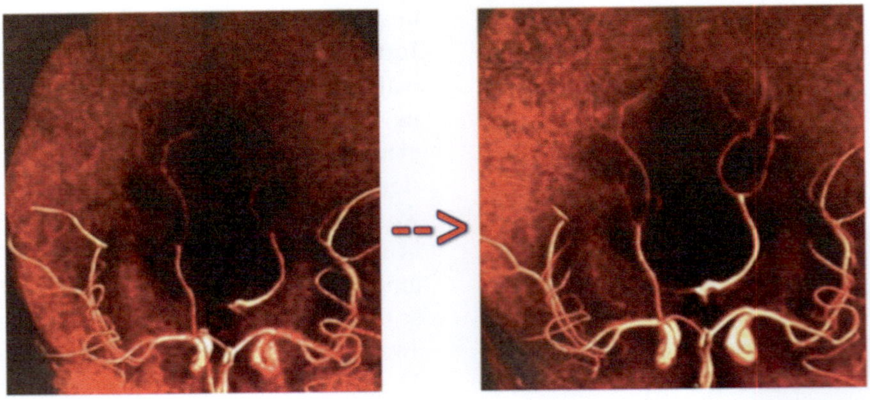

Fig. 3.46 Oral contraceptive-related thrombotic occlusion of the left posterior cerebral artery branches successfully treated by IV tPA

sustained suggested the possibility of acute stroke and prompted immediate evaluation by MR with MRA followed by IV tPA resulting in normalization of vision by the third hospital day (Fig. 3.46).

3.11 IV tPA Contraindicated with Anticoagulation

An 88-year-old male with acute left hemiparesis on Coumadin—due to prolonged PT INR of 2.79, this patient was unable to be treated by IV tPA. CT angiography reveals right ICA occlusion, presumed to be chronic, with focal thrombosis of cross-filling right MCA M1 segment producing tenuous flow into right hemisphere (prolonged time to peak measurements, as above) with presumed right lenticulostriate artery territory ischemia producing a pure motor deficit of left arm>face>leg motor weakness (Fig. 3.47).

Stroke Mimics: an important clinical concept especially as it relates to emergent decision-making in the ED with regard to possible use of tPA. Consider the following study on 512 patients treated with tPA for suspected stroke at a major medical center over a 4-year period: "... 14 % of all patients treated emergently for suspected stroke were actually later found to represent stroke mimics with 21 % of this stroke mimic group representing conversion disorder.... The most common etiologies were seizure, complicated migraine, and conversion disorder" [32].

3.11.1 Common Normal Developmental Variations

In the cerebral vasculature, benign congenital variations are noted versus other rare variants that can be lethal such as carotid agenesis: Persistent trigeminal artery can be identified on MRA or CT angiography and is a benign variant (Fig. 3.48) as is left vertebral ending as PICA (Fig. 3.49). However, congenital absence of common carotid arteries simulating bilateral dissections can result in fatal outcomes, as seen in a 36-year-old female, and shown in Figs. 3.50 and 3.51.

Congenital absence of the right MCA with secondary ischemic changes in 30-year-old female who had developed extensive collaterals is shown in Fig. 3.52.

In older patients with chronic hypertension and advanced cerebrovascular disease the major vessels such as the basilar and MCAs may be thread-like in nature; it becomes hard to know in these cases how much is due to congenital maldevelopment (Fig. 3.53).

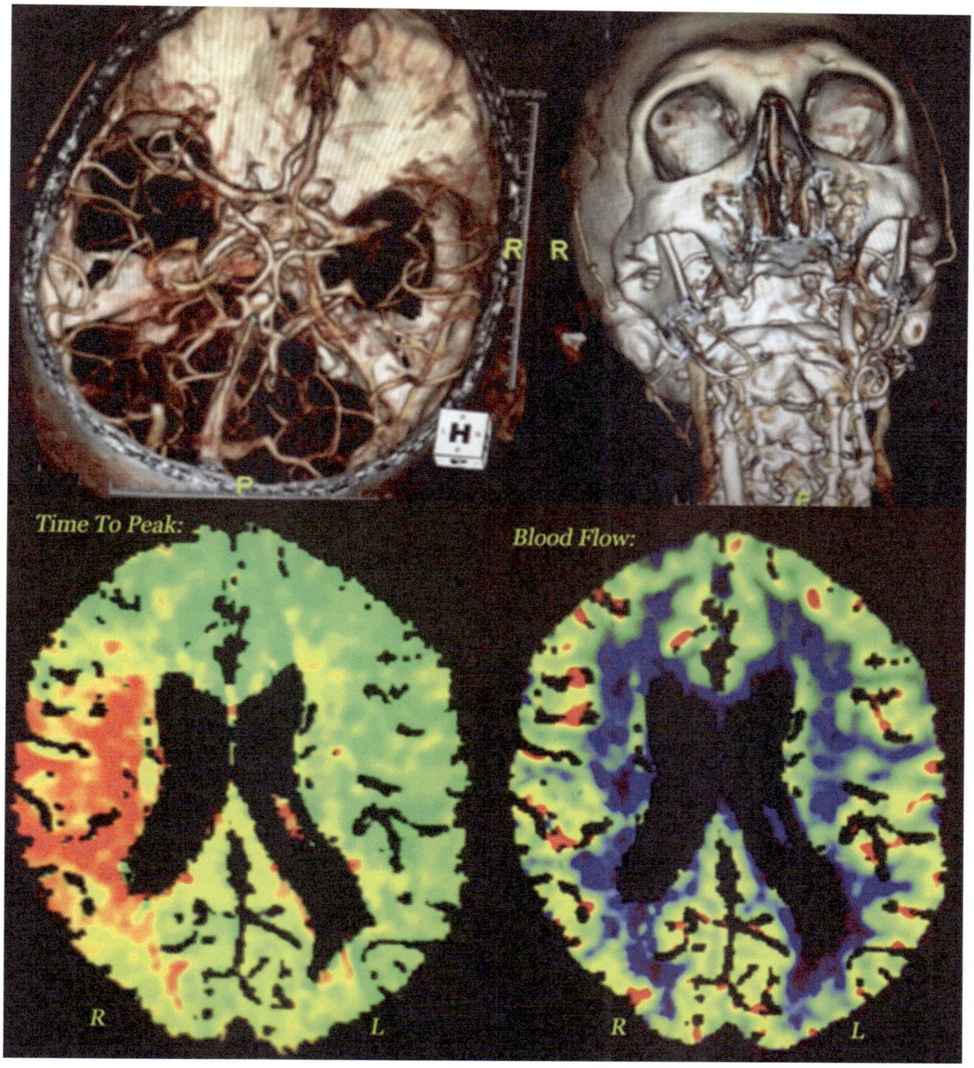

Fig. 3.47 Right MCA ischemia due to occlusion of right ICA complicated by right MCA stenosis as revealed by CT angiography (*upper panels*) with CT perfusion shown in *lower panels*

3.12 New Developments in Acute Stroke Care

New developments in acute stroke care include the CT ambulance concept to reduce time to thrombolytic therapy with the hope of improving outcomes, investigators in Berlin equipped an ambulance with a portable CT scanner in an attempt to administer iv tPA for acute stroke as soon as possible. As noted by the investigators, "….the ambulance was staffed with a neurologist, paramedic, and radiographer and equipped with a CT scanner, point-of-care laboratory, and a teleradiology system. It was deployed by the dispatch center whenever a specific emergency call algorithm indicated an acute stroke situation… 45 (58 %) had an acute ischemic stroke and 23 (51 %) of these patients received tPA. The mean call-to-needle time was 62 min…. This new approach using prehospital tPA may be effective in reducing call-to-needle times, but this is currently being scrutinized in a prospective controlled study" [33].

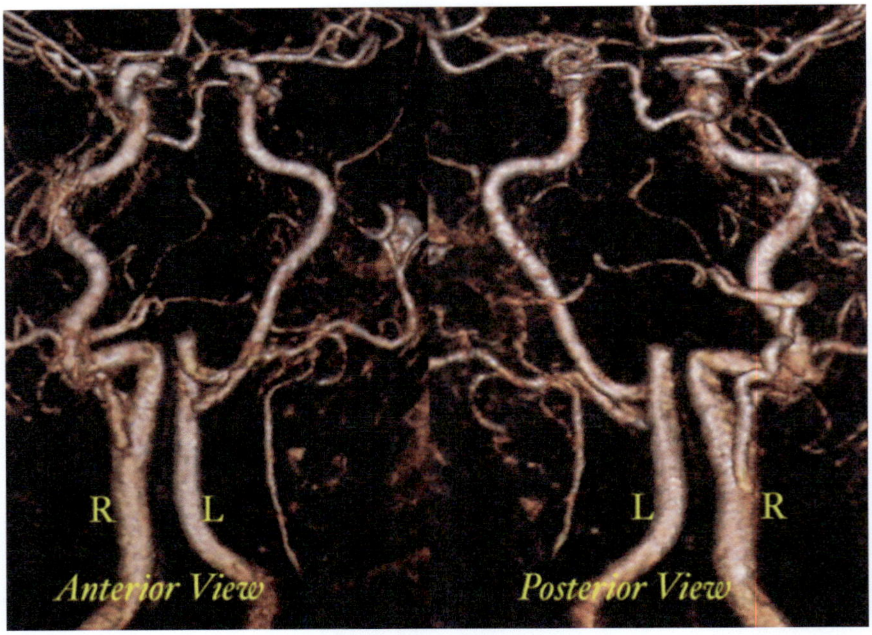

Fig. 3.48 Congenital vascular anomalies: persistent trigeminal artery

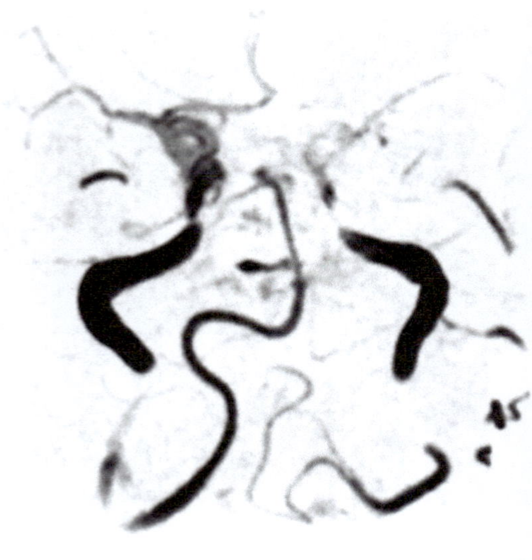

Fig. 3.49 Normal variants: vertebral ending as PICA

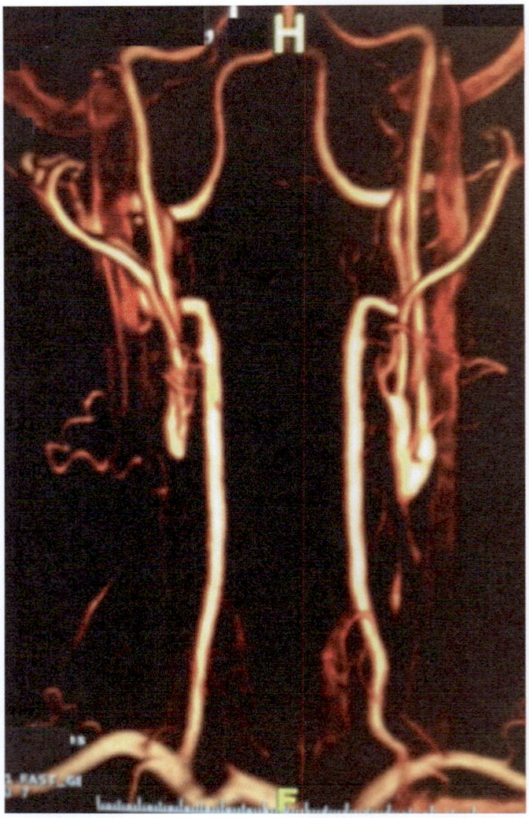

Fig. 3.50 Rare lethal congenital variants: common carotid agenesis

3.13 Stroke in Special Populations

Unusual causes of acute stroke-like changes need to be considered in special patient populations, and include but are not limited to: posterior reversible encephalopathy syndrome amongst hypertensive pregnant females suspected to have eclampsia, oral contraceptive-related stroke in young females, Herpes Zoster Ophthalmicus Followed by Contralateral Hemiparesis due to Granulomatous Arteritis with secondary infarction, delayed radiation vasculopathy in a former cancer patients, Cerebral Fat Embolism as in hip fracture, Cerebral air embolism as in central line removal.

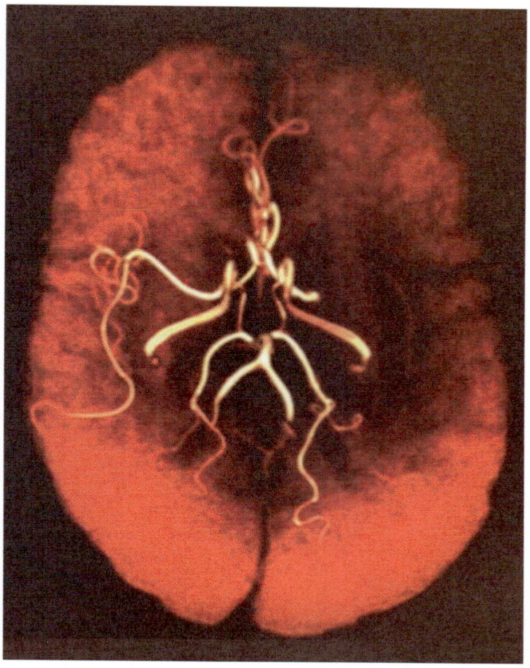

Fig. 3.51 Fatal stroke event for young patient with thrombotic occlusion of left MCA

Case Example
A 64-year-old hospitalized patient had a central venous catheter removed by a nurse without the use of prophylactic Valsalva type maneuvers or Trendelenburg positioning and then had the sudden development of acute complete blindness; CT revealed vascular profiles suggesting the presence of air and MR revealed complex posterior signal hyper-intensities on FLAIR exam. The patient underwent treatment in a hyperbaric chamber and subsequently made a full recovery (Fig. 3.54).

Stroke in young women is an important consideration with regard to Oral Contraceptives as a Major Risk factor (Fig. 3.55). This important topic has been extensively reviewed in a major 2012 Danish study, titled: Thrombotic Stroke and Myocardial Infarction with Hormonal

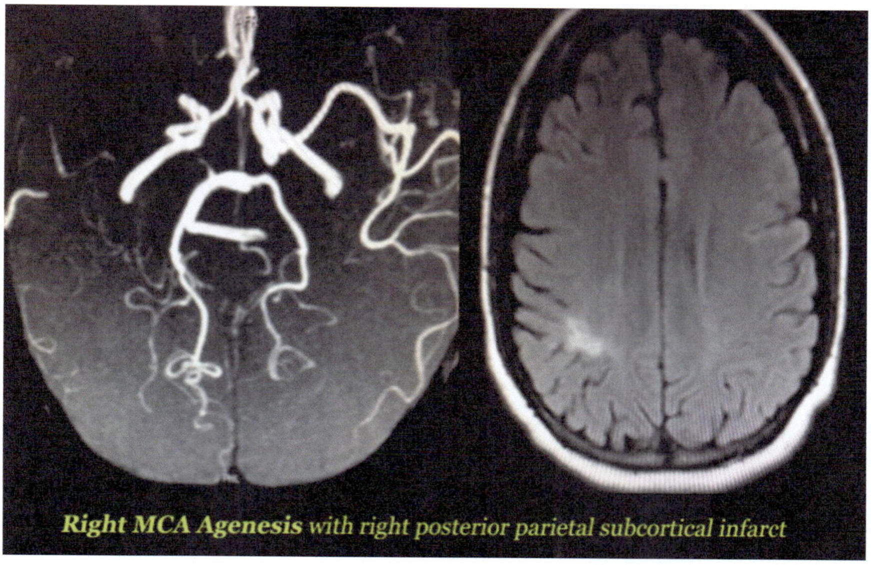

Fig. 3.52 Congenital absence of right MCA complicated by compromise of fine collateral circulation due to cocaine use

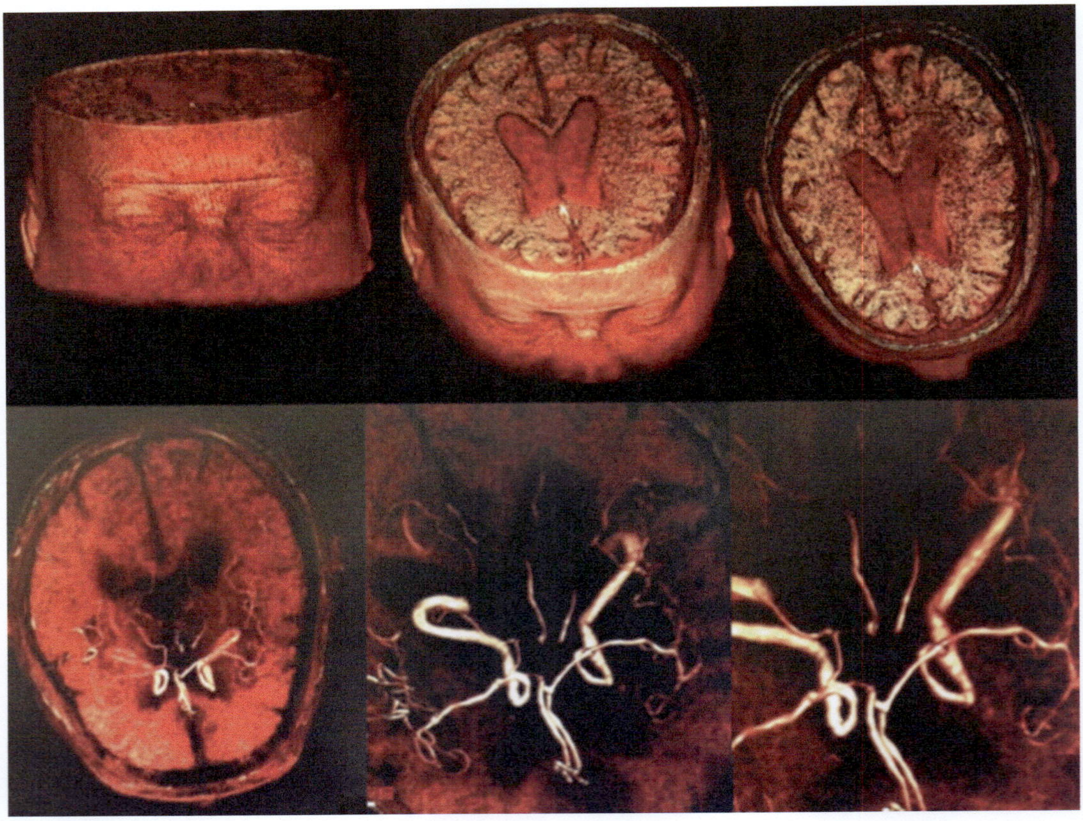

Fig. 3.53 Congenital maldevelopment of bilateral MCAs, basilar and PCAs

Contraception. This study concluded, "Although the absolute risks of thrombotic stroke and myocardial infarction associated with the use of hormonal contraception were low, the risk was increased by a factor of 0.9–1.7 with oral contraceptives that included ethinyl estradiol at a dose of 20 μg and by a factor of 1.3–2.3 with those that included ethinyl estradiol at a dose of 30–40 μg, with relatively small differences in risk according to progestin type" [34].

Case Example

An unfortunate oral contraceptive-related stroke event in a young woman is shown in Fig. 3.55.

Radiation-related vasculopathy is another not uncommon late complication for the unfortunate patient who recovers from cancer, thanks to the use of ionizing external beam radiation therapy, only to suffer a stroke years later via accelerated carotid atherosclerotic changes for the example of neck radiation for lymphoma, or incur a primary stroke event from radiation induced middle cerebral vasculopathy, as shown in the example below for a patient who had recovered from clivus chordoma after external beam radiation (Fig. 3.56).

3.14 Seasonal Fluctuations in Stroke Mortality

Based on an analysis that included all fee-for-service Medicare beneficiaries aged ≥ 65 years with a primary discharge diagnosis of ischemic stroke from 1999 to 2006, the authors of the study concluded that "the 30-day RAMR (30-day risk-adjusted mortality rate) decreased overall, but

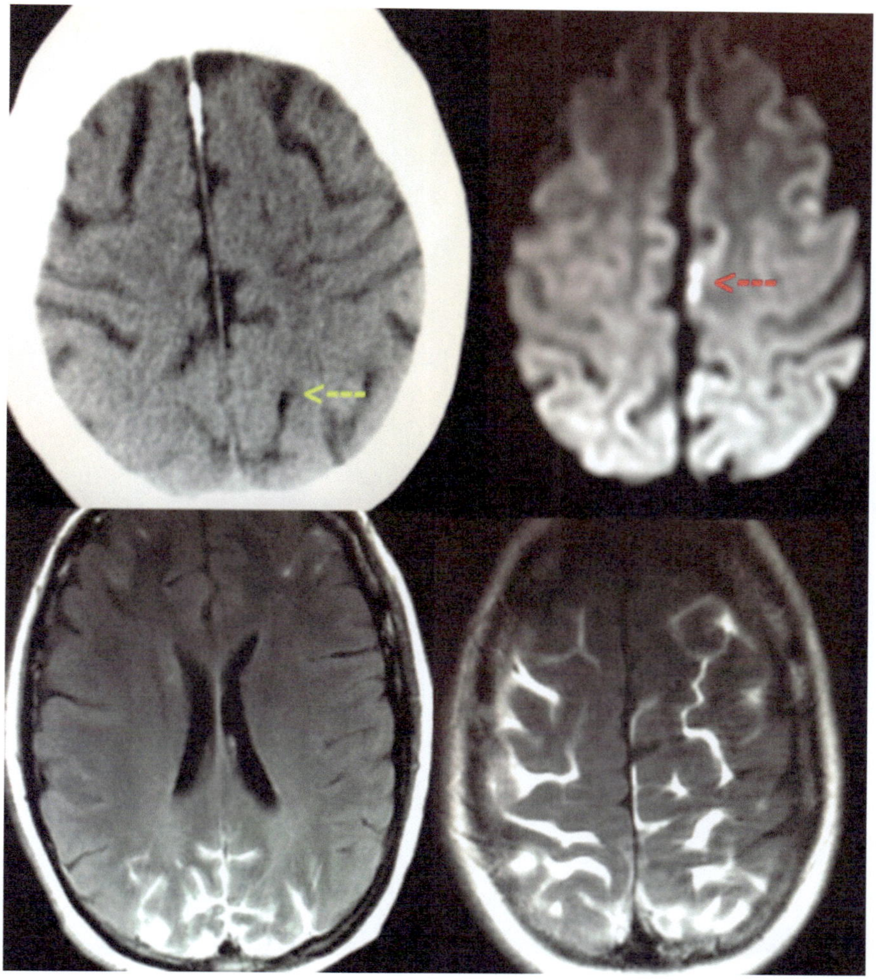

Fig. 3.54 Air emboli appear on CT as *black spots* (*upper left*) with negative Hounsfield numbers; this patient recovered her vision with the use of a hyperbaric chamber

seasonal patterns were present, with the highest RAMR in January and a smaller peak in July. Because patterns were similar for teaching and nonteaching hospitals, the July peak cannot be explained by the introduction of new trainees in the beginning of the academic year. The reasons for these seasonal patterns warrant further investigation" [35].

3.15 Circadian Variation in the Timing of Stroke Onset

Onset peaks in the early morning waking hours of 6 to 8 AM as shown by multiple studies [36, 37].

3.15.1 CT Angiography in the Management of Carotid Disease

Clinical examples of this important tool in evaluating cerebrovascular disease in great detail with the aid of three-dimensional reconstruction are shown in Figs. 3.57, 3.58, and 3.59.

Case Example

A 52-year-old male smoker with intraluminal thrombus discovered by CT angiography (Fig. 3.60) after a right MCA stroke event; spontaneous resolution of thrombus after initial heparin infusion then maintained on Clopidogrel (patient elected against medical advise to

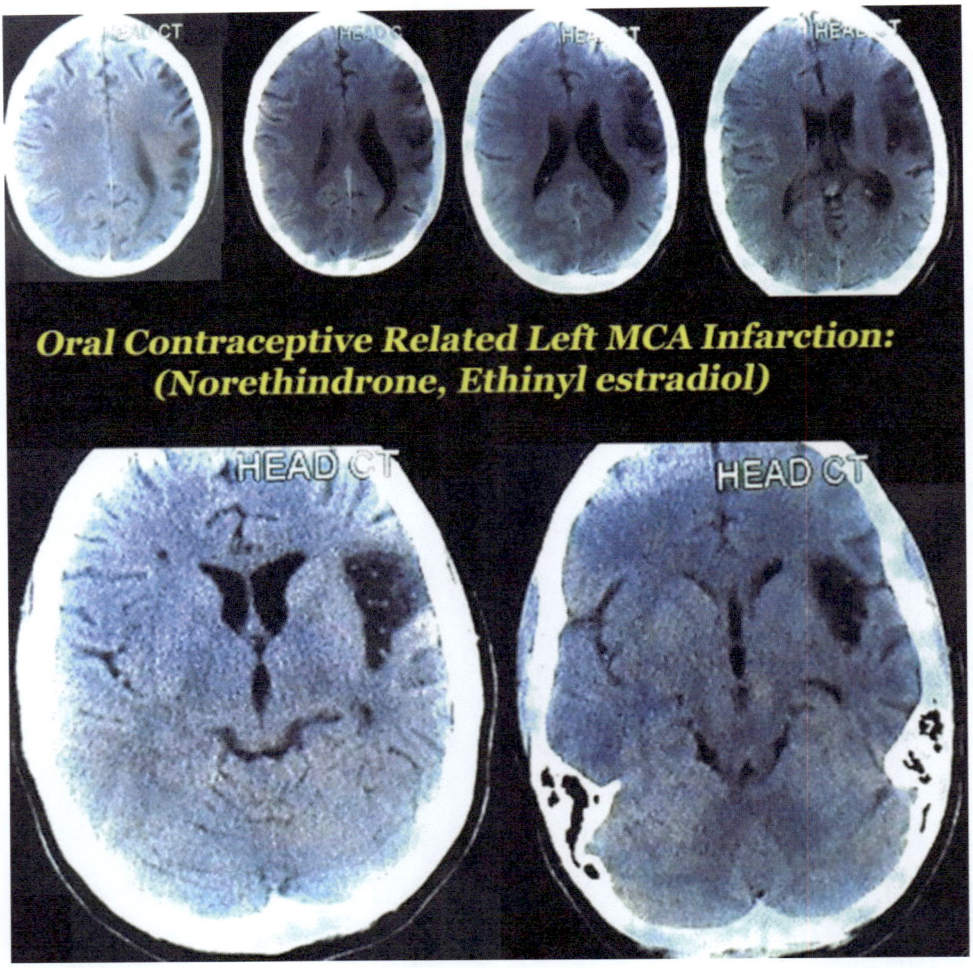

Fig. 3.55 Large left MCA infarction related to oral contraceptive use in a young woman

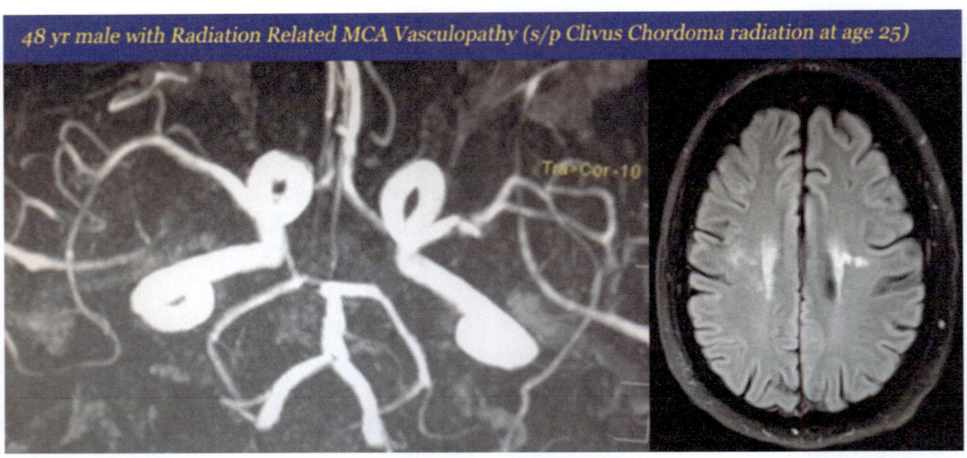

Fig. 3.56 Radiation vasculopathy in 48 years male with acute right lenticulostriate artery area infarction

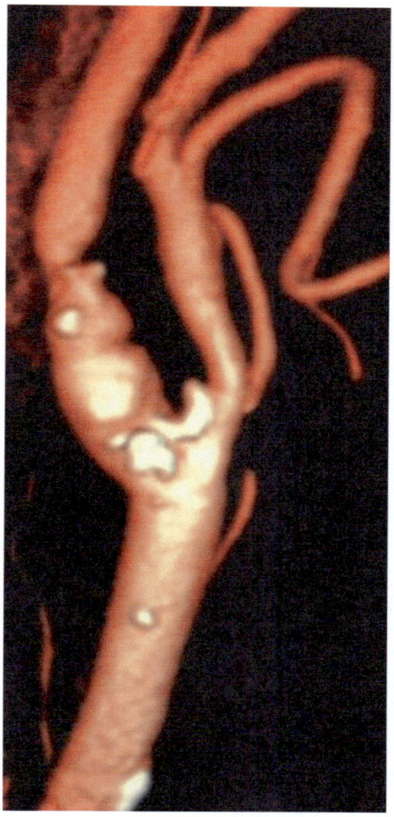

Fig. 3.57 Fine anatomic 3D detail can be gained about the carotid bifurcation using CT angiography

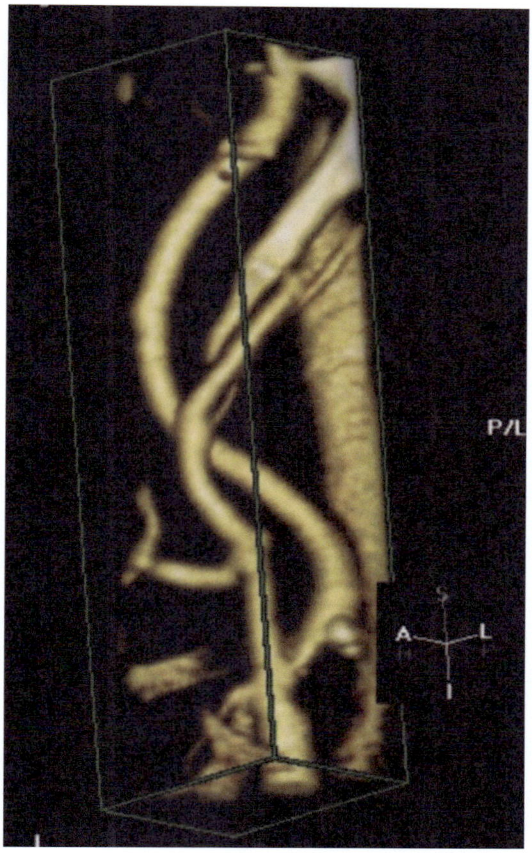

Fig. 3.58 CT angio can depict carotid stenosis in relation other nearby structures, such as the styloid process

continue to smoke). This difficult "time bomb" scenario of intraluminal thrombus has been addressed by a recent 2013 study [38], where the authors concluded, "Results of this study suggest that initial anticoagulation for symptomatic ICAT leads to a low rate of recurrent ischemic events and that carotid revascularization, if indicated, can be safely performed in a delayed manner."

3.15.2 Circle of Willis Is Crucial in Maintaining Flow in Setting of Unilateral ICA Disease

Crescendo Recurrent TIA events leading to the discovery of Left ICA occlusion, chronic, as above in a 61-year-old smoker requiring lung biopsy of an indeterminate nodule (Fig. 3.61).

Despite MRA evidence for left ICA occlusion from its origin as a chronic finding, with secondary reduced left MCA regional cerebral blood flow (rCBF) with prolonged mean transit times (MTT), there was a fairly symmetric pattern of glucose metabolism as assessed by 18F-FDG PET imaging (axial view shown above, lower right panel), shown in Fig. 3.61. Symptomatic ICA occlusion can result in ischemic changes in a watershed distribution with a "string of pearls" sign on MR diffusion.

Case Example

As suggested by the case example in Fig. 3.62, significant vertebrobasilar disease carries a high risk for stroke. Supporting data for this includes a recent study [39] that concluded: "In patients with posterior circulation events, ≥50 % vertebral

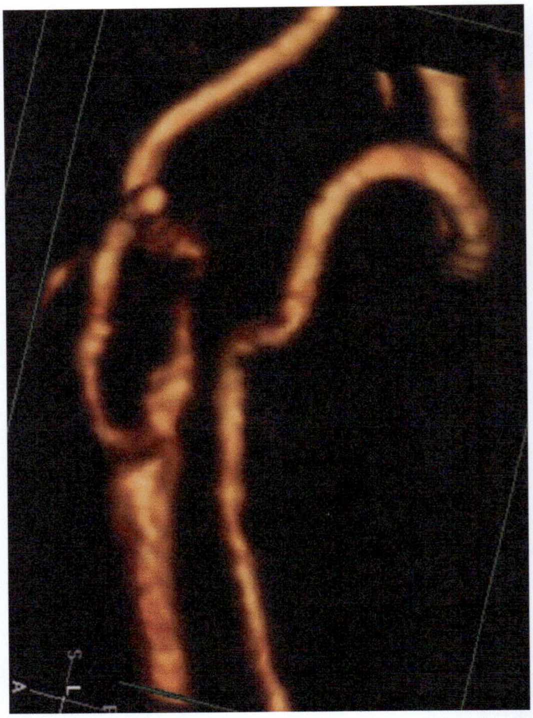

Fig. 3.59 Critical ICA stenosis seen on CT angio prior to successful stenting

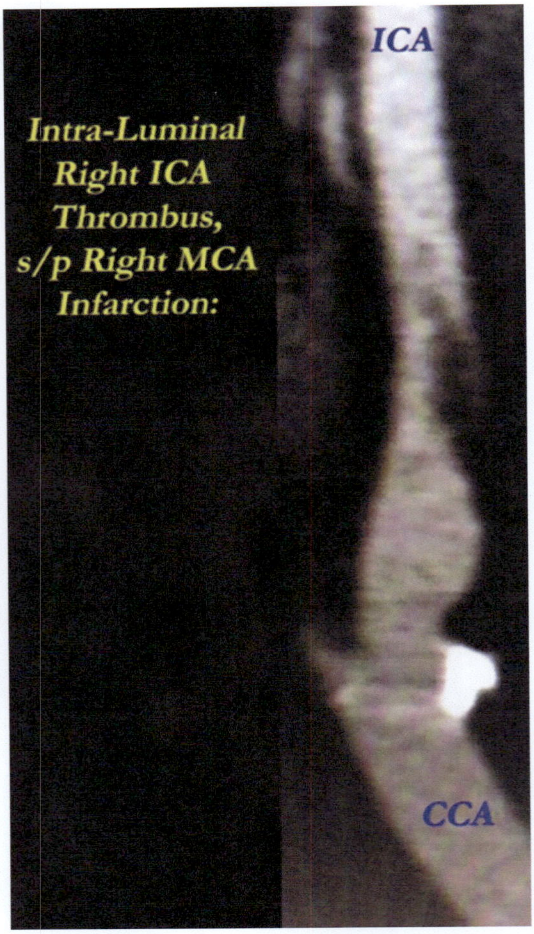

Fig. 3.60 Intraluminal thrombus within right ICA seen on CT angio after right MCA infarction; this thrombus spontaneously resolved and disappeared over 2 weeks without further complication

and basilar stenosis was associated multiple transient ischaemic attacks at presentation (22 % vs. 3 %; OR = 9.29; $p < 0.001$) and with a significantly higher 90-day risk of recurrent events (OR = 3.2; $p = 0.006$), reaching 22 % for stroke and 46 % for transient ischaemic attack and stroke." Figure 3.62 portrays distal embolization from a focal left distal vertebral atherosclerotic lesion in a 78-year-old male presenting with gait ataxia and veering off to the left, consistent with an area of acute left cerebellar ischemia.

Special Circulations: Anterior Spinal Artery infarction (Fig. 3.63). As shown in Fig. 3.62, the anatomy of spinal arteries including artery of Adamkiewicz can be revealed by CT angiography imaging of a patient suspected of having acute spinal cord ischemia. As noted in a recent review [40], "The largest intradural blood supplier to the anterior part of the thoracolumbar spinal cord is called the Adamkiewicz artery (AKA; diameter, 0.5–1.0 mm), named after its discoverer. The AKA is the largest of multiple supplying Anterior Radicular Arteries (ARA). Each ARA derives from a posterior branch of a segmental (i.e., intercostal or lumbar) artery, which is a direct branch of the aorta, and the ARA intradurally continues as the ASA. In approximately 70 % of cases, the AKA originates from an intercostal or lumbar artery on the left side of the vertebral column and most frequently between the vertebral levels T8 to L1."

Case Example

Extensive Carotid Dissection. As shown in Fig. 3.64, CT angiography is also useful in evaluating intimal dissection as a cause of stroke. CT

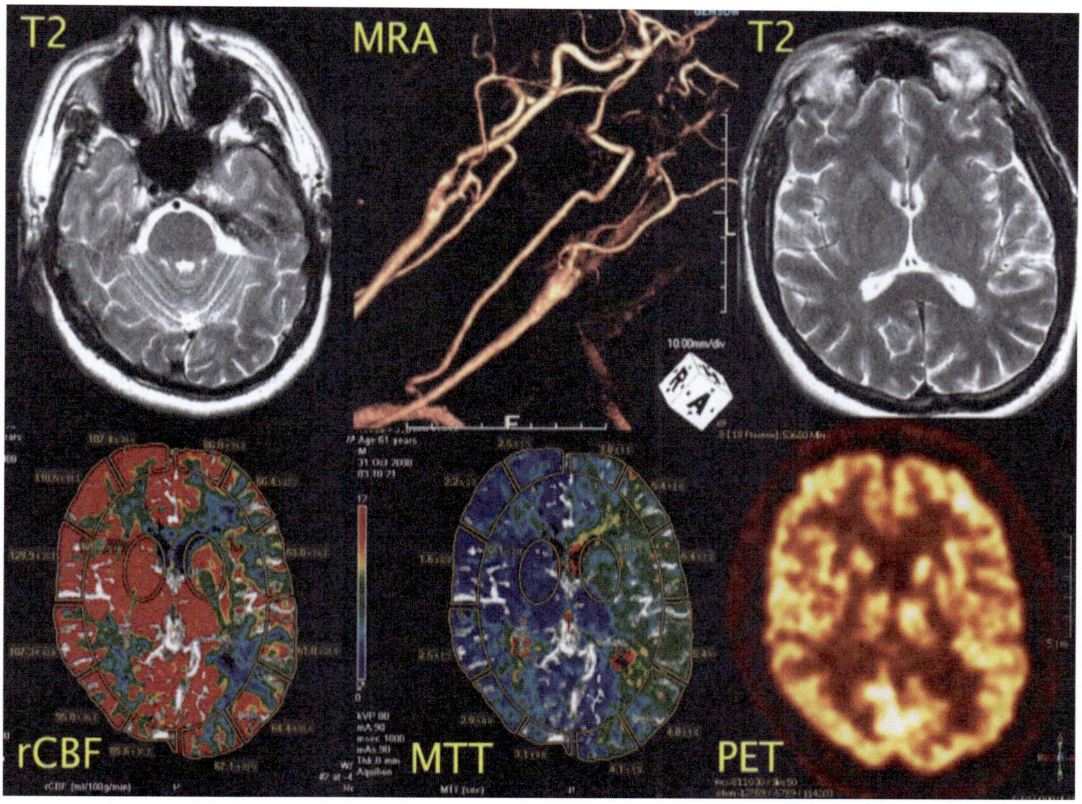

Fig. 3.61 Depressed left hemispheric blood flow (*lower left*) in a patient with a chronic left ICA occlusion yet maintains normal cerebral glucose metabolism (*lower right*) by PET imaging

angiography discloses extensive aortic dissection (c) extending into the cervical carotids (b), with auscultation of the right carotid being distinctly unusual with a double beat very evident on clinical exam corresponding to biphasic changes recorded on carotid Doppler (a).

Case Example of Focal Carotid Dissection due to Fibromuscular Dysplasia

Neurologic history revealed a 3 h right amaurosis fugax event occurred in a 66-year-old female who dismissed her transient visual loss until initial neurologic review many months later for incidental and unrelated radicular symptoms. Comprehensive review also found an asymptomatic splenic artery aneurysm in addition to fibromuscular dysplasia for the left carotid and focal dissection of the right carotid (Fig. 3.65). No recurrent neurologic events were noted after being placed on clopidogrel.

Case Example of Vertebral Dissection (Fig. 3.66)

Brain stem stroke in a young adult with hyperdense thrombus within the basilar that extended into the right PCA (a–d) with extensive diffusion changes seen within the right greater than left pons as well as bilateral cerebellar hemispheres (e). Initial angiogram showed absence of normal flow into the vertebral—basilar system (f), which improved after endovascular procedures (h) with eventual restoration of flow into the right vertebral and basilar as well as both PCAs (j).

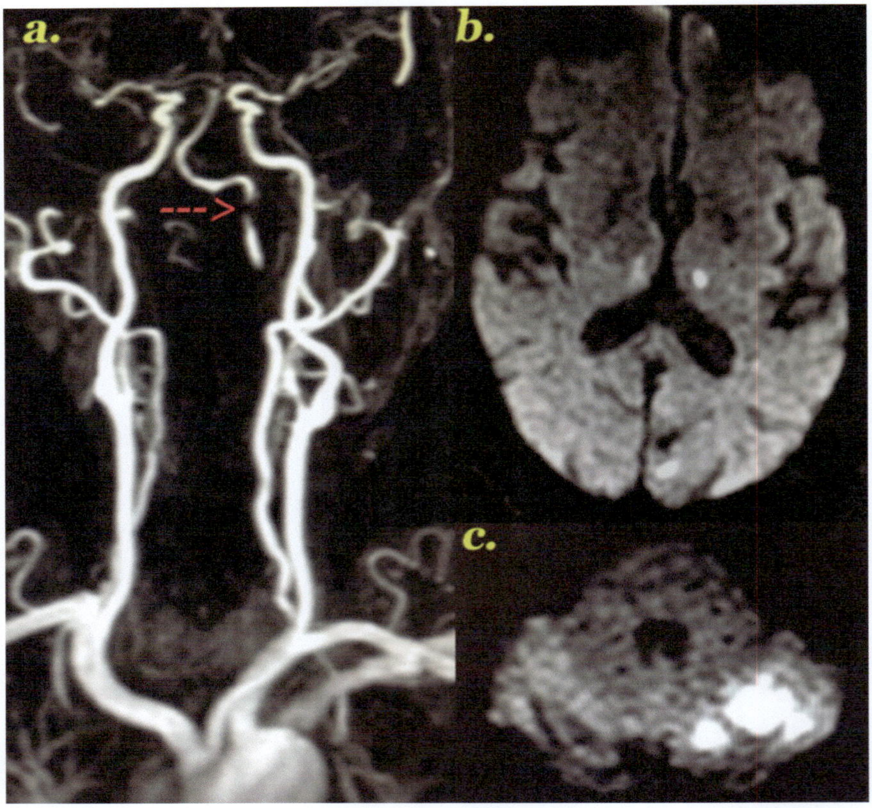

Fig. 3.62 Focal atherosclerotic left vertebral lesion (**a**) with distal embolic ischemic changes (**b**, **c**)

Case Example (Fig. 3.67)
Post-traumatic left vertebral dissection with occlusion in a young adult who was found to have a left-sided Horner's syndrome after being observed overnight in the hospital after a motor vehicle crash with the car flipping over. When significant cerebellar infarction occurs, a decompressive craniectomy may need to be performed for relief of the mass effect incurred from the associated secondary cerebellar infarction; this is a consideration to be made for all acute major cerebellar infarctions and may be a critical procedure in some cases to prevent life-threatening compression of the brain stem.

- Massive cerebellar infarction:
  - Surgical decompression with removal of infracted tissue
  - Identify mechanism: evaluate for serious vertebral-basilar stenosis/ulceration, exclude cardio-embolic factors, vertebral dissection
  - Neuro ICU

Decompressive Hemicraniectomy (DHC) for major MCA infarcts can be beneficial as well; this approach has recently been reviewed by Staykov and Gupta, who concluded: "Predictive models of patients who may require DHC are improving through volumetric analysis based on MRI and serum markers to assess for neuronal injury… DHC is a life-saving surgery that appears to benefit younger patients the most. Further study is required to better elucidate quality-of-life outcome measures, timing of surgery, and treatment of the dominant hemisphere" [41].

Vertebral artery dissection have become increasingly more apparent as a serious form of stroke in young adults accounting for up to 1/4th

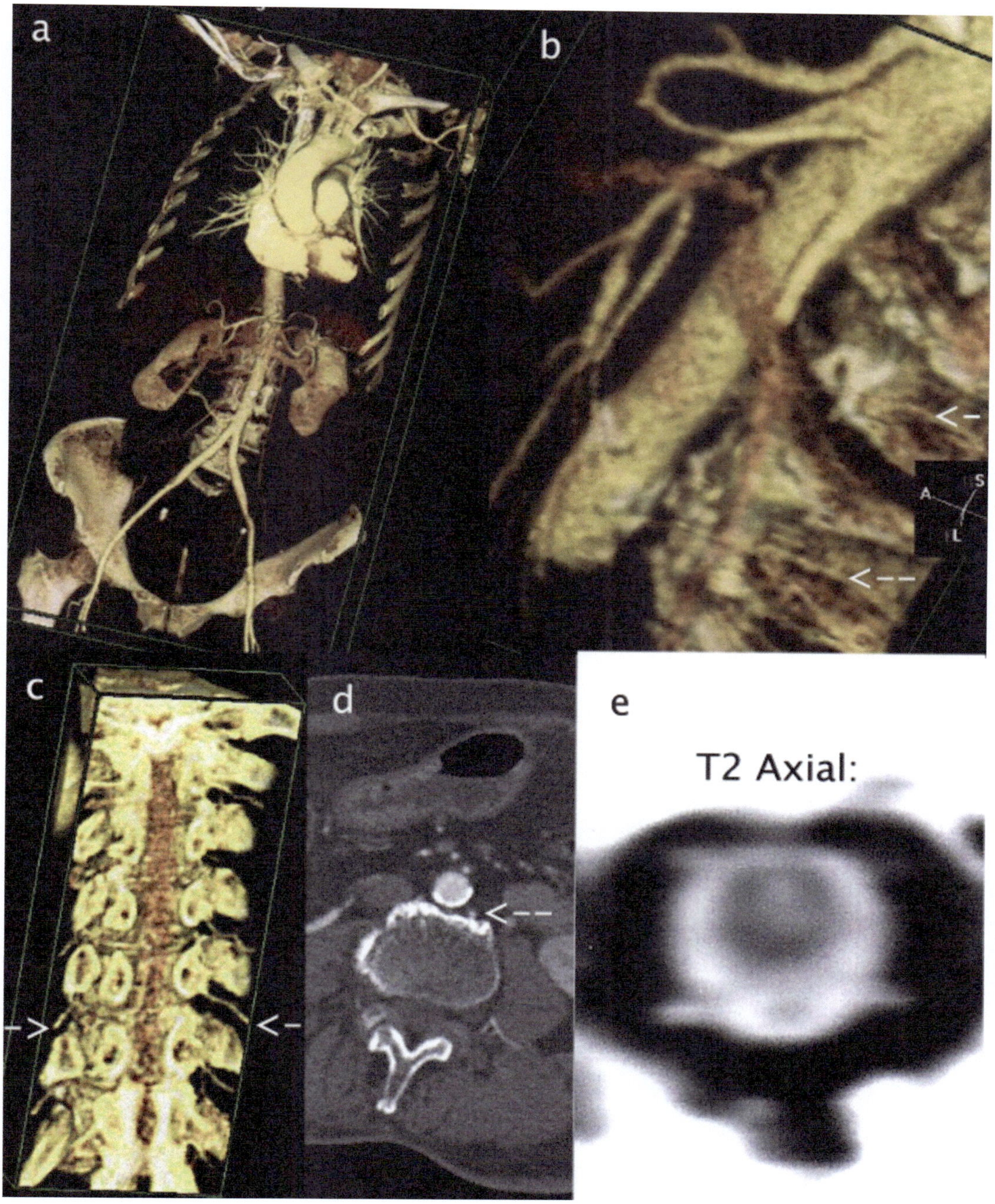

Fig. 3.63 Anterior spinal artery ischemic change evident on axial T2 MRI with demonstration of radicular arteries

of all strokes in the 25–45 year age group, with mortalities ranging from 19 to 83 % [42, 43]. Risk factors include neck trauma and excessive neck stretch or strain as may occur in chiropractic cervical manipulation. Alternatively, it may arise spontaneously with relation to fibromuscular dysplasia. Typical presentations include local pain, headache, and ipsilateral Horner's syndrome.

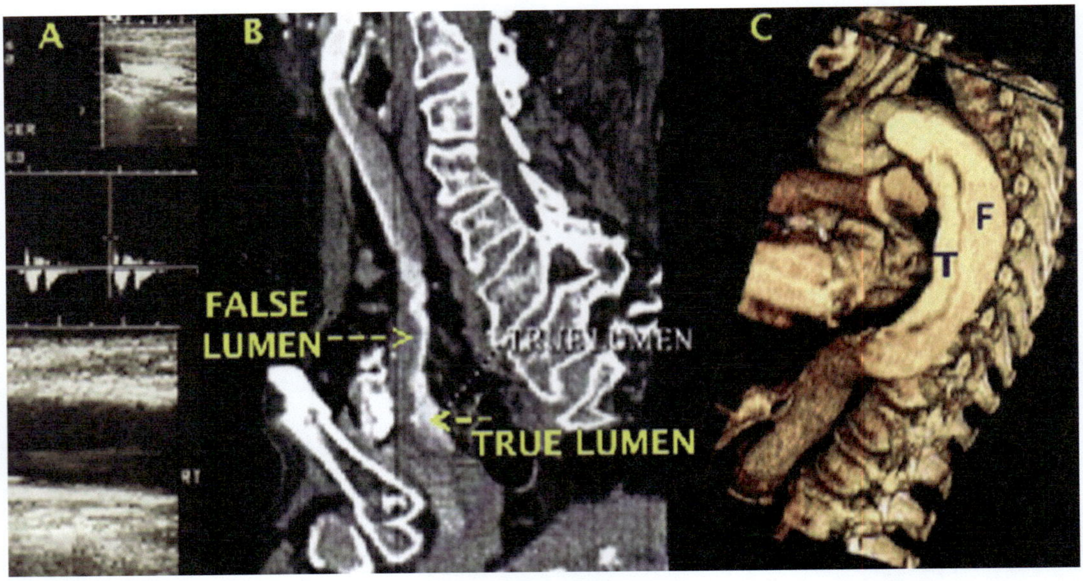

Fig. 3.64 Extensive aortic dissection ascending up into the right carotid

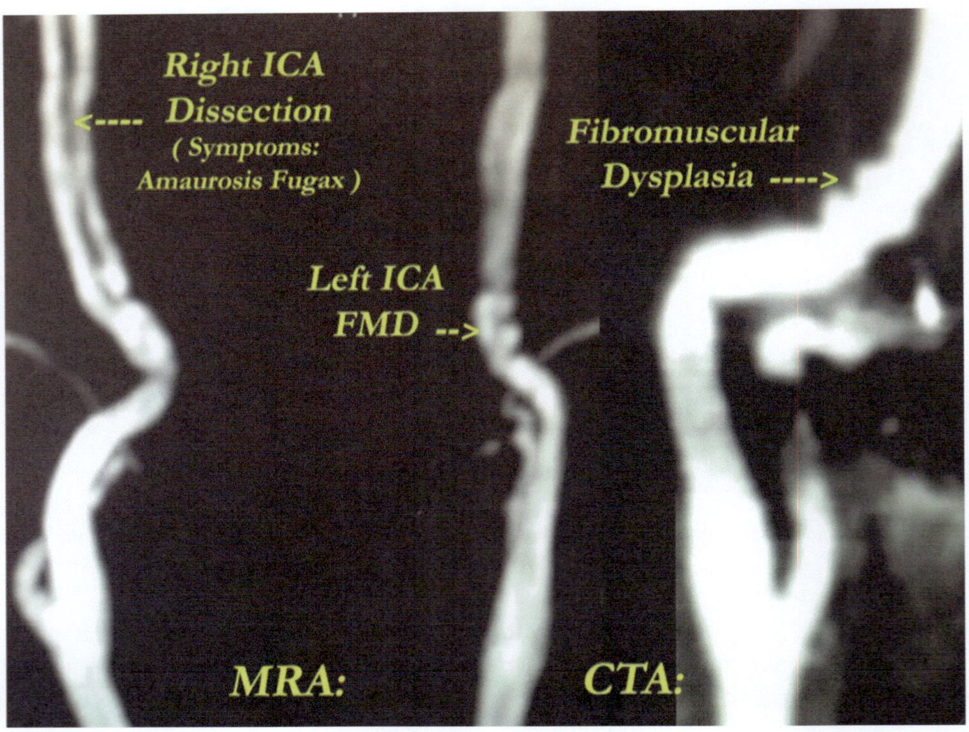

Fig. 3.65 Amaurosis fugax event led to the discovery of right ICA dissection due to fibromuscular dysplasia

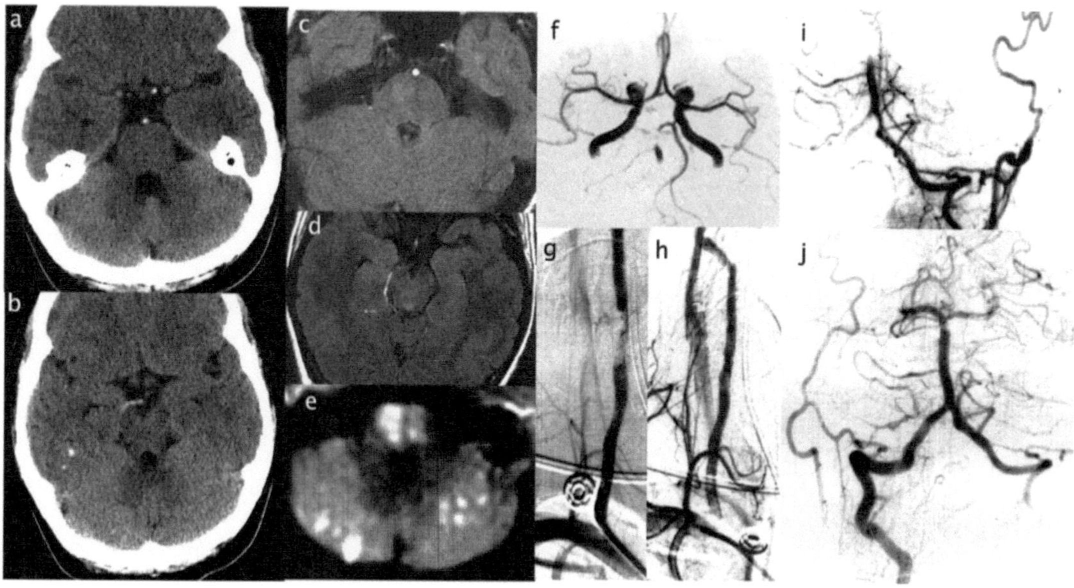

Fig. 3.66 Acute vertebral dissection with distal basilar and right PCA embolic occlusion (**f**), urgently reversed by endovascular approach using stents (**j**)

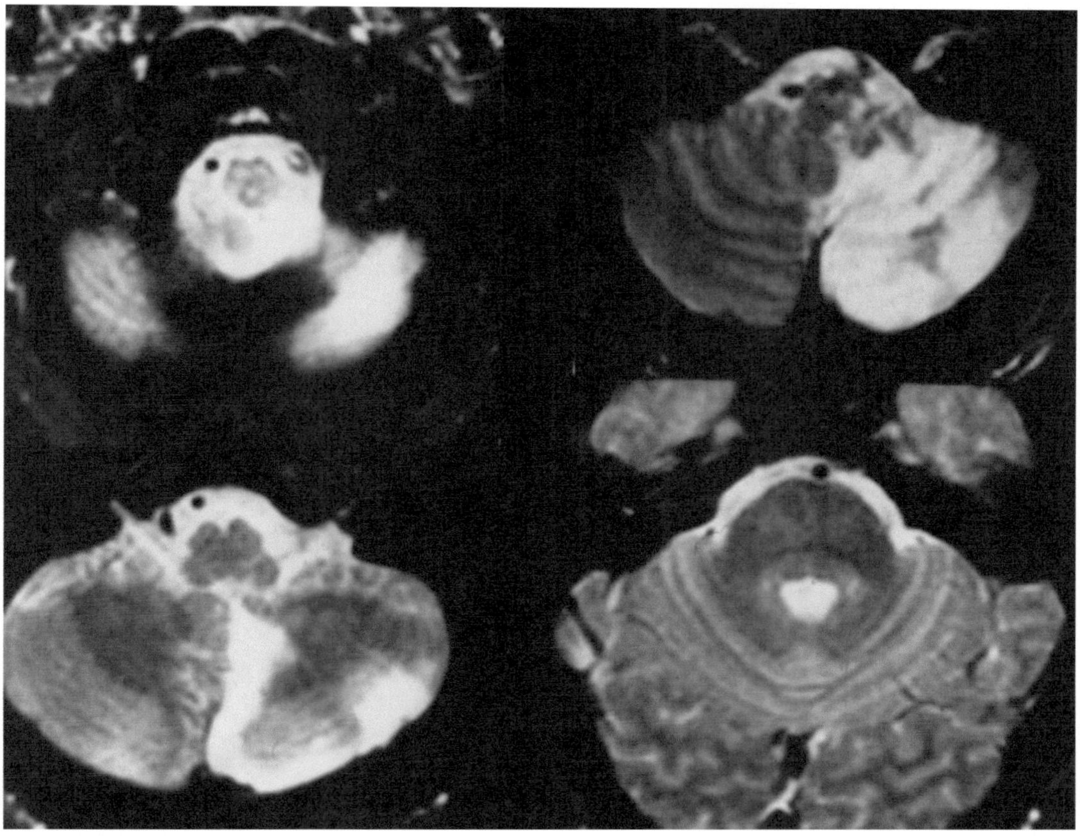

Fig. 3.67 Post-traumatic vertebral dissection in a young adult, producing left cerebellar infarction

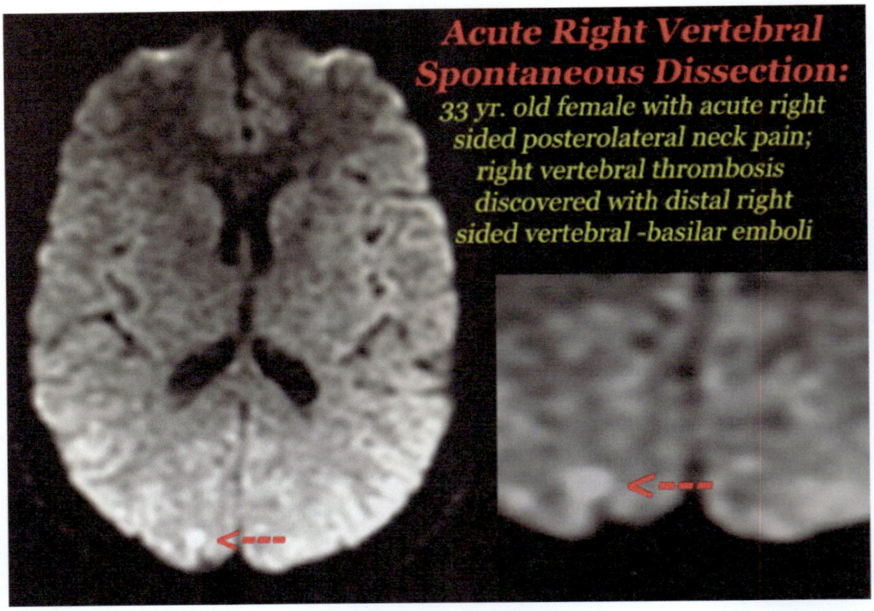

Fig. 3.68 Distant posterior circulation emboli found in a young woman with an acute right vertebral dissection

Distal emboli into the posterior circulation can be seen in cases of vertebral dissection (Fig. 3.68).

Case Example of Cardio-Embolic Etiology of Stroke (Fig. 3.69)

A 77-year-old male with a new diagnosis for atrial fibrillation who developed severe nose bleeds with a INR of 8 two weeks after prophylactic coumadin therapy had been initiated. Three weeks after stopping Coumadin, he was found be very confused. Neurologic exam revealed a right homonymous hemianopsia with MRA confirming a left PCA embolic occlusion and diffusion-weighted MR imaging (DWI) showing a complete left PCA infarction with a small peri-ventricular change as well within the left lenticulostriate artery distribution, with the multifocal changes further confirming the suspected cardio-embolic mechanism.

Case Example of Atrial Fibrillation in a Frequent Cause of Stroke (Fig. 3.70)

MRI images are shown for a 58-year-old male with chronic persistent atrial fibrillation who suffered a recurrent cardio-embolic stroke with left posterior parietal infarction after reducing Pradaxa anticoagulation dosing in half after noting minor bleeding at gum margins.

Atrial fibrillation-related stroke rises with age: only 1.5 % of stroke patients in their 50s have had an atrial fibrillation-related event versus about 20 % for those in their 80s [44]. Recent studies show that without prolonged monitoring, paroxysmal atrial fibrillation may be missed in those with cryptogenic stroke [45]. Over 90 % of atrial fibrillation-related embolic strokes are thought to arise from clots originating in the left atrial appendage; with the use of transesophageal echocardiography, over 90 % of thrombi can be found in the left atrial appendage in non-valvular atrial fibrillation patients. Anticoagulation is the treatment of choice and reduces the risk of stroke by 60 %.

Case Example (Fig. 3.71)

A 49-year-old male with psychiatric history was not heard from for 48 h and found to have what EMS described as “altered mental status” and brought to the emergency room where neurologic exam revealed agitation, and expressive aphasia. EKG revealed acute MI with CT

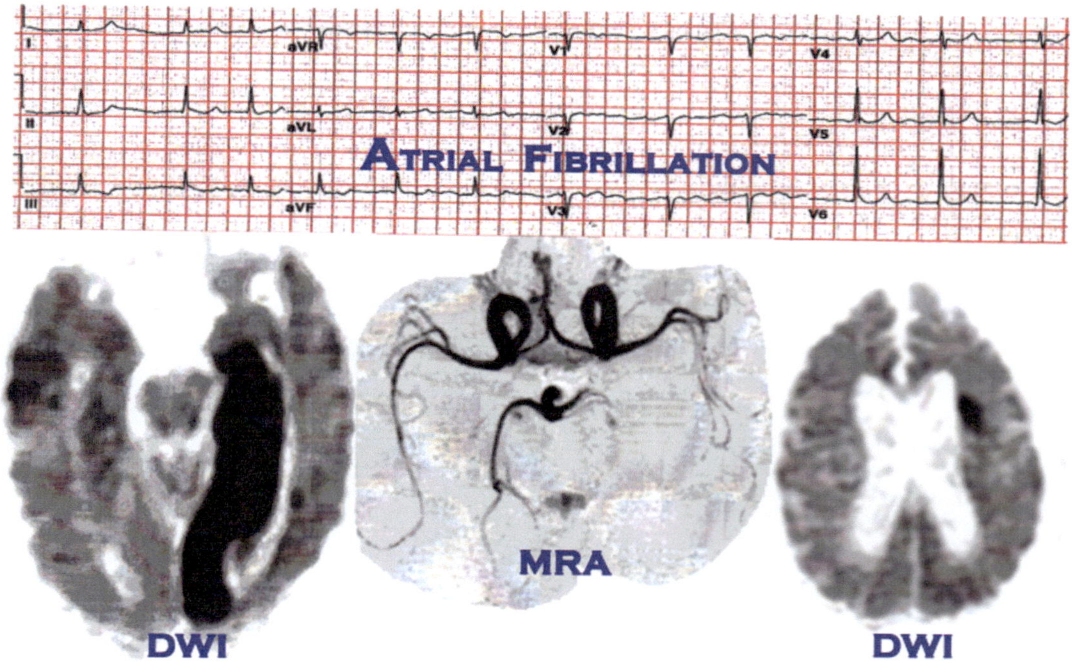

Fig. 3.69 Case example of atrial fibrillation-related acute multifocal ischemic infarcts

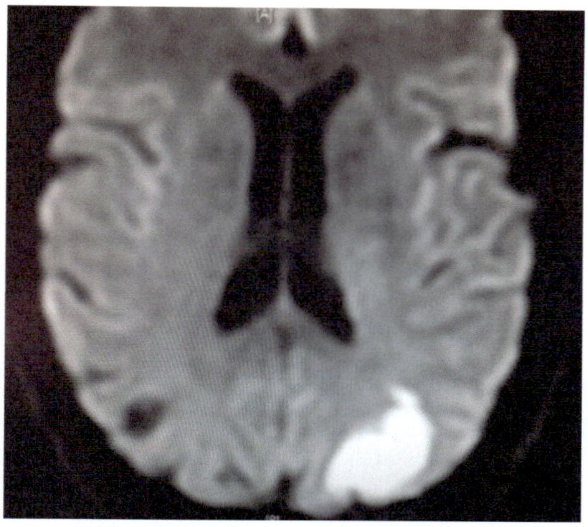

Fig. 3.70 Case example: recurrent atrial fibrillation-related infarct due to transient and brief suboptimal anticoagulation

angiography revealing a left MCA M3 branch occlusion; MR diffusion revealed hyper-intense changes within peri-sylvian language areas. ECHO revealed localized akinetic segments with formation a post-MI mural thrombus.

3.16 Functional Recovery After Stroke: New Insights Using MRI and PET

Recovery after stroke has been extensively reviewed in the medical literature, with recent updates on rehabilitation discussed by Brewer et al. [46]. Novel therapies in stroke rehabilitation now include noninvasive brain stimulation, robotics and pharmacological augmentation as well as the use of stem cells to induce repair of tissue damage. With regard to the latter, it is important to note that a series of small trials have already been conducted with stem cells, including a study from Brazil involving the intra-arterial infusion of autologous bone marrow mononuclear cells into stroke damaged middle cerebral artery territories of 30 patients. At the 3-month mark, satisfactory clinical improvement was found in 6 of the 20 patients [47, 48].

Functional aspects of stroke recovery can be explored using PET imaging of cerebral perfusion with 13N-ammonia (Fig. 3.72) or PET imaging

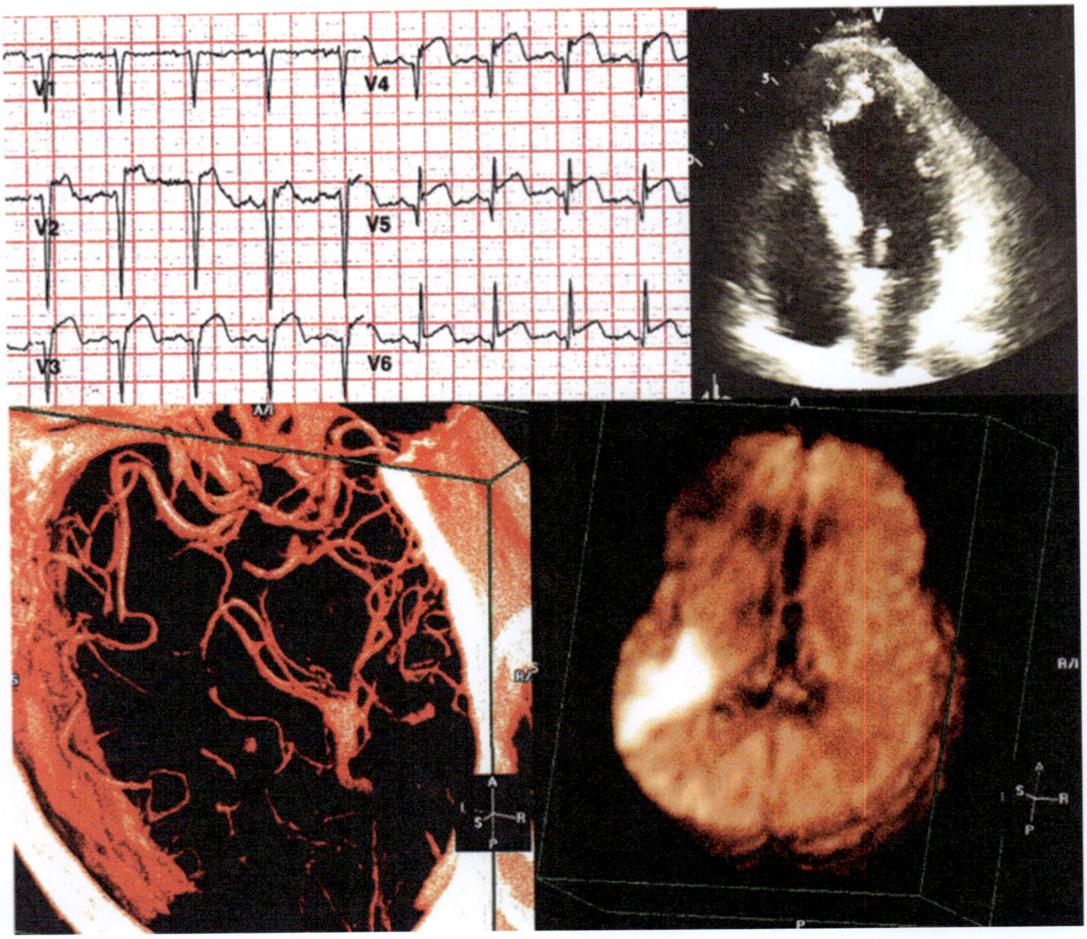

Fig. 3.71 Cardio-embolic ischemic stroke after myocardial infarction

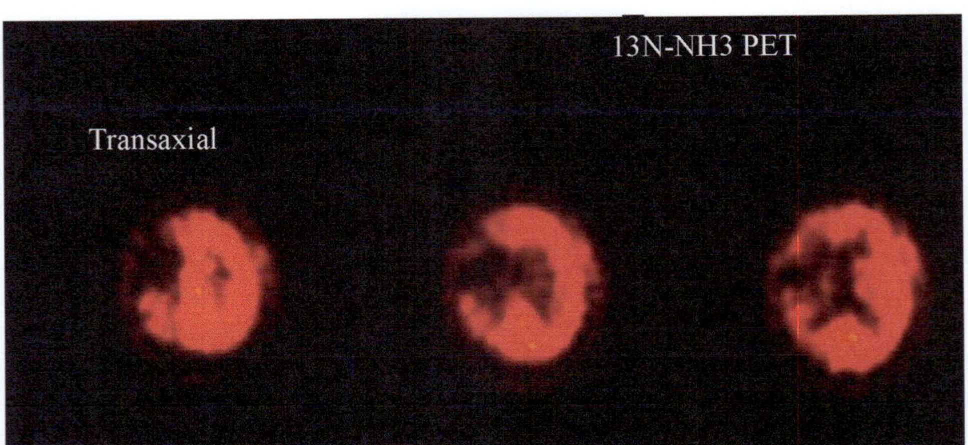

Fig. 3.72 Cerebral perfusion imaging of right MCA ischemia with 13N-ammonia using PET. Right MCA infarction

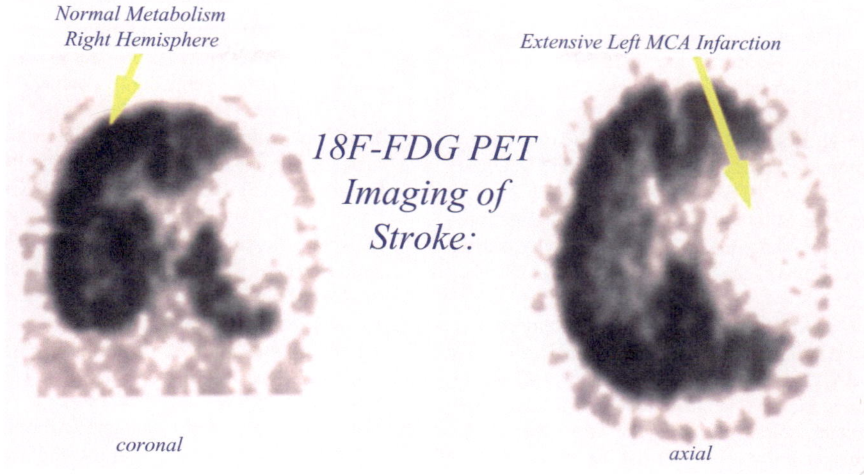

Fig. 3.73 18F-FDG PET scan of a patient with a left MCA infarction

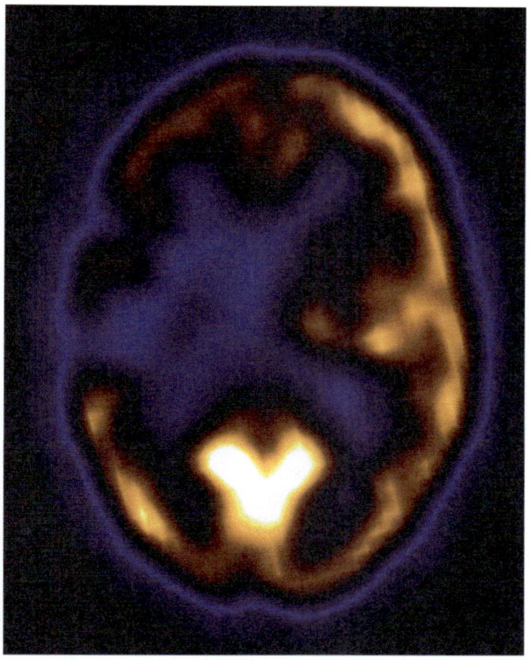

Fig. 3.74 Metabolic imaging of FDG uptake using PET in a patient with an old distant right hemispheric stroke who made a remarkably good functional recovery without focal deficits on neurologic exam

of cerebral metabolism using 18F-FDG after infarction of the middle cerebral artery territory (Figs. 3.73 and 3.74).

References

1. Centers for Disease Control and Prevention. Stroke maps and data sources. http://www.cdc.gov/stroke/maps_data.htm.
2. Clifford FR. The history of migraine from Mesopotamian to Medieval times. Cephalalgia. 1995; 15 Suppl 15:1–3.
3. Nobel L, Mayo NE, Hanley J, Nadeau L, Daskalopoulou SS. MyRiskStroke calculator: a personalized stroke risk assessment tool for the general population. J Clin Neurol. 2014;10(1):1–9.
4. Davis SM, Donnan GA. Secondary prevention after ischemic stroke or transient ischemic attack. N Engl J Med. 2012;366:1914–22.
5. O'Donnell MJ, Xavier D, Liu L, et al. Risk factors for ischaemic and intracerebral haemorrhagic stroke in 22 countries (the INTERSTROKE study): a case-control study. Lancet. 2010;376(9735):112–23.
6. PROGRESS Collaborative Group. Randomised trial of a perindopril-based blood-pressure-lowering regimen among 6,105 individuals with previous stroke or transient ischaemic attack. Lancet. 2001; 358(9287):1033–41.
7. Sandercock PA, Counsell C, Tseng MC, Cecconi E. Oral antiplatelet therapy for acute ischaemic stroke. Cochrane Database Syst Rev. 2014;3:CD000029.
8. Wang Y, et al. Clopidogrel with aspirin in acute minor stroke or transient ischemic attack. N Engl J Med. 2013;369(1):11–9.
9. Furlan AJ, et al. Closure or medical therapy for cryptogenic stroke with patent foramen ovale. N Engl J Med. 2012;366:991–9.
10. Chimowitz MI, et al. Stenting versus aggressive medical therapy for intracranial arterial stenosis. N Engl J Med. 2011;365(11):993–1003.

11. Berkhemer OA, Fransen PS, Beumer D, et al. A randomized trial of intraarterial treatment for acute ischemic stroke. N Engl J Med. 2015;372:11–20.
12. Grotta JC. Carotid stenosis. N Engl J Med. 2013;369:1143–50.
13. Rerkasem K, Rothwell PM. Carotid endarterectomy for symptomatic carotid stenosis. Cochrane Database Syst Rev. 2011;4:CD001081.
14. Silver FL, et al. Safety of stenting and endarterectomy by symptomatic status in the Carotid Revascularization Endarterectomy vs. Stenting Trial (CREST). Stroke. 2011;42:675–80.
15. Caceres JA, Goldstein JN. Intracerebral hemorrhage. Emerg Med Clin North Am. 2012;30(3):771–94.
16. Sakamoto Y, et al. Systolic blood pressure after intravenous antihypertensive treatment and clinical outcomes in hyperacute intracerebral hemorrhage: the stroke acute management with urgent risk-factor assessment and improvement-intracerebral hemorrhage study. Stroke. 2013;44(7):1846–51.
17. Morgenstern LB, et al. Guidelines for the management of spontaneous intracerebral hemorrhage. Stroke. 2010;41:2108–29.
18. Fong WC, et al. The benefit of prothrombin complex concentrate in decreasing neurological deterioration in patients with warfarin-associated intracerebral haemorrhage. Hong Kong Med J. 2014;20(6):486–94.
19. Friedlander RM. Arteriovenous malformations of the brain. N Engl J Med. 2007;356:2704–12.
20. Galletti F, et al. Brain arteriovenous malformations and seizures: an Italian study. J Neurol Neurosurg Psychiatry. 2014;85:284–8.
21. Mohr JP, et al. Medical management with or without interventional therapy for unruptured brain arteriovenous malformations (ARUBA): a multicentre, non-blinded, randomised trial. Lancet. 2014;383(9917): 614–21.
22. Brisman JL, Song JK, Newell DW. Cerebral aneurysms. N Engl J Med. 2006;355:928–39.
23. Juvela S, et al. Natural history of unruptured intracranial aneurysms: a long-term follow-up study. Stroke. 2013;44(9):2414–21.
24. Broderick JP, et al. Greater rupture risk for familial as compared to sporadic unruptured intracranial aneurysms. Stroke. 2009;40:1952–7.
25. Pereira JL, et al. Importance of recognizing sentinel headache. Surg Neurol Int. 2012;3:162.
26. Molyneux AJ, et al. The durability of endovascular coiling versus neurosurgical clipping of ruptured cerebral aneurysms: 18 year follow-up of the UK cohort of the International Subarachnoid Aneurysm Trial (ISAT). Lancet. 2015;385(9969):691–7.
27. Fukushima Y, et al. Ptosis as partial oculomotor nerve palsy due to compression by infundibular dilatation of posterior communicating artery, visualized with three-dimensional computer graphics: case report. Neurol Med Chir (Tokyo). 2014;54:214–8.
28. Rothwell PM, et al. Effect of urgent treatment of transient ischaemic attack and minor stroke on early recurrent stroke (EXPRESS study): a prospective population-based sequential comparison. Lancet. 2007;370(9596):1432–42.
29. Tissue plasminogen activator for acute ischemic stroke. The National Institute of Neurological Disorders and Stroke rt-PA Stroke Study Group. N Eng J Med. 1995;333:1581–7.
30. Hacke W, Kaste M, Bluhmki E, et al. Thrombolysis with alteplase 3 to 4.5 hours after acute ischemic stroke. N Engl J Med. 2008;359:1317–29.
31. Meyer MA. Stroke Quick Score: a visual aid in scoring neurologic deficits for acute stroke with National Institutes of Health Stroke Scale. Am J Emerg Med. 2008;26(2):189–90.
32. Chernyshev OY, Martin-Schild S, Albright KC, et al. Safety of tPA in stroke mimics and neuroimaging negative cerebral ischemia. Neurology. 2010;74(17): 1340–5.
33. Weber JE, Ebinger M, Rozanski M, et al. Prehospital thrombolysis in acute stroke: results of the PHANTOM-S pilot study. Neurology. 2013;80(2): 163–8.
34. Lidegaard O, Lokkegaard E, Jensen A, et al. Thrombotic stroke and myocardial infarction with hormonal contraception. N Engl J Med. 2012;366:2257–66.
35. Lichtman JH, et al. Seasonal variation in 30-day mortality after stroke: teaching versus nonteaching hospitals. N Engl J Med. 2013;44(2):531–3.
36. Elliott WJ. Circadian variation in the timing of stroke onset: a meta-analysis. Stroke. 1998;29:992–6.
37. Argentino C, et al. Circadian variation in the frequency of ischemic stroke. Stroke. 1990;21(3): 387–9.
38. Vellimana AK, et al. Symptomatic patients with intraluminal carotid artery thrombus: outcome with a strategy of initial anticoagulation. Stroke. 2013;118(1):34–41.
39. Marquardt L, Kuker W, Chandratheva A, et al. Incidence and prognosis of ≥50% symptomatic vertebral or basilar artery stenosis: prospective population-based study. Brain. 2009;132:982–8.
40. Backes WH, Nijenhuis RJ. Advances in spinal cord MR angiography. AJNR Am J Neuroradiol. 2008;29:619–31.
41. Staykov D, Gupta R. Hemicraniectomy in malignant middle cerebral artery infarction. Stroke. 2011;42:513–6.
42. Ali MS, Amenta PS, Starke RM, et al. Intracranial vertebral artery dissections: evolving perspectives. Interv Neuroradiol. 2012;18(4):469–83.
43. Thanvi B, et al. Carotid and vertebral artery dissection syndromes. Postgrad Med J. 2005;81(956):383–8.
44. Landmesser U, Holmes DR. Left atrial appendage closure: a percutaneous transcatheter approach for stroke prevention in atrial fibrillation. Eur Heart J. 2012;33:698–704.

45. Gladstone DJ, Spring M, Dorian P, et al. Atrial fibrillation in patients with cryptogenic stroke. N Engl J Med. 2014;370:2467–77.
46. Brewer L, Horgan F, Hickey A, Williams D. Stroke rehabilitation: recent advances and future therapies. QJM. 2012;106:11–25.
47. Friedrich MA, et al. Intra-arterial infusion of autologous bone marrow mononuclear cells in patients with moderate to severe middle cerebral artery acute ischemic stroke. Cell Transplant. 2012;21 Suppl 1:S13–21.
48. Willis T. Cerebri Anatome. 1664.

4 Epilepsy

4.1 Introduction

Epilepsy and the phenomenon of seizure activity is a fascinating area of neurology—the variety of seizure activity is wide and in some cases very complex and also sometimes very bizarre. Seizure activity is surprisingly common, and found in patients with multiple types of medical illness—almost any field of medicine will have the issue of seizure activity to contend with as it is also part of daily evaluations seen in almost any hospital Emergency Department. Epilepsy is thought to affect 45 million people worldwide and has a prevalence of 3–6 individuals per 1000 worldwide.

4.2 Historical Aspects of Epilepsy

The history of epilepsy is remarkable for an amazing transformation in the diagnosis, care, and treatment of the disorder, where primitive bromides were first used 100 years ago; after the 1953 introduction of Phenytoin (Figs. 4.1 and 4.2), a new era for effective epilepsy care began. Despite some side effects with ataxia and long-term toxicity to the cerebellum, it still remains in use as an effective anticonvulsant. As shown in Fig. 4.2, a wide spectrum of anti-seizure medications now exist, including the now widely used leviteracetam. Of additional note, gabapentin had been designed as an anticonvulsant with structural similarities to the inhibitory endogenous neuro-transmitter GABA (Fig. 4.2). Carbamazepine has an established and preferred role for temporal lobe epilepsy, whereas valproic acid also shares structural similarities to GABA but is used more for generalized seizures and also has a prophylactic role in the low-dose form for stabilizing and controlling migraine recurrences.

Historical figures have interesting epilepsy histories as well including Julius Caesar who had absence type seizures in his youth in the setting of a strong family history for epilepsy. Post-infarction seizure recurrences plagued Lennin, who died in status epilepticus. Alcohol-related seizure activity was suspected for Van Gogh. The writer Fyodor Dostoyevsky was severely affected by epilepsy, and described what the events were like in his writing [1].

The key to treatment is to understand the mechanism to the patient's seizures (Fig. 4.3). This approach to evaluating seizure activity is heavily based on obtaining a detailed history from not only the patient but also from eyewitnesses and family to help determine factors that can predict whether the seizure originated in a focal manner, as may occur with patients who have simple motor events of convulsive jerking of one limb representing a discharge from a focal spot within the motor cortex, or arose without warning and came on in a generalized fashion,

M.A. Meyer, *Neurologic Disease*, DOI 10.1007/978-3-319-39581-4_4

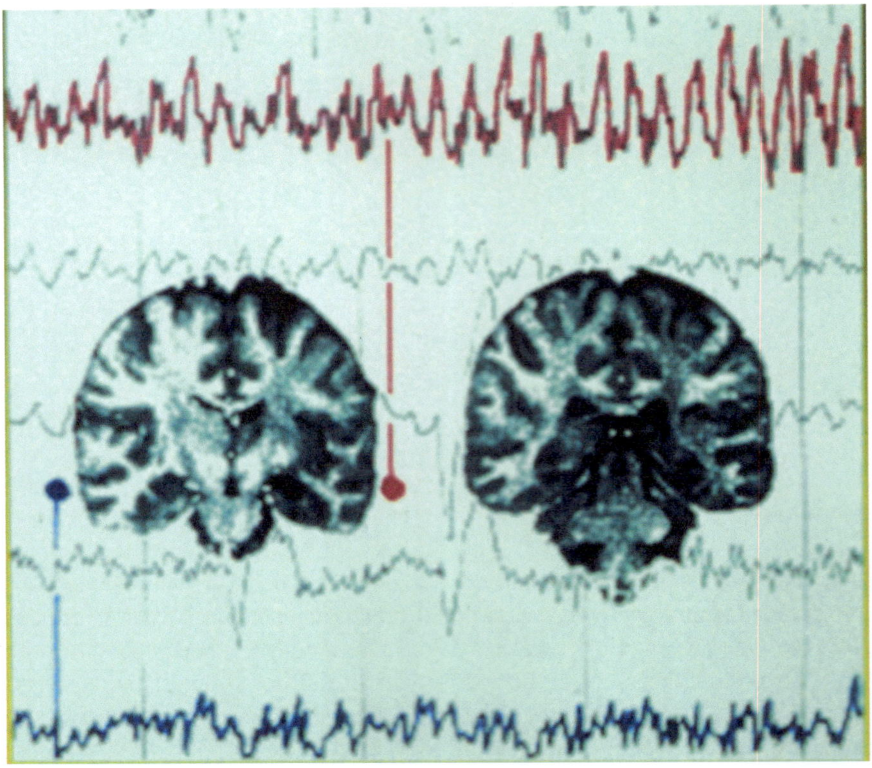

Fig. 4.1 Treatment decisions for epilepsy requires careful consideration of the history and examination findings, coupled with EEG and imaging findings

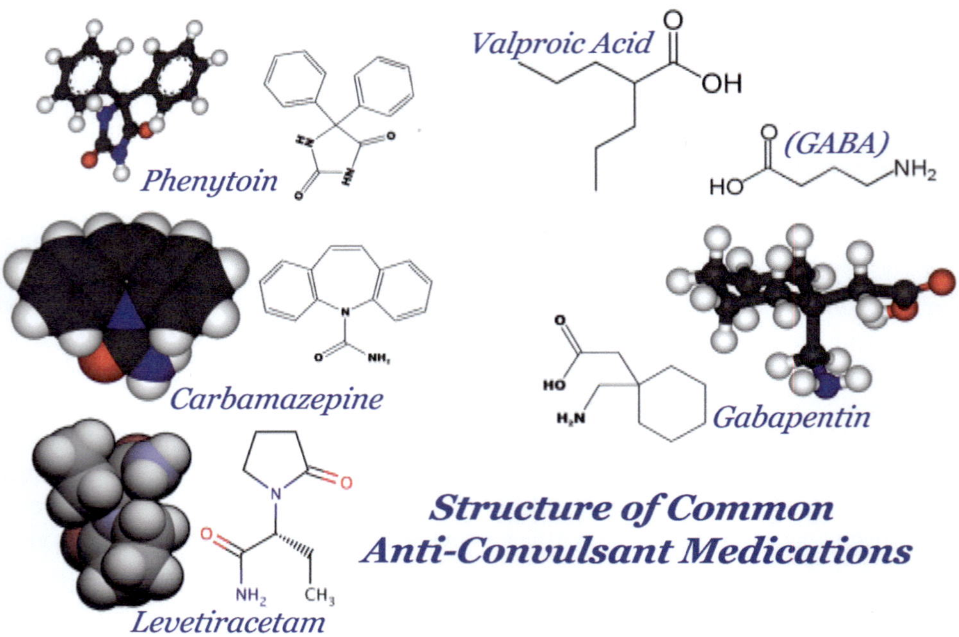

Fig. 4.2 Major anticonvulsant medications with their structures

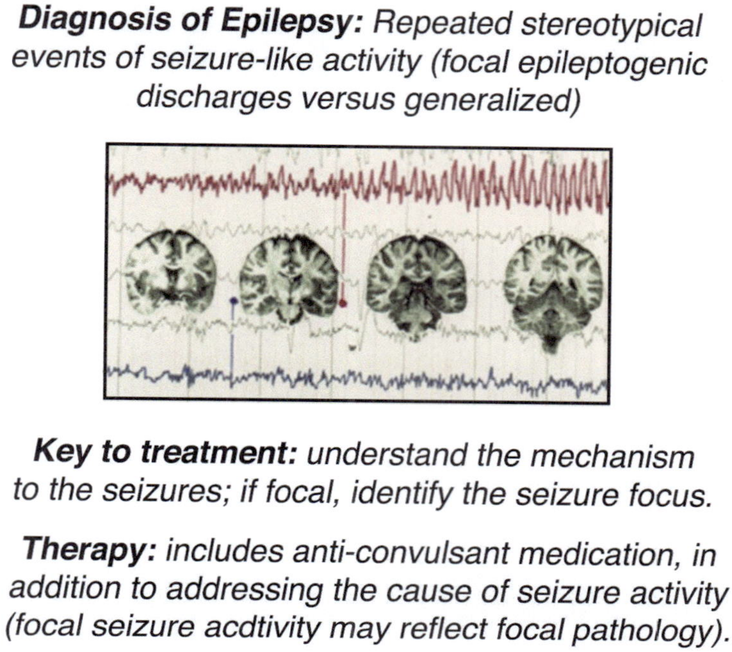

Fig. 4.3 The key to forming a safe and effective treatment plan is to understand the mechanism to the patient's seizures

which may reflect an intrinsic defect within neuronal sodium channels for example, or was a diffuse event related to drug withdrawal to cite another example. Post-ictal weakness focally or of a diffuse nature may give similar clues to the seizure focus and its causation. Although CT head examination is a good basic screen to exclude obvious pathology such as an intracerebral bleed or subdural hematoma, most if not all patients gain further benefit from undergoing brain MRI to exclude other pathology such as hippocampal scar or gliosis (mesial temporal sclerosis linked to complex-partial seizures), or for example possibly reveal an arterio-venous malformation to cite another example (occult AVM not obvious on a non-contrast CT but well seen as a tangle of T2 flow voids on MRI).

New onset of seizure activity at any age requires close attention as it may reflect serious focal pathology, including brain neoplasm. A good rule to remember in this regard is that focal seizure activity may be linked to focal pathology—a dedicated search is required. For new onset of epilepsy in adults, it has been estimated that about 70 % of cases were related to focal epilepsy. In this regard, the case shown below illustrates the challenges in identifying other types of focal epilepsy where the focal discharges produce complex events. This is well illustrated by the case of a 48-year-old female, with a history of "panic attacks", who had a sudden new onset of generalized seizure activity while traveling in a car—the MRI shown in Fig. 4.4 was initially read as "negative" by Radiology; it was not until she presented to the Neurologist that the "panic attack" events were recognized in actuality to be complex-partial seizure events arising from the left temporal lobe, as the MR study of the brain was in fact diagnostic for left-sided mesial temporal sclerosis, with the right hippocampal formation fully intact but very small and atrophic on the left with high T2 signal intensity (best seen in the coronal plane as shown in Fig. 4.4). Examination findings were unremarkable with normal cognition and objectively normal recall, yet review of systems was positive for being forgetful. This patient responded well to levetiracetam on a 500 mg bid basis along with carbamazepine and had no further recurrent spells while on this dual medication regimen to combat temporal lobe epilepsy.

Another complex-partial epilepsy patient is shown in Fig. 4.5 with MR revealing abnormally high T2 signal within the right hippocampus that

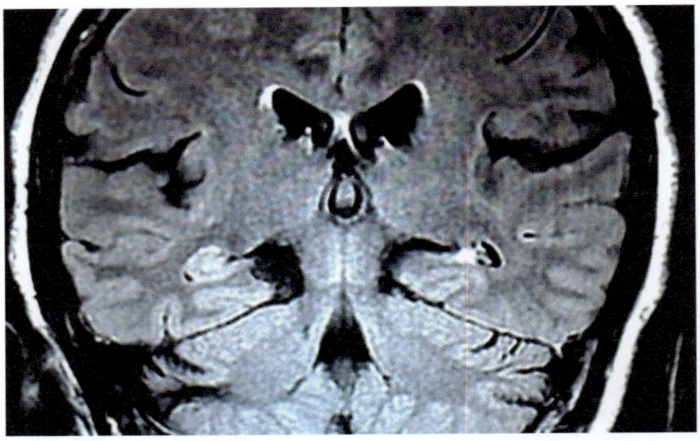

Fig. 4.4 Coronal brain MRI showing left mesial temporal sclerosis

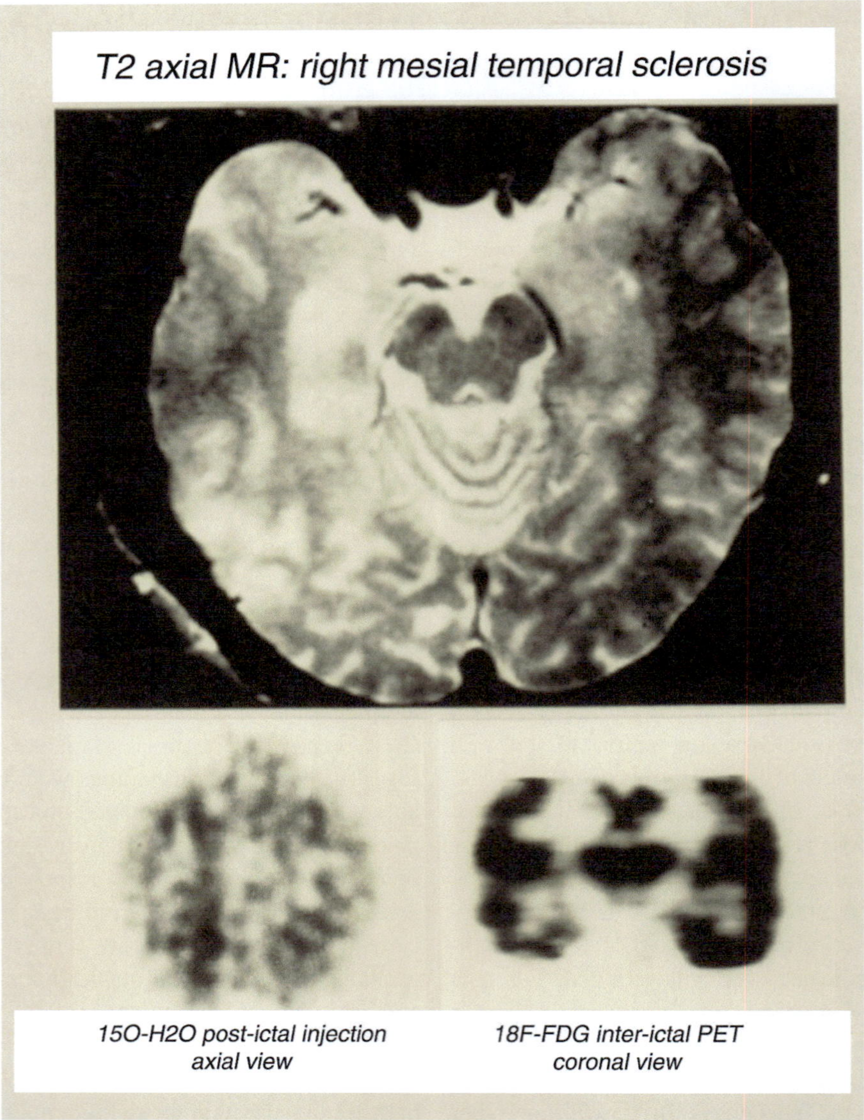

Fig. 4.5 Ictal versus inter-ictal PET imaging studies in a patient with right mesial temporal sclerosis

functionally correspond to depressed metabolism inter-ictally between seizures, and a post-ictal hyperemia with higher levels of perfusion captured by PET imaging very shortly after a spontaneous recurrent seizure.

MR obtained in the coronal plane is the most sensitive way to detect abnormally high T2 signal within the hippocampus of complex-partial seizure patients who harbor a highly focal area of hippocampal scarring, other known as mesial temporal sclerosis (MTS) as shown above in the preoperative evaluation that included 18F-FDG imaging as well to confirm site of suspected inter-ictal metabolic depression (Fig. 4.6; PET confirms inter-ictal left temporal hypometabolism concordant with the left hippocampal area of MTS seen on MRI).

Quantitative PET is another helpful clinical tool where imaging is performed in the dynamic mode to construct time–activity curves for uptake

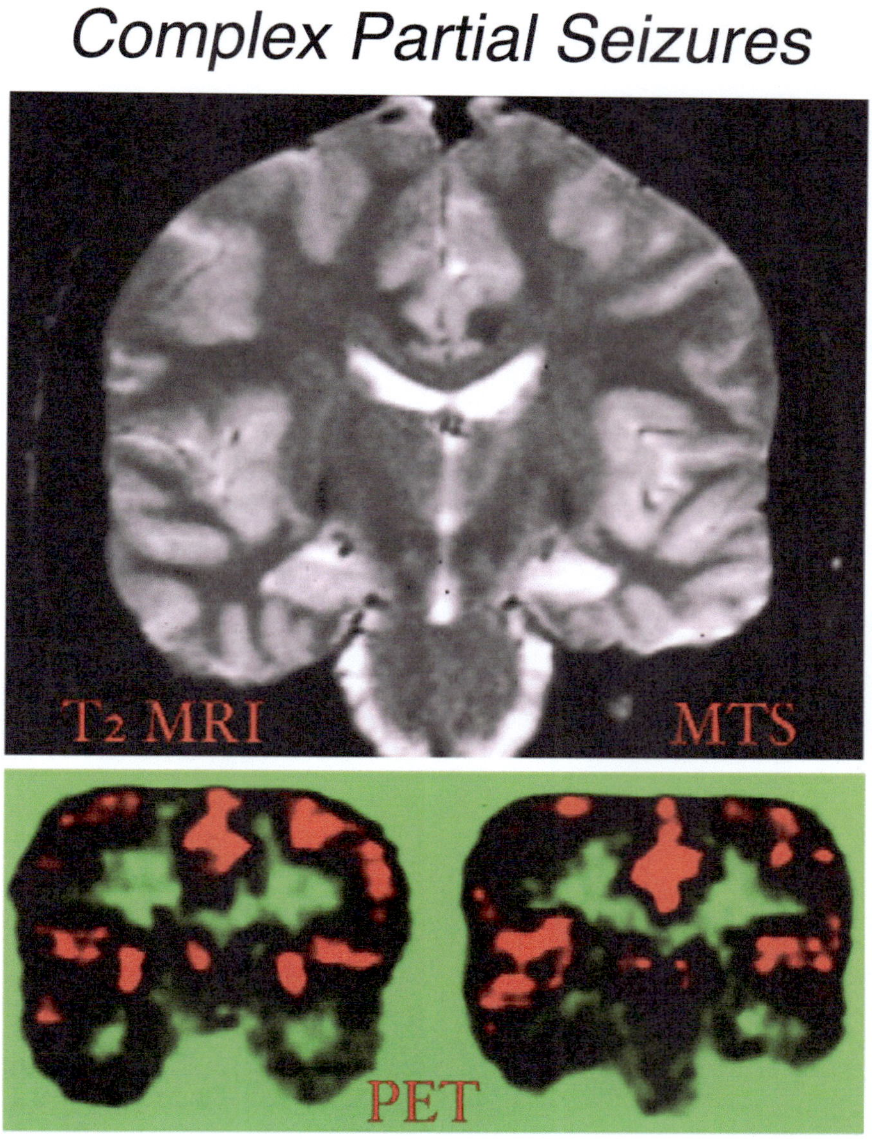

Fig. 4.6 Left mesial temporal sclerosis: coronal MR versus PET findings

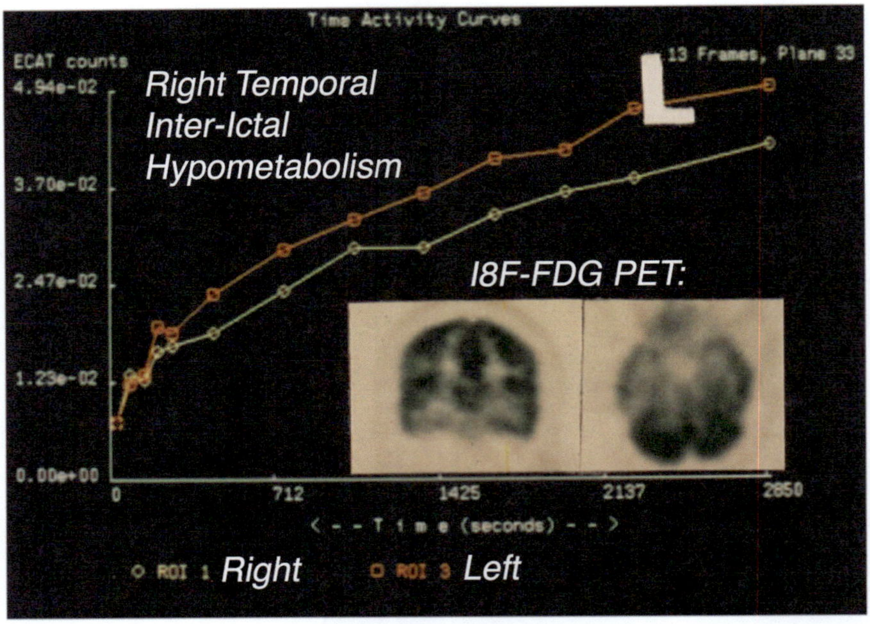

Fig. 4.7 Dynamic PET imaging of 18F-FDG uptake in a complex-partial seizure patient

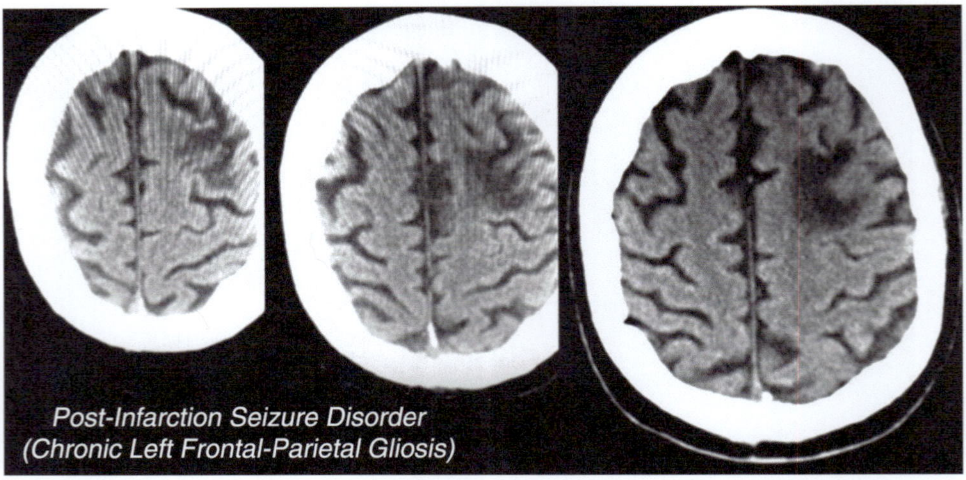

Fig. 4.8 Post-infarction epilepsy: CT findings

to help further confirm the seizure focus; the case example in Fig. 4.7 illustrates identification of the right temporal lobe as the inter-ictal focus of metabolic depression for the complex-partial epilepsy case in question.

Nearly three out of four patients with new onset of seizures have a focal origin for the epileptogenic discharges. Although tissue at the margins of an old ischemic infarct can be epileptogenic and is known to commonly serve a seizure focus (Fig. 4.8), the cause may still be unknown for 25 % of patients 65 years and older with new onset of seizures. With regards to diagnostic testing, EEG may show epileptiform discharges in as many as one out of four cases of new onset of seizure activity. For those with chronic medically refractory epilepsy that may be amenable to surgery, prolonged in-patient video-EEG

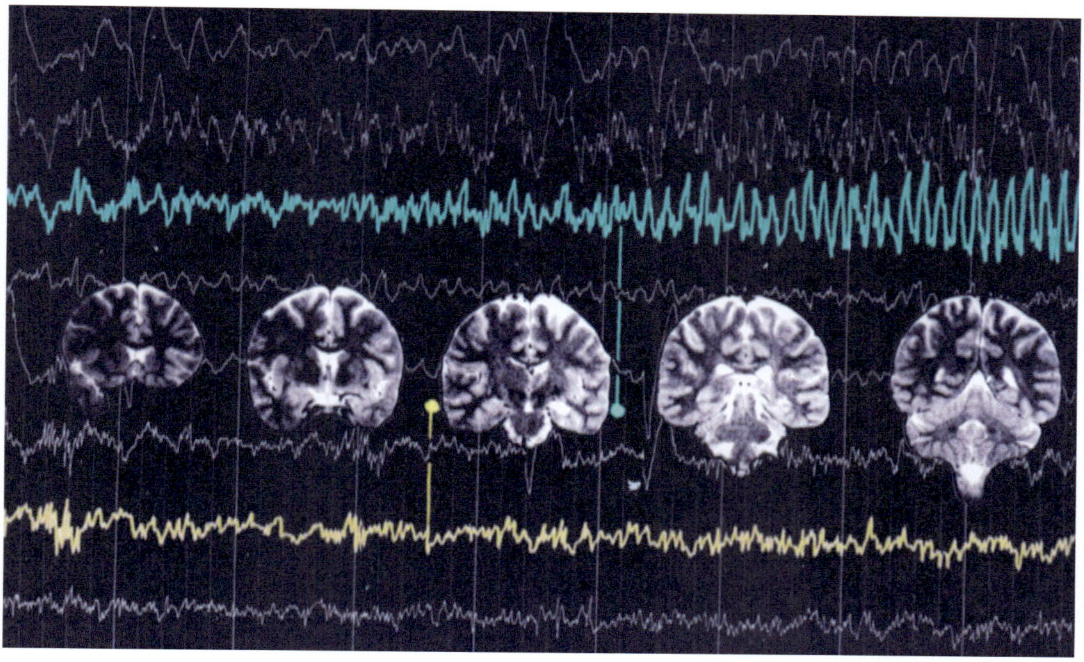

Fig. 4.9 Ictal EEG demonstrating left temporal discharge at onset

monitoring in a pre-arranged state of drug withdrawal is also very helpful in capturing the ictal focus on EEG, as shown in Fig. 4.9 [2].

One out of four patients without obvious predisposing factors for recurrent seizures will in fact experience a seizure recurrence within 2 years of the initial event; for those with predisposing factors, the recurrence rate is 40 % within 2 years. It therefore appears that the old clinical practice of not treating the first seizure does not make sense, especially in view of the fact that randomized trials show up to a 60 % reduction in the risk for seizure recurrence after starting treatment. Studies show that with a single anticonvulsant monotherapy regimen, half of all patients can be rendered seizure free. When two anticonvulsant medications are needed, about two out of every three patients on a dual medication regimen become seizure free. Those unfortunate patients who fail to respond even to triple medication regimens are clearly felt to have uncontrolled epilepsy; one study from France estimated that about 22 % of patients with epilepsy have drug-resistant epilepsy. A more formal definition of drug-resistant epilepsy has been given as "as a failure of adequate trials of two (or more) tolerated, appropriately chosen, and appropriately used antiepileptic drug regimens (whether administered as monotherapies or in combination) to achieve freedom from seizures" [3].

For those patients with uncontrolled epilepsy, a number of complications can occur, including sudden unexpected death, and traumatic body injuries, and suffer adverse effects from multiple medications; also, depression is a comorbid factor found in about half of the patient population with uncontrolled epilepsy. A key principle of management for those felt to have uncontrolled epilepsy is ruling out pseudoresistance, as there are a number of epilepsy mimics including vasovagal syncope, cardiac arrhythmias, as well as psychogenic disorders; the latter has been estimated to account for at least 25 % of what may appear to be drug-resistant epilepsy in adults [4]. Other factors to consider when seizures recur or worsen despite medication might be the drug itself. In this regard, it is important to remember that phenytoin, carbamazepine, gabapentin, oxcarbazepine, vigabatrin, tiagabine, and pregabalin can worsen absence epilepsy and myoclonic seizures; lamotrigine can also aggravate and actually worsen some myoclonic epilepsy syndromes.

With regards to adverse effects from polypharmacy in those with uncontrolled epilepsy, it is important to note that loss of bone density may occur with phenytoin, carbamazepine, and possibly with other hepatic enzyme-inducing antiepileptic drugs, and may require monitoring of bone mineral density with calcium supplementation as needed. These hepatic enzyme-inducing antiepileptic drugs, which also include topiramate and oxcarbazepine, increase the clearance of oral contraceptives and potentially reduce effectiveness, leading to unwanted risks to a developing fetus for adverse drug effects. In this regard, it is important to note that babies born to women with epilepsy have an increased rate of congenital malformations, attributable mainly to antiepileptic drugs.

With regards to other adverse effects from antiepileptic drugs, hyponatremia can result from treatment with carbamazepine or oxcarbazepine; reduced anticoagulation effects from warfarin can occur with phenytoin or carbamazepine due to increased warfarin clearance. Weight gain can be another important adverse effect to consider, which can be modest with carbamazepine or gabapentin but more substantial for valproate or pregabalin, where weight gain of 10–50 lb may occur in about one-third of patients.

Some patients find adverse effects intolerable and elect to come off medication after becoming seizure free; in doing so, the incidence of seizure recurrence after drug withdrawal after a 2-year seizure-free period ranges from 12 to 66 %.

Non-pharmacologic approaches to uncontrolled epilepsy include the ketogenic diet, which is a high-fat, low-protein, low-carbohydrate regimen useful for pediatric cases. One randomized, controlled study revealed that half of the children on the diet experienced a drop in seizures by more than 50 % [5]. Other non-pharmacologic approaches to uncontrolled epilepsy include surgery, as outlined below.

When all medications fail, and the seizure focus is identifiable with confidence, surgical removal of the seizure focus may be a reasonable alternative. As shown in Fig. 4.10, the Montreal Neurologic Institute did pioneering work in this

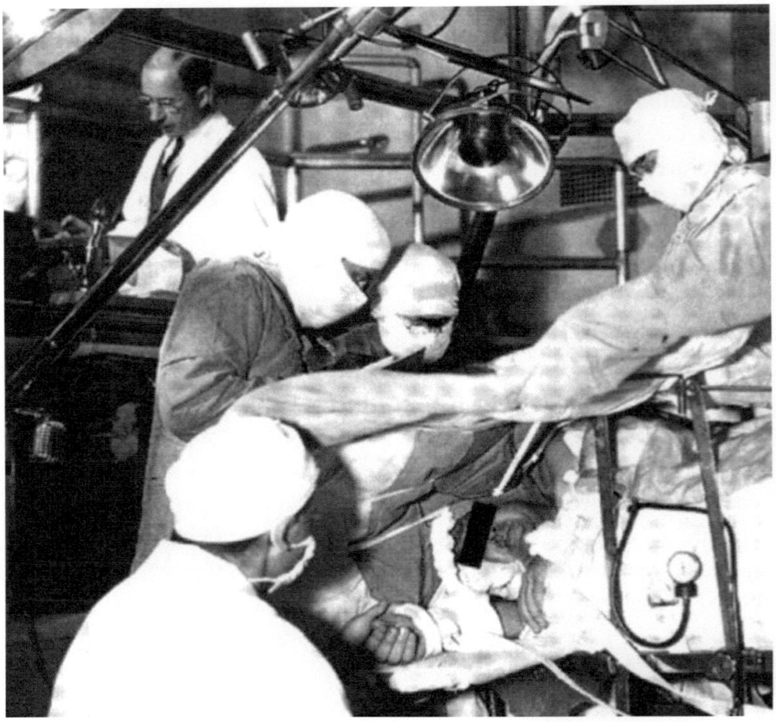

Fig. 4.10 Epilepsy surgery had its beginnings at the Montreal Neurologic Institute

regard, with an example of a surgical case with EEG monitoring performed by epilepsy pioneer, Dr. Herbert Henri Jasper in the upper left of the photo. Currently, the preoperative set of required studies employ not only MRI and video-EEG to identify the focus, but also inter-ictal PET and ictal SPECT are used as well; language dominance is also identified preoperatively with amytal Wada testing.

A recent review by the government of Ontario revealed that six systematic reviews on surgical approaches to epilepsy reported pooled seizure-free rates that ranged from 43 to 75 %. Eight retrospective cohort studies with long follow-up periods ranging from a mean of 2–7 years reported on the safety of epilepsy surgery: only three deaths were noted out of the 2725 patients included in these studies; other complications included hemiparesis, infection, and visual field defects [6].

Another surgical option is the use of vagal nerve stimulator placement, which has been demonstrated to be safe and effective in medically refractory epilepsy. The vagal nerve stimulator that is implanted in the upper chest delivers electrical current to the vagus nerve [7]. Although approved for use as an adjunctive therapy for partial-onset seizures resistant to medication, the response overall is felt to be modest. Although well described in the adult population, recent data suggest a use for this as well for pediatric epilepsy [8].

Patients who meet the criteria for having drug-resistant epilepsy might be candidates for surgery, particularly if they have a focal lesion, such as unilateral hippocampal sclerosis which may be amenable to anterior temporal lobectomy; studies show this to be superior to medical management in up to 70 % of adults with drug-resistant temporal-lobe epilepsy [9]. For intractable temporal lobe seizures, surgery has been known to be an effective and safe option for those who qualify and meet presurgical criteria with appropriate testing for language dominance using the Wada test.

Promising results are now found with the newly developed implanted responsive neurostimulator that delivers stimulation to one or two seizure foci via chronically implanted electrodes. Randomized blinded controlled studies show median percent seizure reduction to be 44 % at 1 year and 53 % at 2 years for a patient population that had a median preimplant frequency of disabling partial or generalized tonic–clonic seizures of 10.2 seizures a month [10].

Surgical approaches to epilepsy include biopsy of atypical focal seizure foci that actively discharge despite medication and might represent a potentially lethal condition (i.e. neoplasm). To establish the underlying cause, benefits to surgical biopsy may exceed the risks and lead to a definitive diagnosis. As shown in Figs. 4.11 and 4.12 that illustrate the case of a child with uncontrollable focal epilepsy, focal right parietal hypermetabolism (Fig. 4.11) was seen on PET imaging, correlated subsequently to biopsy proven focus of epileptogenic cortical dysplasia (Fig. 4.12).

Other developmental malformations causing severe epilepsy include schizencephaly as shown in the case example illustrated in Fig. 4.13. In consideration of a possible surgical solution, a profoundly impaired 20-year-old with left hemispheric open lip schizencephaly was referred for

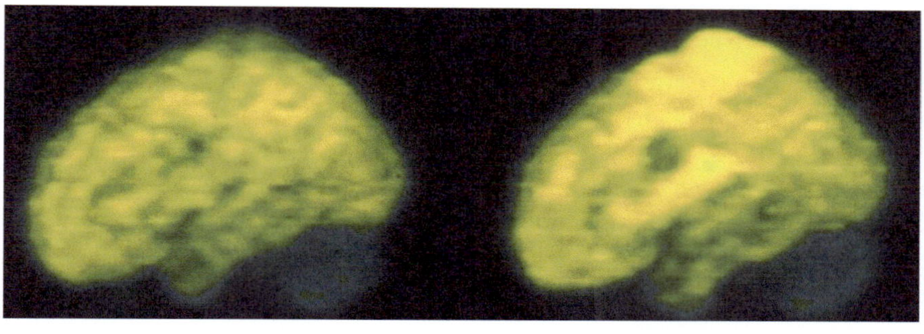

Fig. 4.11 Childhood epilepsy due to cortical dysplasia: PET findings

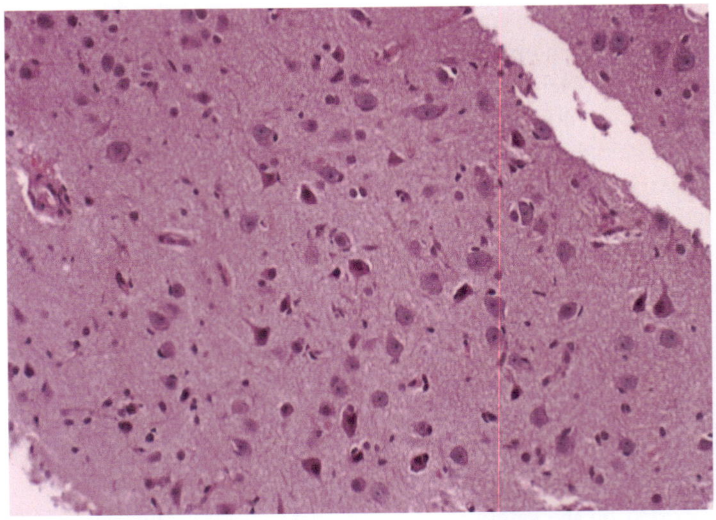

Fig. 4.12 Microscopic examination of cortical dysplasia biopsy showing disorganized collection of neurons

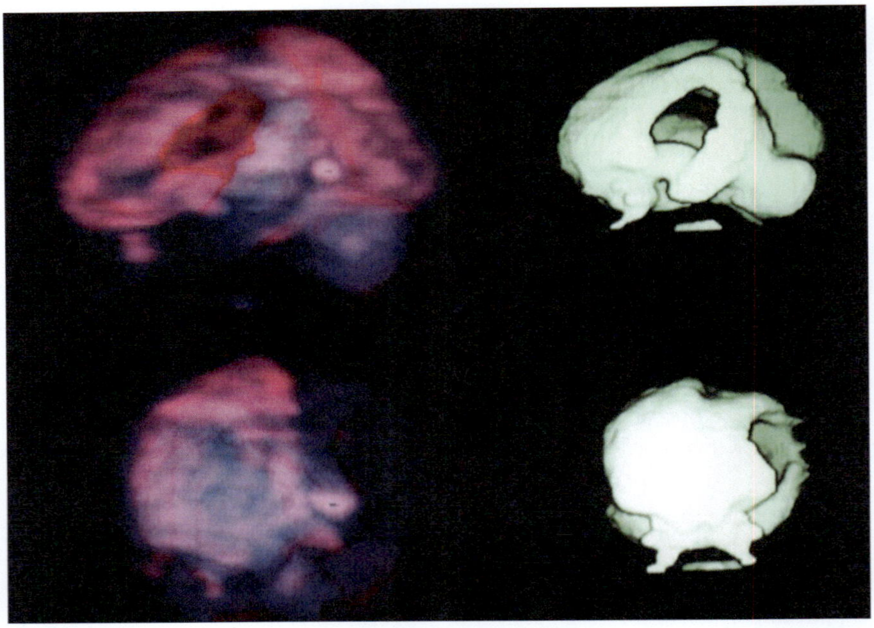

Fig. 4.13 PET findings for severe epilepsy due to open lip schizencephaly

PET to help understand the cause of intractable seizure activity. As revealed by the three-dimensional reconstructions, the metabolic pattern for the right hemisphere was normal yet remarkably impaired for the left hemisphere, which appeared to be nonfunctional except for an intense solitary focus in the region of the left splenium and occipital cortex region, suggesting that surgical isolation of this area as the presumed seizure focus would be of benefit; he was lost to follow-up.

MRI is a very sensitive tool in evaluating seizure patients with closed lip schizencephaly, as shown in Fig. 4.14, MRI can more accurately diagnose subtle cortical malformations in epilepsy patients that may be missed on axial CT brain examinations (Fig. 4.15). Multiple case reports have shown that mutations in the human

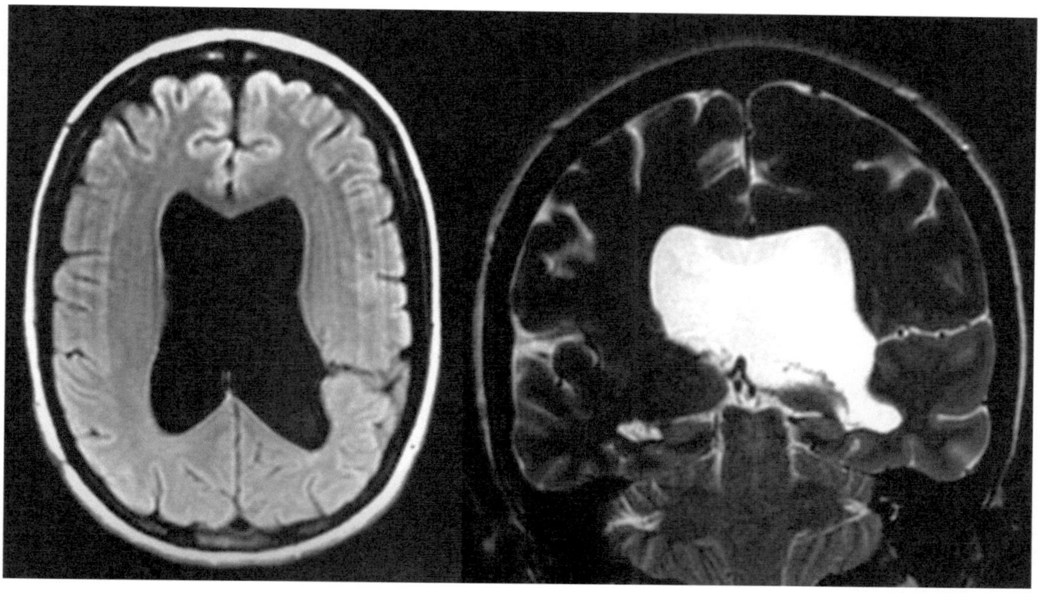

Fig. 4.14 Seizures secondary to parietal schizencephaly. MR revealing closed lip schizencephaly

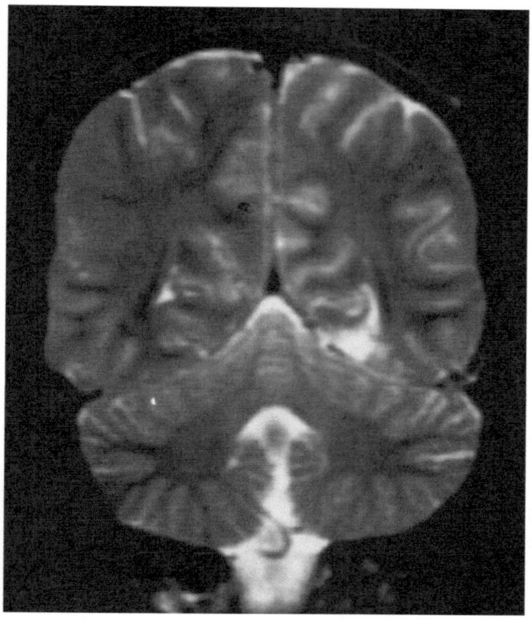

Fig. 4.15 Focal left occipital-temporal cortical maldevelopment: visual prodrome reported by epilepsy patient in advance of generalized seizure activity corresponding to focal left inferior occipital-temporal cortical lesion seen on coronal T2 MRI

Sonic Hedgehog gene can result in cortical maldevelopment and other severe brain malformations, including schizencephaly [11].

As shown in Fig. 4.16, hemispherectomy can be of great value in certain children with extreme forms of drug-resistant hemispheric focal epilepsy. Removal of the dysfunctional right hemisphere for this young child at age 4 was very beneficial in relieving constant and intractable seizure activity. PET at age 9 was negative for any obvious seizure focus (Fig. 4.16); the sequential scans were completed at different times in two different states of unilateral leg activity (patient was cognitively normal and fully ambulatory and able to run without obvious defects).

Patients with generalized seizures that are idiopathic and have normal MRI examinations are generally not surgical candidates, and best managed by medication. A fascinating discovery about these patients who do fall into this group of generalized epilepsy is that many individuals have this problem on a genetic basis that affects proper ion channel currents within neuronal membranes, which predisposes them to aberrant epileptogenic discharges. In this regard, absence seizures of childhood characterized by brief diffuse 3 Hz spike and wave discharge on EEG (which can persist into adulthood) has been linked to mutations within the gene encoding a certain type of calcium channel (T-type) involved in burst firing of neurons. Displaying a lower

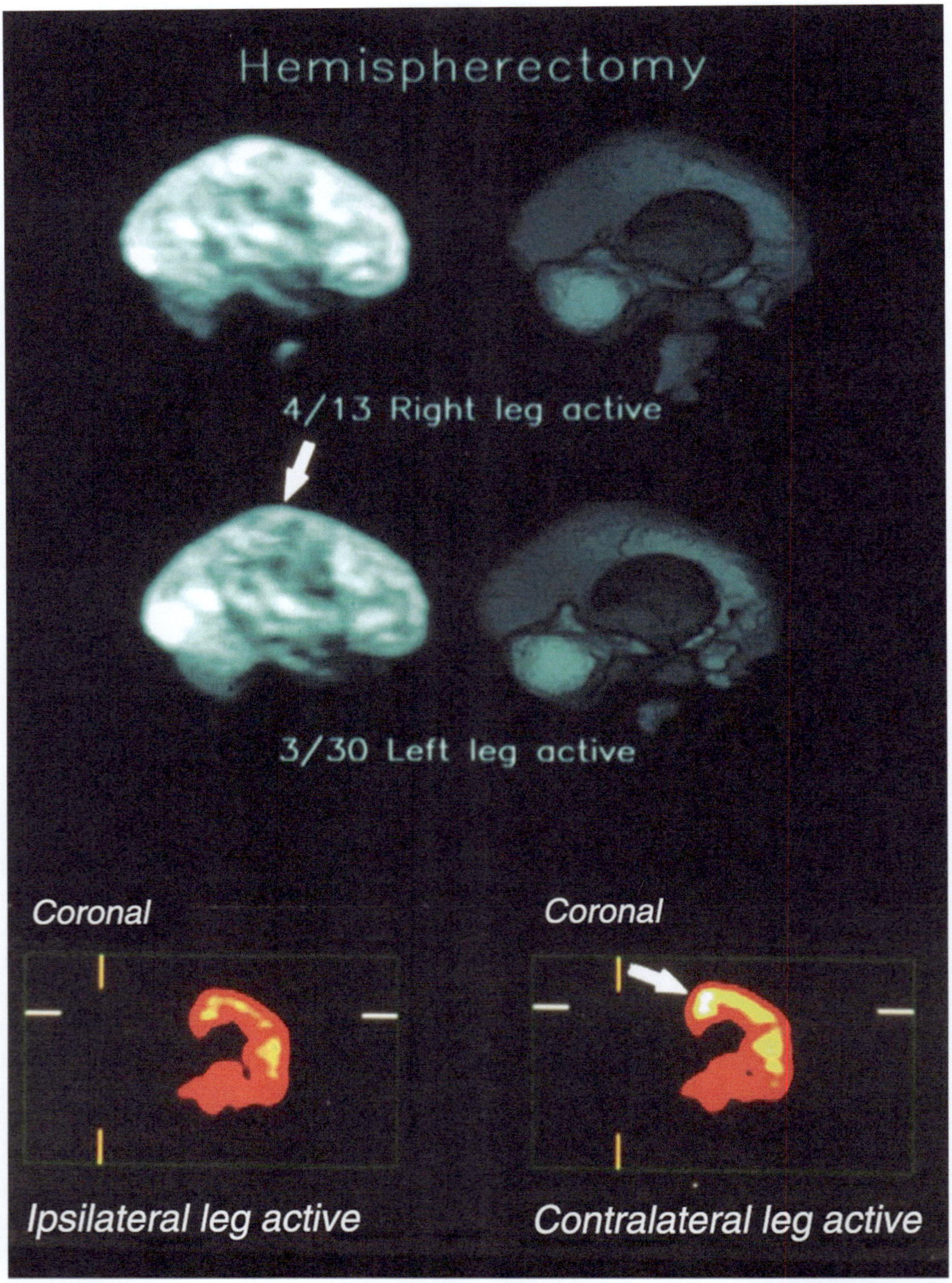

Fig. 4.16 PET findings after hemispherectomy

threshold for activation, T-type channels also inactivate faster, leading to a transient surge in calcium within the neuron that then predisposes to burst firing [12]. Calcium entry through the T channels encoded by the CACNA1H gene generate low-threshold current spikes that lead to bursts of sodium-dependent action potentials [13]. Mutations in the encoding CACNA1H gene have been widely reported in patients with childhood absence epilepsy [14].

The link between absence epilepsy and CACNA1H gene mutations becomes more evident in considering that ethosuximide, which blocks all three T-type calcium channels, is considered as first choice drug for treating absence seizures [15]. Ethosuximide can dramatically improve absence epileptic spells, which consist of brief staring and unresponsiveness, often with brief, mild eyelid fluttering or myoclonic jerks; duration is typically no more than 10 s but can recur hundreds of times per day with patient perceiving small "gaps in time". Ethosuximide and valproic acid are more effective than lamotrigine in the monotherapy approach to treatment of childhood absence epilepsy; ethosuximide has fewer adverse effects upon attention. Absence epilepsy is the most common form of pediatric epilepsy and accounts for up to 17 % of all cases of childhood-onset seizures [16].

Aside from absence epilepsy, juvenile myoclonic epilepsy (Janz syndrome) is the most common type of idiopathic generalized epilepsy, accounting for approximately 12–30 % of all epilepsies. Characterized by both absence and myoclonic seizures as well as generalized tonic–clonic seizures, it has been linked to alterations in the BRD2 gene. Although its exact role is not yet clear, BRD2 is felt to be a transcriptional regulator that may influence brain development; it has been hypothesized that epilepsy-associated mutations of this gene may result in disorganized neuronal connectivity and neocortical hyperexcitability [17].

Whereas absence seizures are at one end of the epilepsy spectrum with very brief events under 10 s and generally not associated with any structural lesions, other types of epilepsy at the other end of the spectrum can predispose to prolonged repetitive seizure activity and produce the most feared complication of status epilepticus. Estimated to occur in about 150,000 individuals annually in the US, convulsive status epilepticus can have a high mortality rate with significant morbidity leading to cognitive decline after an event [18].

The incidence of status epilepticus peaks in two extreme age groups: one in infancy and the other for those over 60 years. The overall case fatality rate varies and tends to be higher at 38 % for the elderly compared to 14 % for younger adults. Although no clear cause cannot be found in about half the cases, epileptogenic tissue around the margins of an old prior cortical ischemic stroke is a leading cause for status epilepticus, with other causes linked to degenerative conditions, metabolic derangements, low anticonvulsant levels, hypoxia, alcohol, tumors, trauma, and CNS infections. The underlying cause generally dictates or predicts the mortality rate, being highest at 72 % for post-anoxic encephalopathy versus only 4 % with seizures traced to a provocative cause such as low anticonvulsant drug levels. Seizure duration is a major factor influencing outcome, with a mortality of 2.6 % for status epilepticus lasting under 30 min versus 19 % for over 30 min [19].

Management strategies for status epilepticus must focus on the ABCs of critical care medicine: airway, breathing, circulation must be optimized as hypoxia will induce a downward spiral of worsening seizure activity that becomes more difficult to terminate with medication. If seizures persist despite IV lorazepam, loading doses of IV leviteracetam, or related medications must be given such as phos-phenytoin or valproic acid, with anesthesia on hand for possible intubation for the use of propopfol. EEG is helpful in managing these cases as well, as shown in Fig. 4.17, where residual right frontal spike activity was persisting in a mentally retarded young adult who was effectively treated with anticonvulsants for recurrent status epilepticus; although seizure activity was no longer obvious on clinical examination after treatment, clinically silent epileptogenic spiking persisted on the EEG (see top panel of Fig. 4.17).

New drugs for epilepsy that have been recently developed include the sodium-channel blocker known as lacosamide, which has been licensed for use in adults with partial seizures. Rufinamide has shown benefit for the Lennox–Gastaut syndrome in infants and children while Vigabatrin has been approved as an adjunctive treatment for complex partial seizures in adults and as monotherapy for infantile spasms. Although ezogabine is licensed as an adjunctive treatment for refractory partial seizures in adults, serious adverse effects are known for this new drug to include

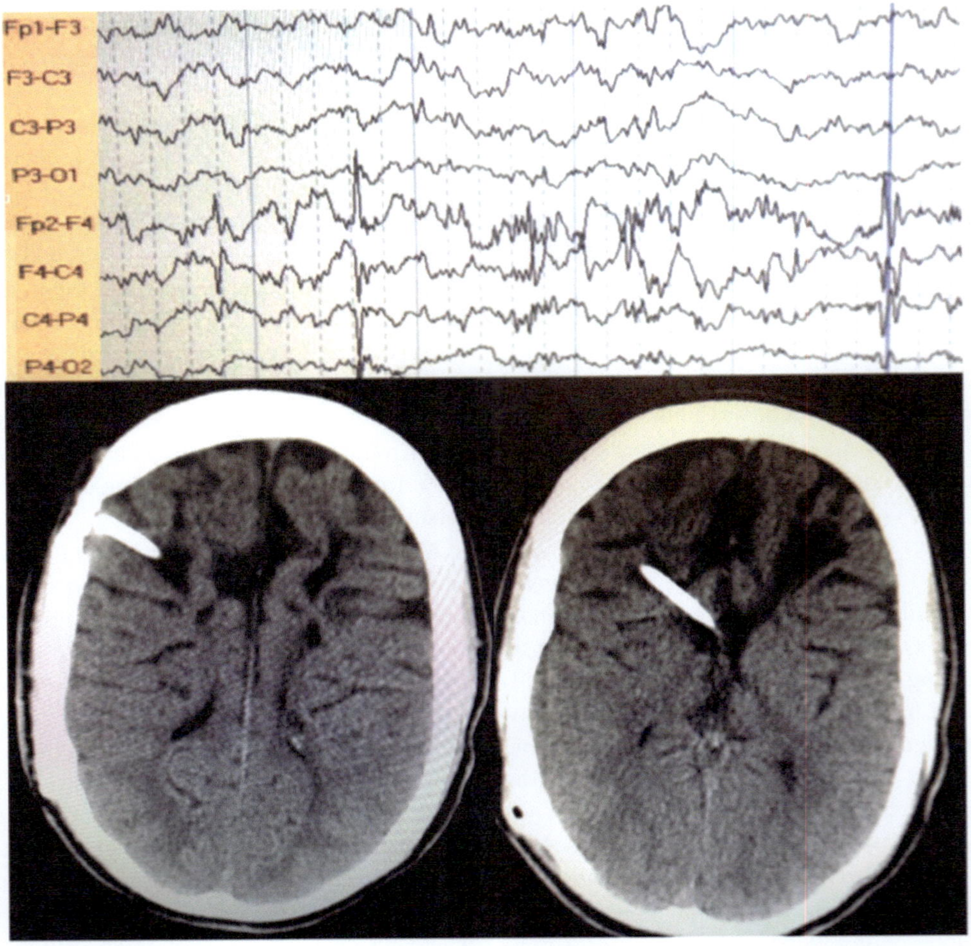

Fig. 4.17 Status epilepticus: recurrent cluster of seizure activity developed over 1 h at home in a 20-year-old with cerebral palsy and a ventriculo-peritoneal shunt with bi-frontal subcortical encephalomalacia evident on CT: he was effectively treated in the Emergency Department with IV Ativan and IV valproic acid; tonic–clonic seizure activity ceased by the time this EEG recording was made which showed episodic right front-central spike discharges

retinal damage with potential vision loss, and blue skin discoloration, all of which may become permanent; this drug acts in a unique manner by opening potassium channels. Other new drugs in development include brivaracetam, which acts similar to levetiracetam by binding to the synaptic vesicle protein 2A molecule. Perampanel is a new selective non-competitive antagonist of AMPA receptors that has an anticonvulsant action by modulating glutaminergic neurotransmission within the brain.

Although most people with epilepsy live full and productive lives, it is important to note that in rare cases, seizures can be unexpectedly suddenly fatal. The incidence of sudden, unexpected death in epilepsy (SUDEP) is probably underestimated as the incidence per 1000 patient-years varies with the sample population, increasing from very low levels in the general population to as low as 1.2 in tertiary care epilepsy centers to 9.3 amongst the epilepsy surgery population [20]. However, the rate of sudden, unexpected death increases with the duration and severity of epilepsy. For epileptic children under 14 years of age, cases of sudden, unexpected death are rare. However, it is also important to note that some seizure-like events are actually due to global cerebral hypoperfusion during potentially lethal cardiac arrhythmias, whereas other authentic epileptic disorders have associated ictal asystole or other ictal cardiac arrhythmias that may predispose to SUDEP [21].

Case Examples: Complex-Partial Seizures
The PET scan shown in Fig. 4.18 was performed to evaluate for mesial temporal sclerosis (MTS) in a 46-year-old female with disabling complex-partial epilepsy, with EEG and PET concordant for a right temporal seizure focus (MRI was unremarkable).

The underlying cause in general for hippocampal gliosis in the form of epileptogenic MTS is still unclear, but in some way relates to the extreme sensitivity to CA1 neurons to any form of hypoxia or metabolic compromise. An interesting idea also relates to viral infections, such as picornavirus [22].

Complex-partial epilepsy can initially present with psychiatric symptoms, such as anxiety and panic attacks in children. For example, a young child with previously unrecognized panic attack spells where she would cry out that she "…. saw the devil" was then found to have an abnormal PET scan (Fig. 4.19) which led to an MR examination

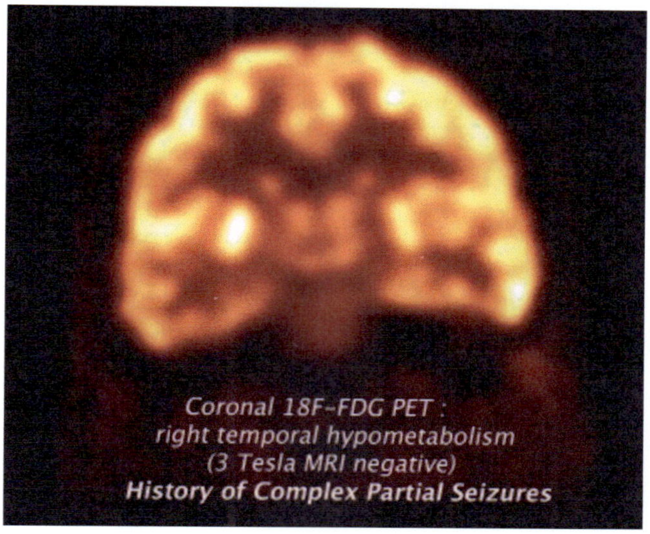

Fig. 4.18 PET findings in temporal lobe epilepsy. Coronal 18F-FDG PET: right temporal hypometabolism (3 T MRI negative). History of complex partial seizures

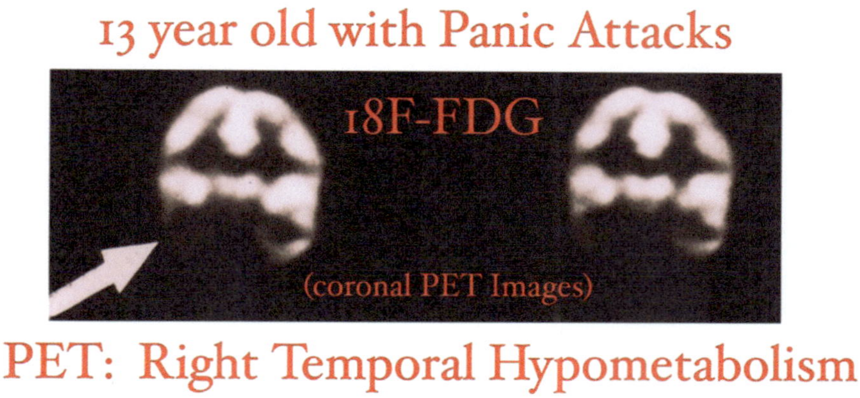

Fig. 4.19 Right mesial temporal sclerosis associated with panic attacks

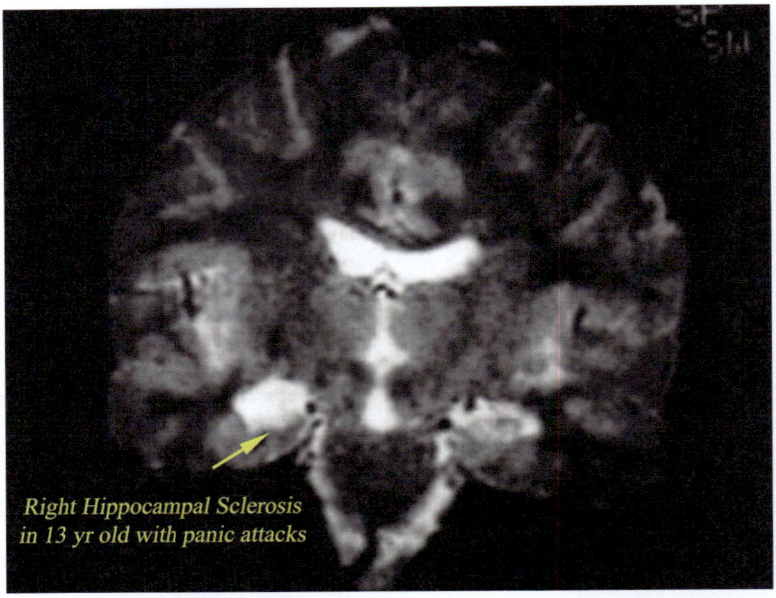

Fig. 4.20 MR findings for case illustrated in Fig. 4.19

Table 4.1 Classification of reflex epilepsy: simple versus complex types

	Simple	Complex
Visual	Photosensitivity	Color induced
	Pattern evoked	Eye closure induced
Auditory	Evoked by nonspecific starting in seconds	Specific but nonverbal sounds without startle; specific voices
Musicogenic	Certain musical notes	Musical themes
Movement induced	Startling passive movement	Active movement or concept of movement
Communications/reading epilepsy	Eye movement or patterns	Due to acquisition of knowledge
Decision-making epilepsy		Sequential decision making under stress
Somatosensory	Startling tap stimulation	Prolonged nonstartle stimulation
Eating	Myoclonic attacks with swallowing	Obscure associated factors with eating

showing ipsilateral mesial temporal sclerosis, predicting a right hippocampal seizure focus (Fig. 4.20). The patient later developed recurrent temporal lobe seizures as a teenager with occasional generalized seizures as well [23].

Unusual forms of epilepsy are known to exist, and may occur with provocative stimuli, as in reflex epilepsy (see tabular summary, Table 4.1); the topic has been reviewed recently [24]. This fascinating area of epilepsy includes rare yet true cases of seizure provoked by specific stimuli that include, but are not limited to visual stimuli, or even music, thinking, music, eating, reading, or being startled; extreme examples of epilepsy triggers are illustrated below that include playing backgammon or hearing the voice of a television celebrity.

Case Examples: Backgammon Epilepsy

An unusual form of decision-making reflex epilepsy. In this regard, the author has encountered and evaluated a young patient who had reproducible generalized epileptogenic discharges in association with playing backgammon. As reproduced in the EEG lab, shortly after engaging in a game of backgammon, myoclonic jerks in association with epileptogenic discharges would selectively develop in this patient who had recently experienced new onset generalized seizure activity; CT head examination was negative [25].

With regards to the unusual provocation of seizure-like activity by backgammon playing (decision-making reflex epilepsy) is another unusual published case: a 76-year-old avid backgammon player who developed epileptogenic discharges from the right frontal area in association with hallucination, and disorientation plus odd behaviors of swinging his hands like throwing large dice and then pretending to move large backgammon pieces from room to room; these behaviors ceased after starting carbamazepine [26].

Case Example of Audiogenic Reflexive Type Epilepsy

A 45-year-old female presented with "black outs" and recurrent episodes of mental confusion triggered by the voice of a female cohost on a popular television entertainment program. Video EEG documented complex partial seizures that were consistently triggered from the right temporal area by a videotape of the specific television show; further testing revealed that the seizures were precipitated only by the voice of the female cohost [27]. The patient remained seizure-free on carbamazepine and valproate.

Case Example of Pilomotor Epilepsy

A 35-year-old female was referred to an epilepsy clinic to evaluate seizure recurring up to 30 times per day. Seizures lasted less than 90 s without loss of consciousness and had bilateral sensations of chill, associated with colored phosphenes in the right hemi-field, nausea, thoracic compression, followed a few seconds later by piloerection involving both arms and legs [28]. Standard EEG recording showed slow waves on the left temporal region and MRI showed increased FLAIR signal intensity of the left hippocampus. Ictal EEG showed rhythmic slow activity in the left central and temporal area; the patient subsequently became seizure-free with carbamazepine.

Case Example of Unusual form of Epilepsy: Gelastic Seizures Related to Hypothalamic Hamartoma

A rare form of epilepsy in association with laughing is illustrated in Fig. 4.21. Known as gelastic seizures, this type of epilepsy is typically found in patients with hypothalamic hamartomas, as shown in Fig. 4.21, which illustrates the metabolic changes associated with a right hypothalamic mass in a 26-year-old gelastic seizure patient. Positron emission tomography (PET) imaging of the brain was performed in the interictal state

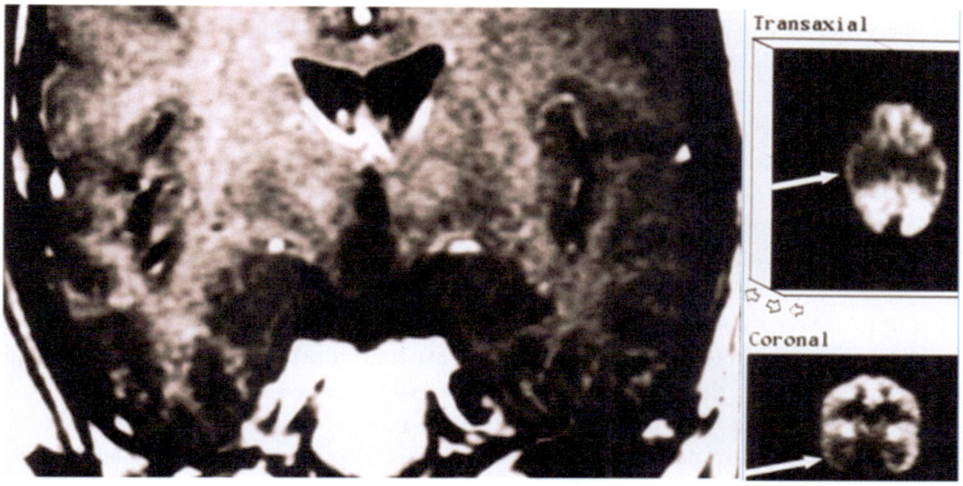

Fig. 4.21 MR and PET findings in gelastic seizure patient

using 18F-fluorodeoxyglucose (18F-FDG) in this patient [29]. Temporal lobe hypometabolism was noted ipsilateral to the hypothalamic lesion; the mass itself had little to no uptake of 18F-FDG. Further studies are needed in other patients to test whether ictal PET imaging may help plan the removal of epileptogenic hypothalamic lesions [30].

Case Example of Limbic Encephalitis

A 71-year-old female presented with the chief complaint of cognitive function decline; she developed increased forgetfulness for names, dates, and places. She was described as becoming irritable and was having difficulty getting along with family members and began making errors with names; her hands would tremble, and that she had progressive difficulty in finding words. By the fourth week of her progressive illness, she could not put together a meal and had fairly significant trouble with short-term memory and word finding. Episodes of confusion and incoherent speech also developed.

Brain SPECT revealed an unusually intense focus of uptake in the left hippocampus and amygdala, which matched an area of abnormally bright T2 signal on subsequent MR images (Fig. 4.22); EEG showed an active seizure focus in the left temporal-occipital region with rhythmic 3–4 Hz left posterior temporal-occipital discharges occurring in 20-s bursts were noted. During hyperventilation, a 35-s 3–4 Hz rhythmic slow discharge with 2 Hz sharp and slow wave complexes were noted, during which time she was mildly dysphasic. Her EEG was considered to be consistent with complex partial seizures. Although diagnosed as limbic encephalitis (which is often a paraneoplastic effect), no underlying malignancy was found [31].

Case Example of Seizure Activity Secondary to Metastatic Foci Within the Brain

Although paraneoplastic limbic encephalitis can at times be found as a remote distant cause of new onset of seizures in patients with non-small cell lung carcinoma [32], direct local epileptogenic secondary effects from metastatic foci are far more common. As shown in Fig. 4.23, metastatic foci from lung cancer can readily induce new onset seizure activity, and is effectively treated with anticonvulsants and steroids. Brain metastases commonly complicate systemic neoplastic disease in about 20–40 % of cancer patients. Although metastatic brain lesions may predispose patients to seizure, studies show that the prophylactic use of anticonvulsants is not effective in preventing this from occurring [33].

Case Example of Post-traumatic Epilepsy

A 51-year-old woman with post-traumatic epilepsy was evaluated for events of ictal asystole. Her initial head trauma was incurred at age 11 after a left occipital skull fracture from a bicycle accident and had only two episodes with loss of awareness between the ages of 13 and 47 years. At age 47 years, she had episodic confusion and left arm tingling as well as convulsive seizures recurring up to once weekly despite medication. MRI revealed focal encephalomalacia in the right inferior frontal gyrus, temporal pole, and anterior parietal lobe (see Figs. 4.24 and 4.25 for CT appearance at age 59); interictal positron emission PET showed these areas to be focally reduced in metabolism, and magnetoencephalography (MEG) showed interictal discharges with a right central dipole. Intracarotid amobarbital test showed exclusive left language lateralization. Hospital EEG monitoring showed not only ictal bradycardia but also episodes of asystole lasting up to 28 s, with EKG activity resuming within one second of the last left hippocampal discharge; there was no preceding per-ictal tachycardia. Surface EEG showed rhythmic left temporal lobe activity starting 23 s after the start of an electrographic seizure recorded by depth electrodes; a cardiac pacemaker was later implanted [34].

Case Example of Epileptogenic Myoclonic Activity Induced by Medication

Provocation of seizure-like activity from medications is a common occurrence, and exemplified by the case of a 66-year-old male who underwent

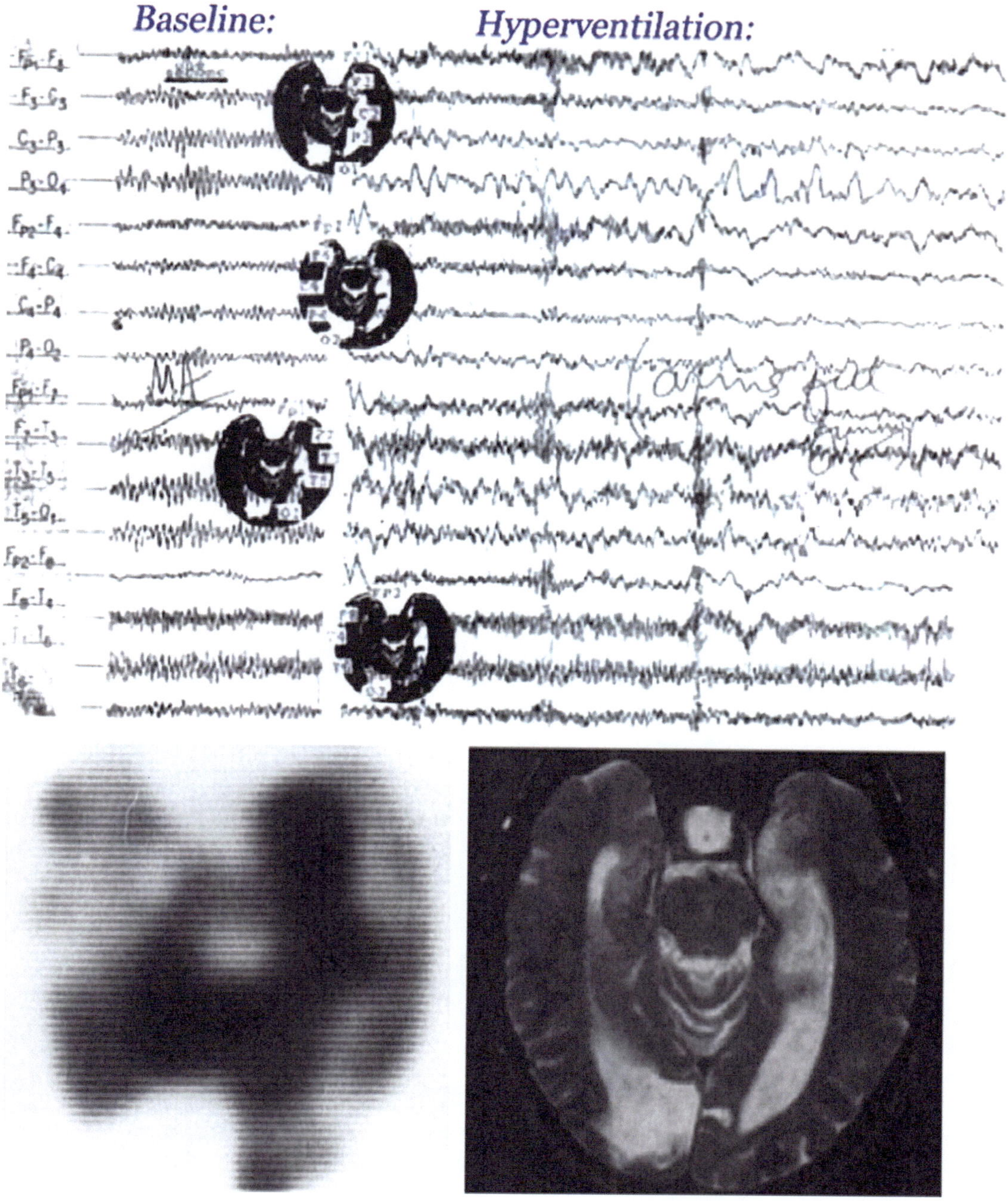

Fig. 4.22 Epileptogenic changes on EEG in limbic encephalitis

a repeat knee prosthesis surgery but developed pain and swelling at the operative site shortly afterward with fever and elevation of white blood count. For the treatment of Staphylococcus warneri isolated from the operative site, intravenous antibiotics were given with vancomycin started initially but then switched to a combination of Nafcillin plus piperacillin/tazobactam. Shortly after starting this regimen, the patient noted the onset of random myoclonic jerks of the extremities, which could be an isolated limb but at other times be all four limbs at once as a single isolated

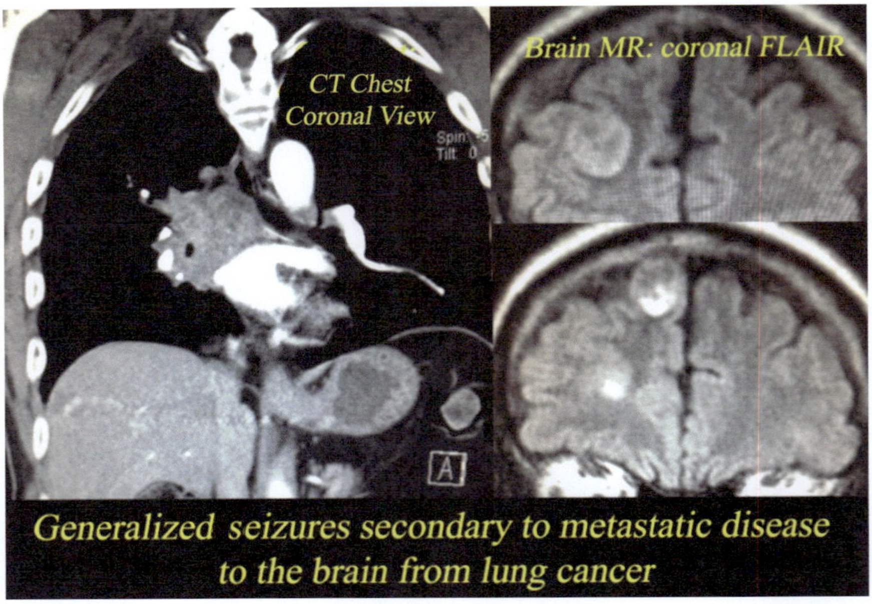

Fig. 4.23 Seizures due to metastatic lesions from lung cancer

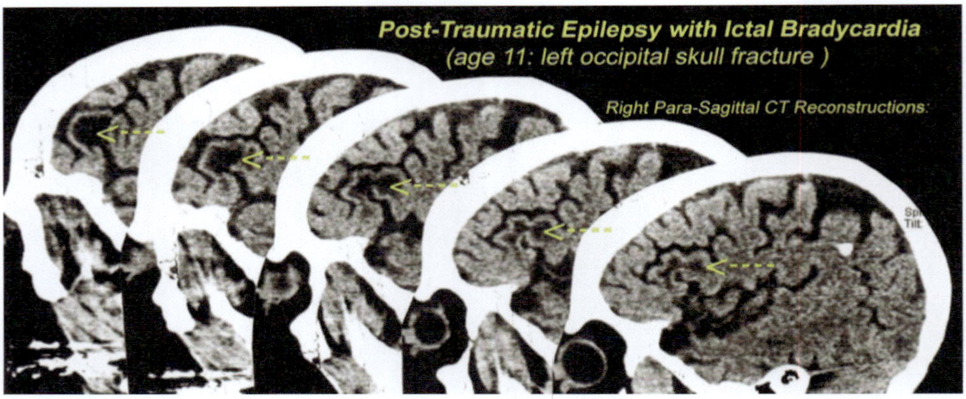

Fig. 4.24 Post-traumatic epilepsy: CT findings

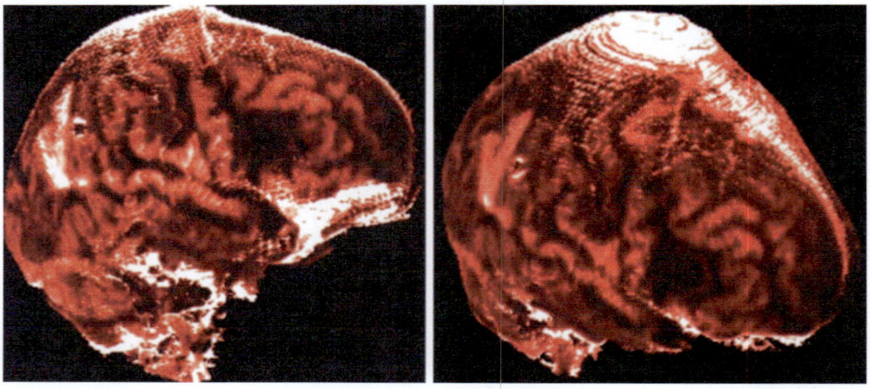

Fig. 4.25 3D reconstruction of CT data from case shown in Fig. 4.25

myoclonic jerk. In addition, the patient reported "something is wrong with my time clock" and felt surprised that long periods of time had passed, and also had a spell of getting up to go to the bathroom, and feeling there was a "gap in time". Approximately 40 random myoclonic jerks were estimated to occur over the course of each day of the 6-week course of the nafcillin/piperacillin combination by his wife, who also noticed random jerks of the extremities during sleep, which would awaken the patients at times. A non-contrast CT head was negative (Fig. 4.26).

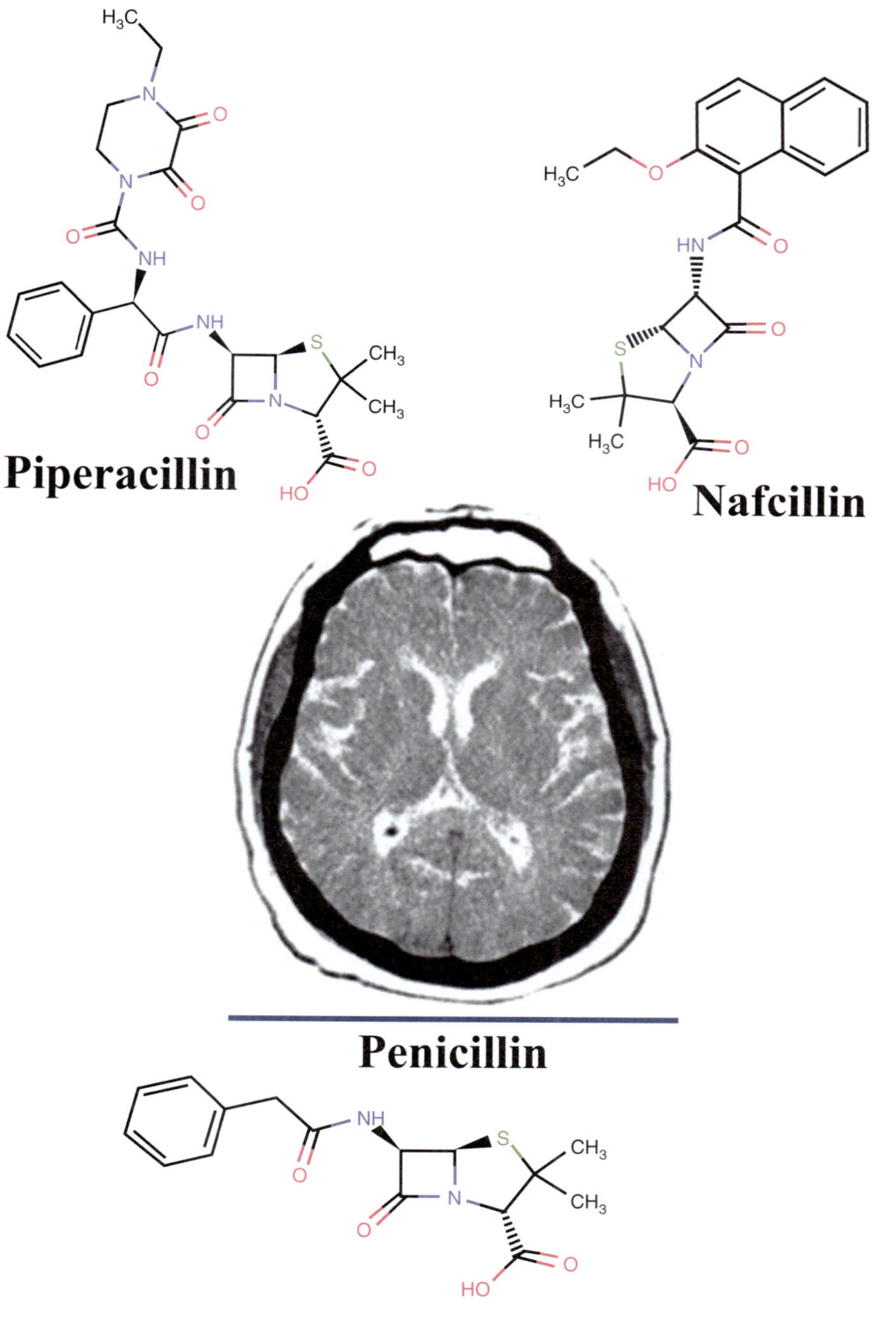

Fig. 4.26 Epileptogenic myoclonic jerks elicited by high-dose antibiotics (see text for case description)

The patient reported complete cessation of the myoclonic jerks after discontinuation of antibiotics, and has been free of this problem afterward [35]. This case illustrates the potential for myoclonic jerks to develop as a secondary adverse effects of piperacillin and/or nafcillin. Given the underlying pathophysiologic interaction of penicillin with the GABA-A receptor chloride channel, it is likely that these two antibiotics may interact in a similar way, and possibly reduce inward inhibitory chloride fluxes into both spinal and supra-spinal neurons [36].

Case Example of New Onset Epilepsy

With regards to the relative value of different testing modalities in relation to EEG normal variants, the following case example is helpful in reminding that radiographic correlation is essential to avoid pitfall in EEG interpretation of physiologic asymmetries, as in fibrous dysplasia of the skull [37].

Case Example

A 22-year-old female with new onset of generalized seizure activity of unknown cause underwent a head CT examination that revealed focal hypo-density within the left frontal bone, consistent with fibrous dysplasia and extended back into the left parietal bone as well (left image within middle panel of Fig. 4.27). Despite anticonvulsant medication, additional nocturnal generalized seizure events recurred, prompting a whole-body bone scan that was negative except for focally elevated 99mTc-MDP uptake in the left frontal-parietal region (upper right of Fig. 4.27). PET imaging failed to reveal any focal metabolic defect within the brain (middle image of middle panel to Fig. 4.27) and displayed a slight diffuse prominence to FDG uptake within the left frontal-parietal bone. MR imaging of the brain also failed to reveal any significant abnormalities but did also show the area of fibrous dysplasia to have mildly prominent T2 signal as seen on the T2-weighted axial section (right-hand image of middle panel, Fig. 4.27).

EEG examination revealed a persistent asymmetry in activity in the left frontal leads, with activity from this region being of higher voltage and better defined (upper part of Fig. 4.27) than right hemispheric activity (lower half of Fig. 4.27). No definite epileptogenic discharges were revealed but did suggest episodic left frontal sharp wave activity compared to the right, but in retrospect, this appears to be of an artifactual nature due to the reduced resistance to current flow across the area of fibrous dysplasia, which apparently conducts EEG potentials with less impedance.

A small number of case reports on the coexistence of fibrous dysplasia with epilepsy are noted with some of these reports suggesting a causative inter-relationship, which clearly seemed not be the case for the patient discussed here, and seemed to be incidental. However, the important unique finding of this case is recognition that misleading EEG interpretations can occur if the electrical conductance properties of focal fibrous dysplasia affecting the skull is not accounted for. In this case, an apparent asymmetry in waveform amplitude and definition appeared from the left frontal leads, similar to the well-known "breach rhythm" phenomenon that occurs over post-surgical skull defects.

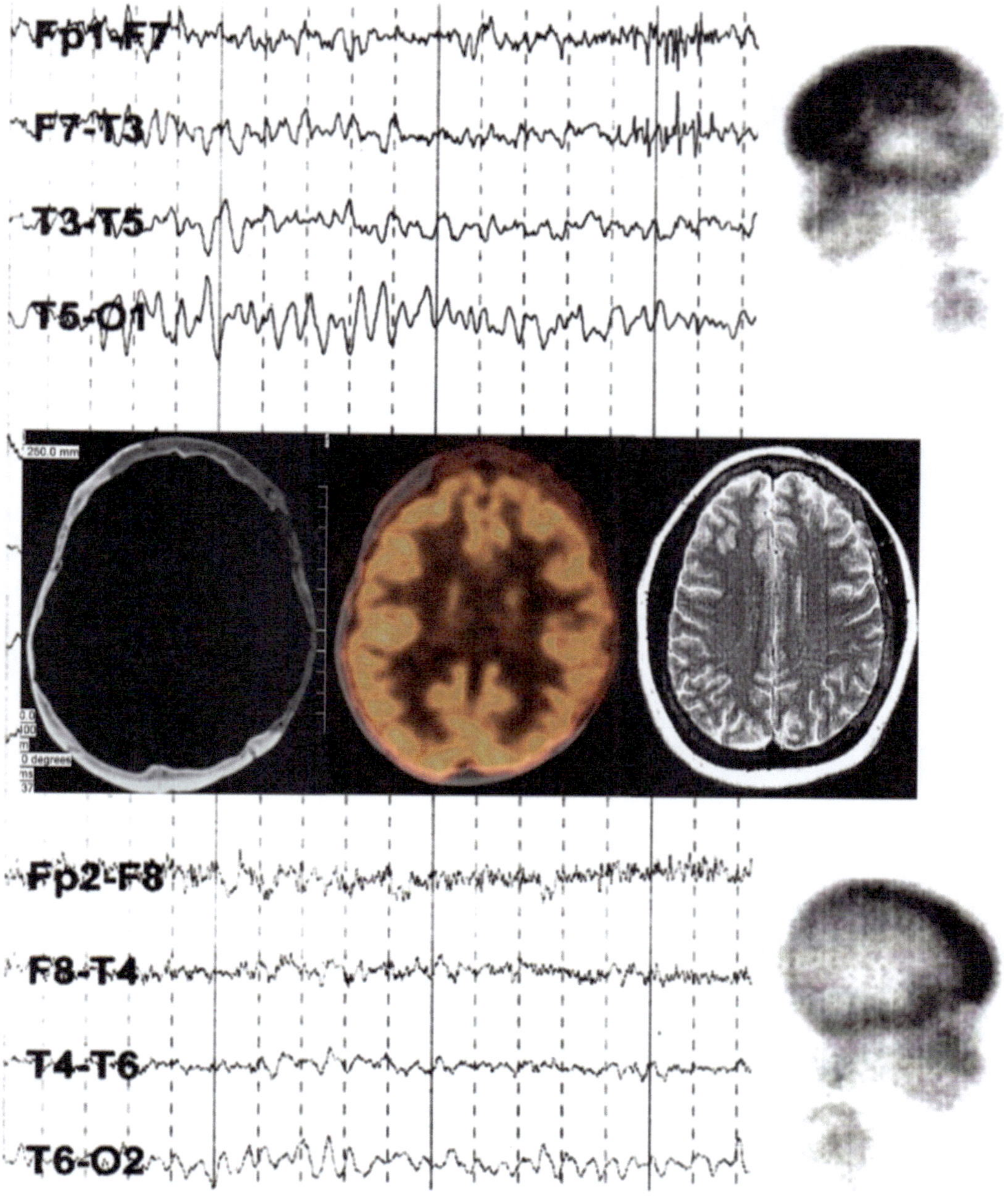

Fig. 4.27 Asymmetry in normal EEG background activity due to left-sided fibrous dysplasia affecting the skull

References

1. Lima AF, Gallian DM. Dostoyevsky and epilepsy: between science and mystique. Arq Neuropsiquiatr. 2010;68(1):140–2.
2. French JA, Pedley TA. Initial management of epilepsy. N Engl J Med. 2008;359:166–76.
3. Kwan P, Arzimanoglou A, Berg AT, et al. Definition of drug resistant epilepsy: consensus proposal by the ad hoc Task Force of the ILAE Commission on Therapeutic Strategies. Epilepsia. 2010;51:1069–77 [Erratum, Epilepsia 2010;51:1922].
4. Smith D, Defalla BA, Chadwick DW. The misdiagnosis of epilepsy and the management of refractory epilepsy in a specialist clinic. QJM. 1999;92:15–23.

5. Neal EG, Chaffe H, Schwartz RH, et al. The ketogenic diet for the treatment of childhood epilepsy: a randomised controlled trial. Lancet Neurol. 2008;7:500–6.
6. Health Quality Ontario. Epilepsy surgery: an evidence summary. Ont Health Technol Assess Ser. 2012;12(17):1–28.
7. Milby AH, Halpern CH, Baltuch GH. Vagus nerve stimulation in the treatment of refractory epilepsy. Neurotherapeutics. 2009;6:228–37.
8. Hauptman JS, Mathern GW. Vagal nerve stimulation for pharmacoresistant epilepsy in children. Surg Neurol Int. 2012;3 Suppl 4:S269–74.
9. Kwan P, Schachter SC, Brodie MJ. Drug-resistant epilepsy. N Engl J Med. 2011;365:919–26.
10. Bergey GK, et al. Long-term treatment with responsive brain stimulation in adults with refractory partial seizures. Neurology. 2015;84(8):810–7.
11. Schell-Apacik CC, Ertl-Wagner B, Panzel A, et al. Maternally inherited heterozygous sequence change in the sonic hedgehog gene in a male patient with bilateral closed-lip schizencephaly and partial absence of the corpus callosum. Am J Med Genet A. 2009; 149A(7):1592–4.
12. Cain SM, Snutch TP. T-type calcium channels in burst-firing, network synchrony, and epilepsy. Biochim Biophys Acta. 2013;1828:1572–8. doi:10.1016/j.bbamem.2012.07.028.
13. Chen Y, et al. The role of T-Type calcium channel genes in absence seizures. Front Neurol. 2014;5:45.
14. Chen Y, et al. Association between genetic variation of CACNA1H and childhood absence epilepsy. Ann Neurol. 2003;54:239–43.
15. Leresche N, Parri HR, Erdemli G, Guyon A, Turner JP, Williams SR, et al. On the action of the anti-absence drug ethosuximide in the rat and cat thalamus. J Neurosci. 1998;18:4842–53.
16. Glauser TA, Cnaan A, Shinnar S, et al. Ethosuximide, valproic acid, and lamotrigine in childhood absence epilepsy. N Engl J Med. 2010;362:790–9.
17. Prasad DKV, et al. Genetics of idiopathic generalized epilepsy: an overview. Neurol India. 2013;61:572–7.
18. Sirven JI, Waterhouse E. Management of status epilepticus. Am Fam Physician. 2003;68(3):469–76.
19. Kinney M, Craig J. Grand rounds: an update on convulsive status epilepticus. Ulster Med J. 2015; 84(2):88–93.
20. Devinsky O. Sudden, unexpected death in epilepsy. N Engl J Med. 2011;365:1801–11.
21. van der Lende M, Surges R, Sander JW, et al. Cardiac arrhythmias during or after epileptic seizures. J Neurol Neurosurg Psychiatry. 2015;2.
22. Howe CL, et al. Hippocampal protection in mice with an attenuated inflammatory monocyte response to acute CNS picornavirus infection. Sci Rep. 2012;2:545.
23. Meyer MA, Zimmerman AW, Miller CA. Temporal lobe epilepsy presenting as panic attacks: detection of interictal hypometabolism with positron emission tomography. J Neuroimaging. 2000;10(2):120–2.
24. Italiano D, Ferlazzo E, Gasparini S, et al. Generalized versus partial reflex seizures: a review. Seizure. 2014;23(7):512–20.
25. Meyer MA, Cascino GD, Hirschorn KA, Westmoreland BF. Seizures evoked by decision making while playing backgammon an unrecognized form of thinking epilepsy. Epilepsia. 1989;30(5):682.
26. Tan E, et al. Playing on an imaginary giant backgammon board: a peculiar ictal behavior. Clin EEG Neurosci. 1990;21:126–8.
27. Ramani V. Audiogenic epilepsy induced by a specific television performer. N Engl J Med. 1991;325: 134–5.
28. Masnou P, et al. Pilomotor seizures associated with sequential changes in magnetic resonance imaging. Epileptic Disord. 2006;8(3):232–7.
29. Meyer MA. Temporal lobe hypometabolism ipsilateral to a hypothalamic mass. Relationship to gelastic seizures. Clin Positron Imaging. 2000;3(2):75–7.
30. Shahar E, Goldsher D, Genizi J. Intractable gelastic seizures during infancy: ictal positron emission tomography (PET) demonstrating epileptiform activity within the hypothalamic hamartoma. J Child Neurol. 2008;23(2):235–9.
31. Meyer MA. Epileptogenic discharges on EEG with neurologic decline: case example. J Nucl Med. 1990; 31:1094–8.
32. Voutsas V, Mylonaki E, Gymnopoulos K, et al. Paraneoplastic limbic encephalitis as a cause of new onset of seizures in a patient with non-small cell lung carcinoma: a case report. J Med Case Rep. 2008;2:270.
33. Mikkelsen T, Paleologos NA, Robinson PD, et al. The role of prophylactic anticonvulsants in the management of brain metastases: a systematic review and evidence-based clinical practice guideline. J Neurooncol. 2010;96(1):97–102.
34. Rosetti AO, Dworetzky BA, Madsen JR, et al. Ictal asystole with convulsive syncope mimicking secondary generalisation: a depth electrode study. J Neurol Neurosurg Psychiatry. 2005;76:885–7.
35. Meyer MA. Myoclonic jerks secondary to piperacillin and nafcillin. Neurol Int. 2014;6(2):5349.
36. Fernández-Torre JL, Santos-Sánchez C, Pelayo AL. De novo generalised non-convulsive status epilepticus triggered by piperacillin/tazobactam. Seizure. 2010;19(8):529–30.
37. Meyer MA. Focal electroencephalography rhythm asymmetry due to focal skull fibrous dysplasia. Neurol Int. 2014;6(2):5347.

5 Demyelinating Diseases of the Peripheral and Central Nervous System: Guillain–Barre and Multiple Sclerosis

5.1 Introduction

A fundamental advance in evolution is the myelination of central and peripheral nerve fibers to enable vertebrates to think, react, and move far more quickly than what had been previously possible with unmyelinated nerve fibers within invertebrates. With the novel addition of myelin sheaths, nerve impulse propagation made a quantum leap forward in terms of the actual conduction velocity attainable by salutatory conduction of an action potential that becomes recharged at the regularly spaced gaps in the myelin insulation known as nodes of Ranvier. A cross section of a peripheral axon insulated by a myelin sheath that wraps repeatedly over and over again is shown by electron microscopy in Fig. 5.1.

5.2 Guillain–Barre Syndrome or Acute Inflammatory Demyelinating Polyneuropathy

When myelination becomes defective within the peripheral nervous system, slowed conduction or actual conduction block develops, producing clinical symptoms of neurologic impairment with decrements in strength and/or sensation for example. When this process is antibody-mediated out in the peripheral nerves where there is no blood–brain barrier to contend with, a severe inflammatory attack occurs upon myelinated nerve fibers which can markedly impair the flow of impulses along motor fibers, leading to paralysis. Otherwise known as the Guillain–Barre syndrome (GBS) or acute inflammatory demyelinating polyneuropathy (AIDP), this antibody-mediated event can be systemic and adversely affect myelinated nerve fibers within both arms and legs as well the phrenic nerves innervating the diaphragm, thereby posing risks for significant mortality and morbidity, prompting the need for intubation and ventilator support in many cases; mechanical ventilation may be needed for those who show hypercarbia, hypoxemia, or a vital capacity below 15 mL per kg of body weight (Fig. 5.2).

Clinical clues to the GBS diagnosis include ascending weakness and numbness affecting both arms and legs; however, one large study showed the weakness to be restricted to the lower extremities in 6 % and to the upper extremities in 1 %. The same study documented that the overwhelming majority had reduced deep tendon reflexes, but in only 15 % was there a mild cerebrospinal fluid (CSF) pleocytosis of 5–50 white cells per microliter (none had more than 50 cells per microliter). Cerebrospinal fluid protein elevation was found in two-thirds of patients but was variable as the elevation became more apparent after 2 weeks than at symptom onset. Clinical nadirs were reached by 2 weeks in 80 % and had

M.A. Meyer, *Neurologic Disease*, DOI 10.1007/978-3-319-39581-4_5

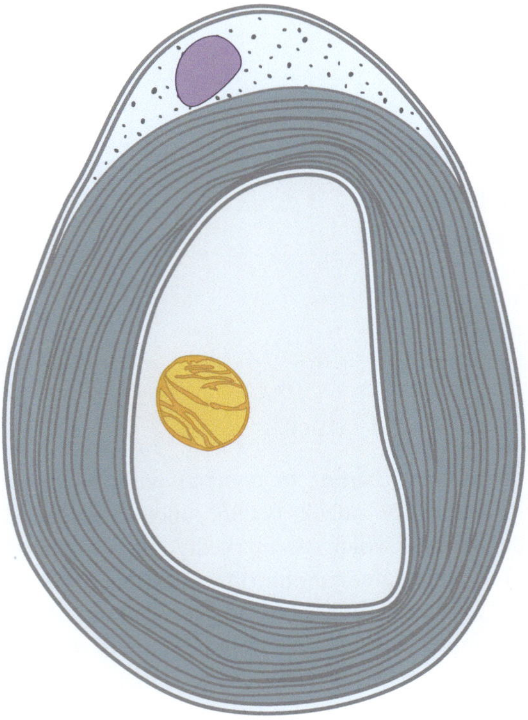

Fig. 5.1 Acute inflammatory demyelinating polyradiculoneuropathy: Guillain–Barre. Cross section of a normal myelinated peripheral nerve axon

been reached within 1 month by 97 % of patients studied [1].

Having an annual incidence of 0.6–4 cases per 100,000, most cases are thought to be post-infectious yet some are clearly post-vaccinal in nature (Fig. 5.3). Approximately two-thirds of GBS patients have had some type of recent infection; although *Campylobacter jejuni* is the most common, other infectious agents include Epstein–Barr virus, and *Mycoplasma pneumonia*; cytomegalovirus has been identified in up to 10 % [2]. Although only 1 in 1000 Campylobacter gastroenteritis cases have GBS as a delayed sequelae (usually within 3 weeks), about 25–40 % of GBS patients are known to have had recent Campylobacter gastroenteritis (Fig. 5.4). Antibody cross reactivity between superficial bacterial sialylated lipooligosaccharide structures and similar ganglioside epitopes within human peripheral nerves seem to account for the intense autoimmune post-infectious attack on the myelin sheath [3].

GBS can result in serious long-term effects, leaving up to 20 % of patients with some form of disability. Age can be a predisposing factor, as the incidence of GBS rises successively by 20 % with every decade after age 10; male to female ratio is 1.78. Although generally monophasic, GBS recurs two or more times in 7 % with the average interval between events being 7 years.

At 1 year, about one-fifth are left with some type of functional disability and almost two-thirds complain of severe fatigue. A recent large study from the Netherlands on 527 GBS patients revealed a 1 year mortality rate of 3.9 %; data at the half year point showed a 2.8 % mortality rate [4]. The study concluded that the factors which more heavily influenced a fatal outcome included age, severity of weakness at the time of diagnosis, mechanical ventilation, delay from onset of weakness to diagnosis, and time to peak disability; two-thirds of those who died within the first 6 months occurred in the recovery phase, usually from respiratory or cardiovascular complications; other medical complications include sepsis, pulmonary emboli, or arrhythmias secondary to GBS-induced autonomic dysfunction that occurs in one-fifth of cases.

Much progress has been made since the disease was first described in 1916 with the main form of modern day treatment regimens being intravenous immunoglobulin that essentially flood the extracellular space of the inflamed nerve fibers and displace and/or block pathogenic antibodies from binding to reactive antigenic sites with nerve neutral pooled antibodies; intravenous immunoglobulin (IVIG) also acts by inhibiting autoantibody-mediated complement activation. Alternatively, plasma exchange (PE) can be used but steroids have been clearly shown not to provide any benefit at all (Fig. 5.5). Large studies demonstrate approximate equivalency in efficacy between PE and IVIG, although IVIG is easier to administer and more likely to be completed in full form than PE [5].

As post-infectious encephalomyelitis is a well established form of central demyelinating disease, and in view of a possible viral etiology or link to multiple sclerosis (MS) in predisposed individuals, the topic of MS has been grouped together in

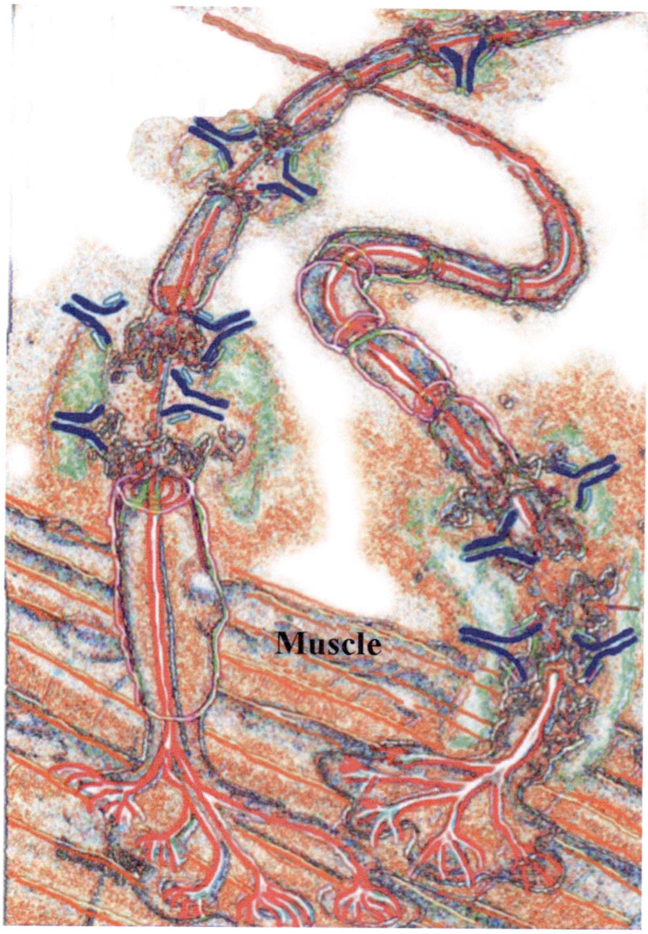

Fig. 5.2 Guillain–Barre syndrome (GBS): Autoimmune attack upon peripheral nerve myelin sheath by antibodies (highlighted in *blue*)

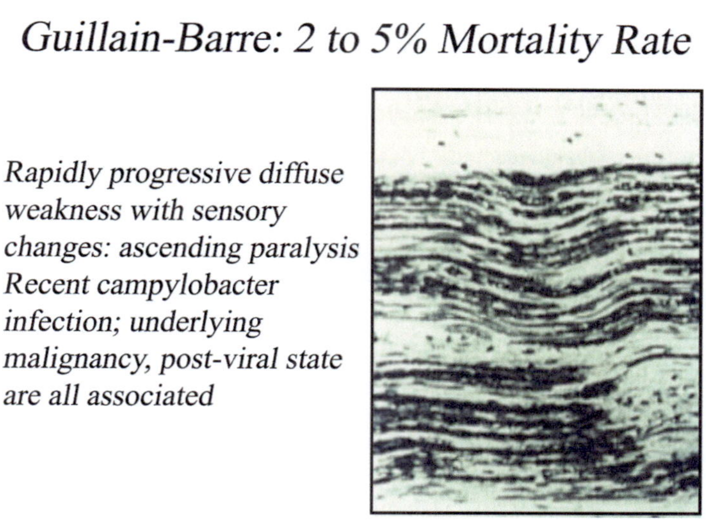

Fig. 5.3 Guillain–Barre syndrome (GBS) can have significant mortality rates of 2–5 %

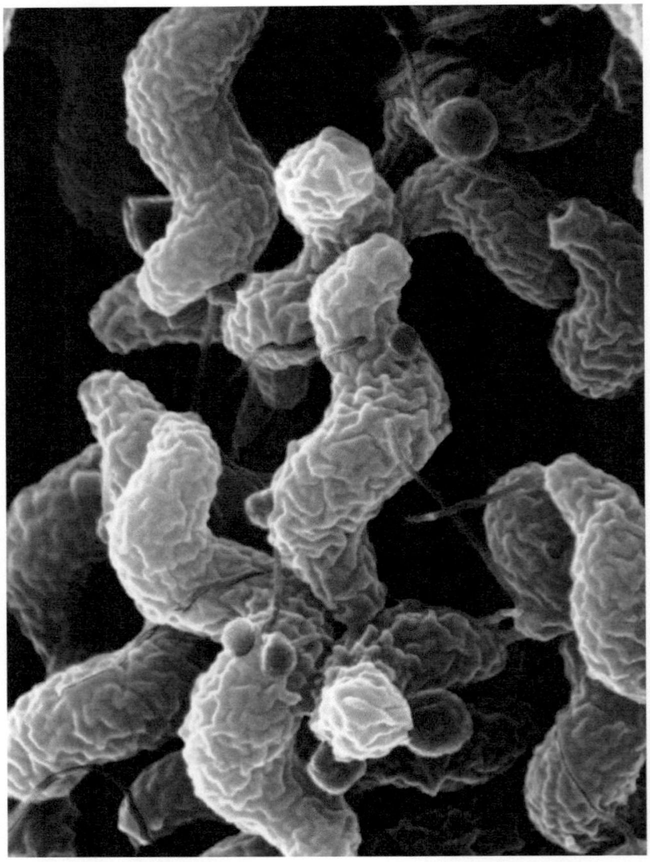

Fig. 5.4 Scanning electron micrograph of campylobacter bacteria, whose surface antigens can play a role in Guillain–Barre syndrome (GBS) pathogenesis (from Wikipedia)

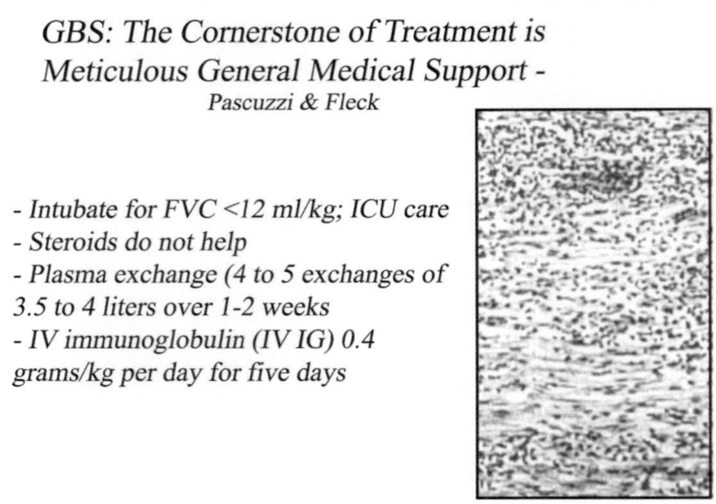

Fig. 5.5 Treatment for Guillain–Barre syndrome (GBS) includes intravenous immunoglobulin (IVIG)

this discussion along with GBS to emphasize the immune-mediated nature of the illnesses and their link to immune reactions against infectious antigens and cross reactivity with myelin sheath components. Although well established for GBS, the immune reaction for the central nervous system is far more complex in MS, especially as antibody molecules do not normally pass through the blood–brain barrier but may pass through thin-walled venules and reach sub-ependymal locations; pathogenic antibodies may also arise instead via intrathecal synthesis and may relate to the recent detection of meningeal B cell follicles in MS patients [6, 7].

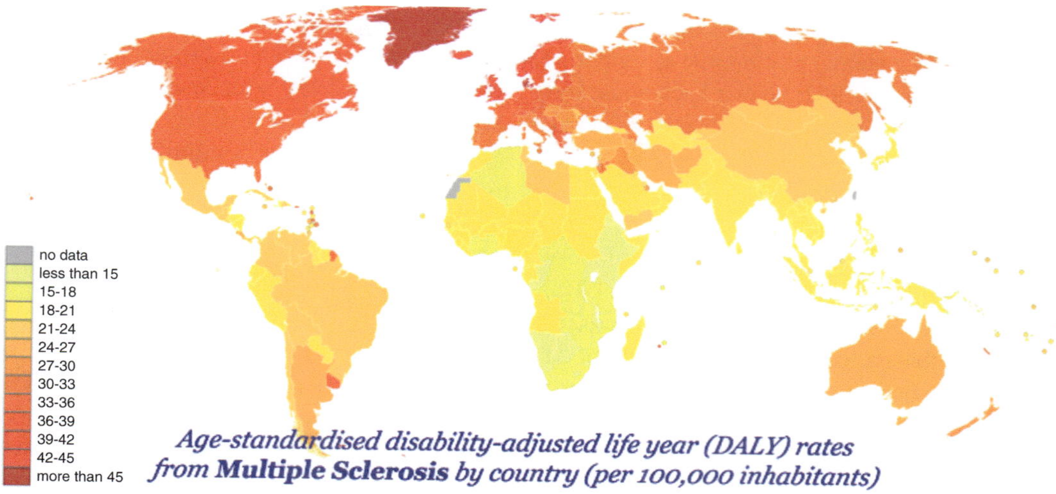

Fig. 5.6 Northern latitude predominance of multiple sclerosis (MS) shown on a global perspective (adapted from Wikipedia)

5.3 Multiple Sclerosis

Multiple sclerosis is an important disease to understand, as it affects 2.3 million people worldwide; in the US alone, the number of people with MS is estimated to be about 400,000, with about 10,000 new cases diagnosed annually. Affecting women more frequently than men, this autoimmune inflammatory process occurs mainly in young adults in the 20- to 45-year age range; uncommonly, it can present for the first time in children as well as older adults. With regards to genetics and epidemiology, those of northern European descent have the highest risk for MS, with more northern latitudes having a higher incidence (Fig. 5.6). Although not considered to be an inherited disease, monozygotic twins are concordant for the disease in 24–30 % of cases, versus 3–5 % for dizygotic twins, which is the same concordance rate for siblings [8].

Initially, the process causes inflammatory demyelination that is capable of repairing itself and leads to remyelination; however, if the attack is intense enough, focal severe inflammation will actually cause irreversible axonal destruction, leading to the appearance of "black holes" on T1-weighted MRI scans, which correlate to long-term disability. Typical modes of presentations include an initial solitary focal demyelinating event, as in the case of a young adult with optic neuritis or transverse myelitis, followed years later by multifocal demyelinating plaque within the brain consistent with relapsing–remitting MS as the most common form of the disease.

Whereas post-infectious immune reactions are clearly defined for GBS, the reader is cautioned that MS pathogenesis is not known for all cases and all types, and MS mimics exist that may relate to genetic causes, or may indeed be viral-mediated as in the case of progressive multifocal leukoencephalopathy (PML). However, to help illustrate a pathophysiologic link for MS being immune-mediated and possibly post-infectious in nature, the following interesting case example of post-vaccinal encephalomyelitis is helpful to review [9].

Case Example

In late February, 1992, while vaccinating hogs, a 52-year-old farmer accidentally injected himself with a hog vaccine containing killed pomona bacteria, parvovirus, leptospira, and Erysipelothrix rhusiopathieae. One month later, he developed a personality change, with agitation, forgetfulness, disorientation, decreased verbalization, and periods of decreased responsiveness; MRI of the brain revealed multifocal demyelinating lesions throughout the semi-centrum ovale white matter. After becoming comatose, a series of eight plasma exchanges were started and within 2 weeks of the treatment, began to improve in being able to follow simple commands, and converse in short sentences. By October 1992, he was back home and living independently but did still display moderate difficulty with concentration and memory, which all improved over the next 3 months.

In the same way that molecular mimicry plays a pathogenic role in post-infectious GBS, such as with cross-reactive immune responses to Campylobacter infections, a similar set of events likely occurred here in this classical case of post-vaccinal encephalomyelitis; a close analogy can be drawn to MS pathogenesis, where the timeline of change is more prolonged, variable yet persistent. As there is a growing body of evidence tying MS to immune reactions to viruses such as the Epstein–Barr virus (EBV), a similar pathophysiologic explanation of antigenic cross reactivity with central nervous system myelin might apply here as well with regards to the formation of multifocal demyelinating plaque. With regards to the EBV, the risk is elevated for those with a history of infectious mononucleosis especially if this occurred after adolescence; conversely, the risk for MS is especially low for those uncommon individuals who happen to be EBV seronegative.

With regards to the variable and unpredictable timeline of MS symptomatology, the majority of cases follow a relapsing–remitting course (Fig. 5.7). Found in 85 % of MS patients, this form is characterized by clinical flare events of transient neurologic deficit (which often respond

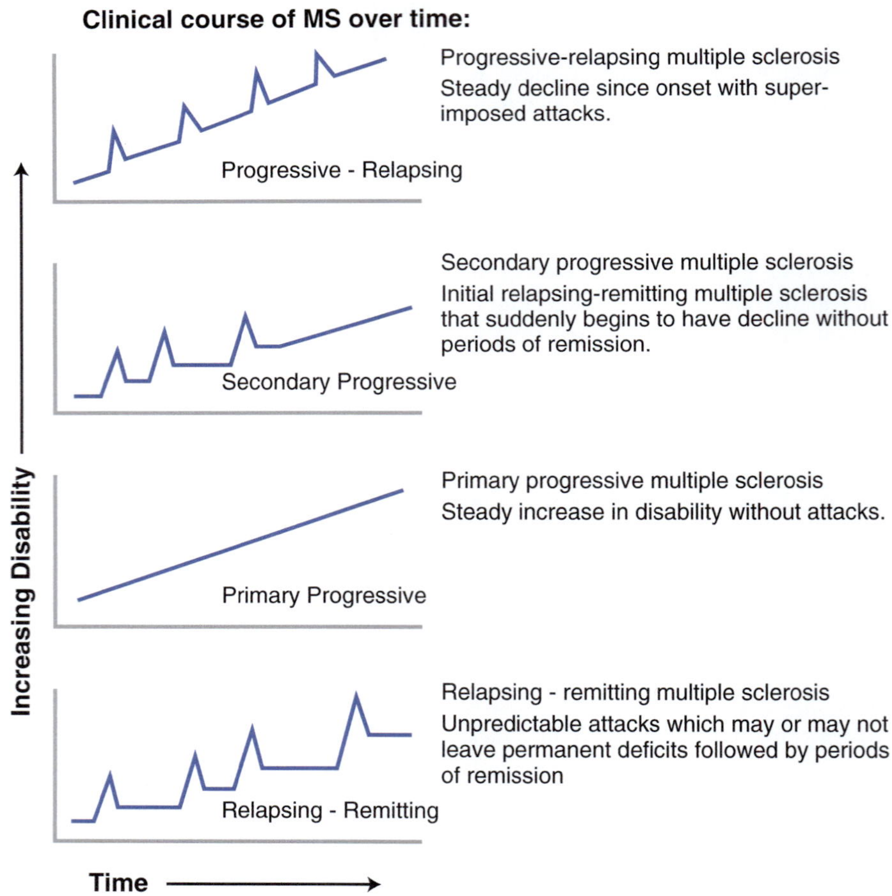

Fig. 5.7 Clinical course patterns of multiple sclerosis (MS) (Adapted from Wikipedia)

Diagnosis of Multiple Sclerosis: Repeated multifocal events of neurologicdeficits (acute to subacute events in young adults may suggest MS)

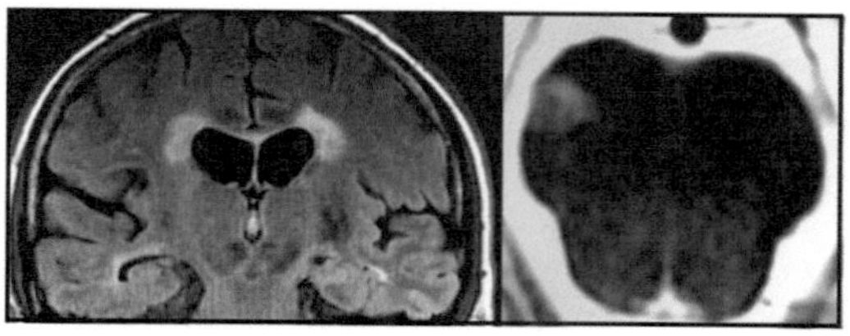

- *Prior optic neuritis makes the diagnosis of MS highly probable in a young symptomatic adult*
- *MR often reveals peri-ventricular demyelinating lesions*
- *Inflammatory demyelinating events are usually responsive to steroids*

Fig. 5.8 Diagnosing multiple sclerosis (MS): typical cases have periventricular lesions

to steroids), followed by variable periods of remission with stabilization, where neurologic symptoms improve remarkably well or fully resolve. Although the secondary progressive form may develop in those with the typical relapsing–remitting symptoms and still respond to treatment, the primary progressive form found in 10 % of MS patients is more difficult to treat and often resistant to medication. The rarest subtype is progressive-relapsing type which is seen in less than 5 % of cases; there are no remissions and only episodic flares as disabling symptoms get steadily worse over time [10, 11].

In order to diagnose MS, criteria have been established that emphasize dissemination in space and time in order to reflect the multifocal nature of the demyelinating events which recur episodically in variable unpredictable ways. Known as the McDonald criteria, and revised in 2010, these guidelines serve as an aid in formally diagnosing MS; for example, the criteria recognize multiple combinations of factors including two or more attacks with objective clinical evidence of two or more lesions as sufficient for diagnosis, or objective clinical evidence of one lesion with reasonable historical evidence of a prior attack [12].

In general, a clinical attack event needs objective support by neurologic exam or MRI. Other supportive testing with regards to MS includes but is not limited to visual evoked potentials, and lumbar puncture; detection of oligoclonal bands unique to the CSF is especially helpful. A classical presentation for MS would be a young adult with multifocal recurrent neurologic events with a prior history for optic neuritis (Fig. 5.8).

Examination clues that can help lead to the diagnosis of MS include hyper-reflexia, as well as the Lhermitte sign, which is an electric shock-like sensation with downward neck flexion, and is due to stretch irritation of hyper-excitable demyelinated fiber tracts of the spinal cord, particularly at the cervical level. Other exam signs characteristic to but not specific to MS include internuclear ophthalmoplegia which is caused by focal demyelination of the medial longitudinal fasciculus, disrupting the connection of the pontine abducens nucleus with the contralateral oculomotor nucleus in the midbrain, resulting in the inability to adduct the eye on lateral abduction of the other eye.

Clinical syndromes reflecting focal demyelination include optic neuritis and transverse myelitis. Acute demyelinating optic neuritis can be the first clinical demyelinating event in patients later diagnosed with multiple sclerosis (Fig. 5.9); one study found that multiple sclerosis was later diagnosed in 38 % of patients with a first episode of optic neuritis. As for recurrences, the Optic Neuritis Treatment Trial showed that during a

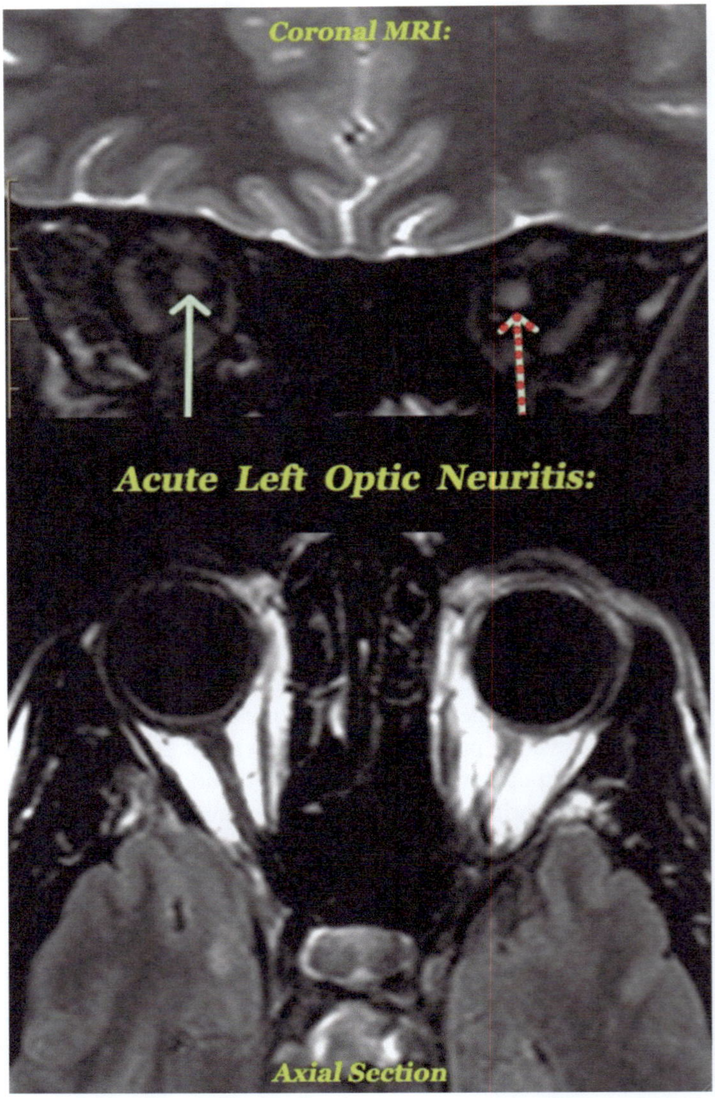

Fig. 5.9 Acute left eye visual loss in a young adult secondary to optic neuritis

10-year follow-up period, the risk of at least one recurrence of visual loss was 48 % in those later diagnosed with MS versus 24 % in those without MS [13].

With regards to the transverse myelitis syndrome, focal demyelination occurs within the spinal cord as a post-infectious or post-vaccinal autoimmune phenomenon (especially in children) and can be part of the spectrum of MS demyelinating diseases including neuromyelitis optica. Although transverse myelitis can develop at any age, bimodal peaks are noted in the 10 to 19 year age group as well as 30–39 years. At least 15–30 % of the cases of transverse myelitis have no known cause but most are felt to represent the possible start of future multifocal demyelinating events. Transverse myelitis is a frequent component of acute disseminated encephalomyelitis in children [14].

Pathologic examination reveals perivenular lymphocytic infiltration into areas that are actively demyelinated (Fig. 5.10); CD68 histochemical staining reveals similarly that macrophages cluster around perivenular locations (Fig. 5.11). Once the inflammatory infiltration recedes, viable oligodendroglia can remyelinate

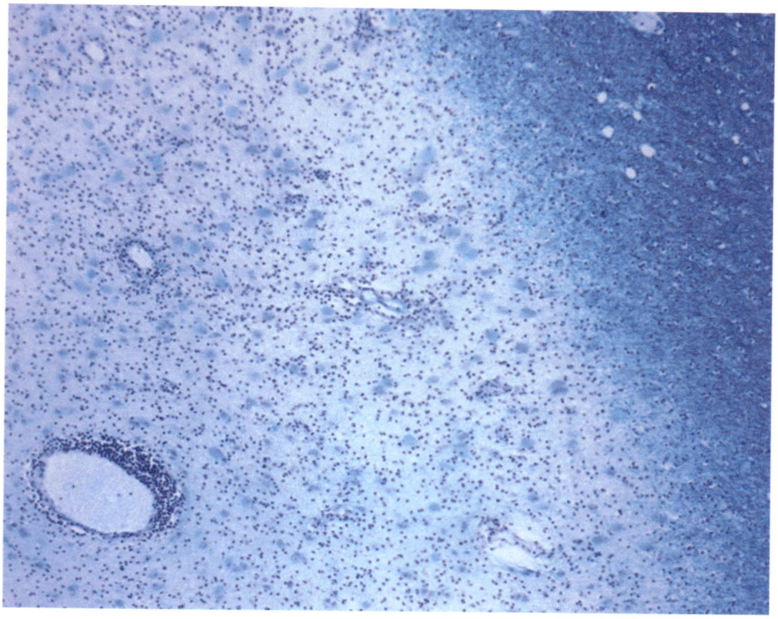

Fig. 5.10 Perivenular lymphocytic infiltration within demyelinated plaques (from Wikipedia)

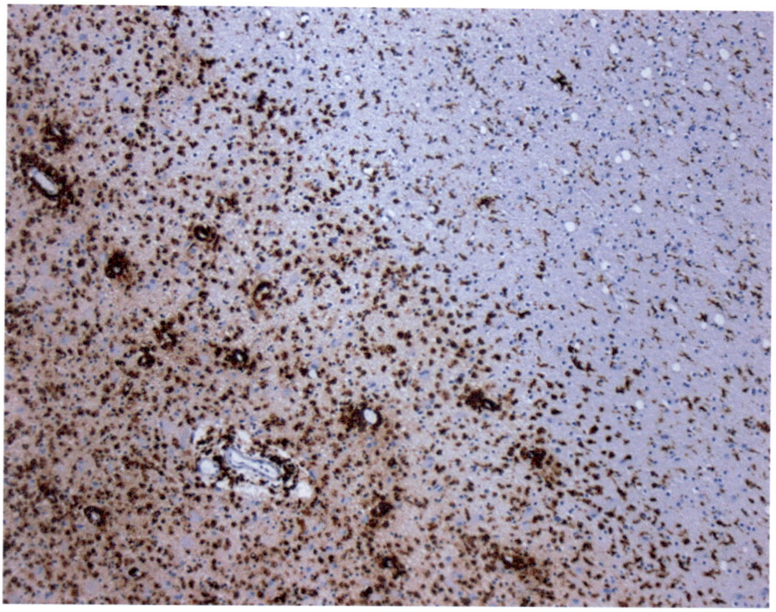

Fig. 5.11 CD68-positive macrophages clustering in perivenular locations within actively demyelinated areas (from Wikipedia)

bare axons and lead toward functional recovery (Fig. 5.12). However, when the disease is aggressive and extensive, little remyelination is possible, especially for those with advanced MS (Figs. 5.13 and 5.14).

Clinical examples of MRI findings in advanced MS are illustrated in Figs. 5.13 and 5.14, emphasizing the periventricular location for most of the plaques; less common are plaques that may be juxta-cortical in location (Fig. 5.15) or a mixture of the two patterns (Fig. 5.16). When demyelinating plaque affects the spinal cord, serious functional impairments may arise; despite a small volume, an isolated unifocal demyelinating plaque within the spinal pyramidal tract can have major effects on ipsilateral motor function (Fig. 5.17).

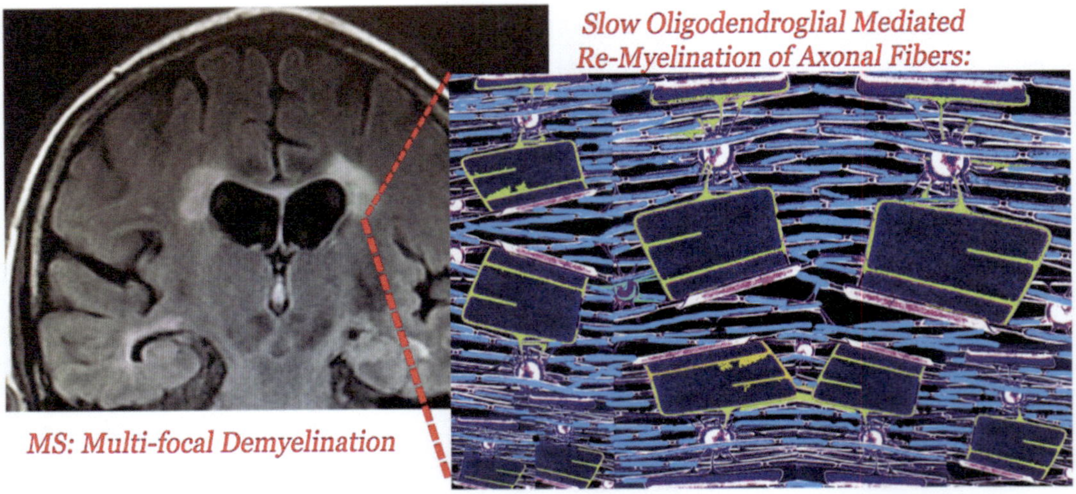

Fig. 5.12 Oligodendroglia can resume the myelination process in the repair phase after a demyelination attack

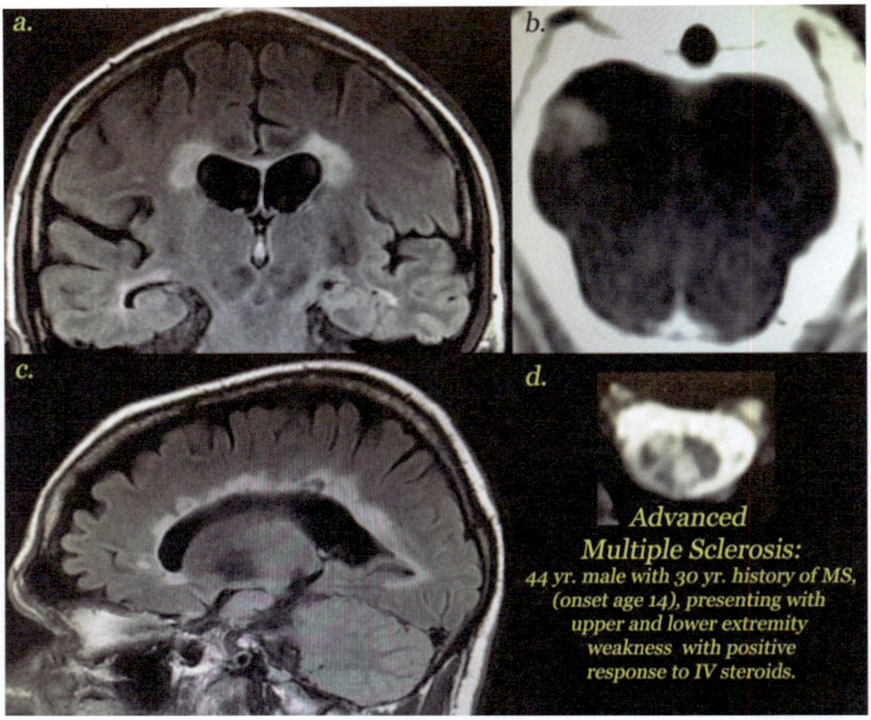

Fig. 5.13 Case example: advanced muscular sclerosis (MS)

With regards to treatment, most flares of MS can be managed in a simple and effective manner with the use of steroids, such as intravenous methylprednisolone. For long-term prophylaxis, interferon beta type medications are helpful and have outcomes approximately equivalent to the use of glatiramer acetate. Considered as first-generation disease-modifying medications,

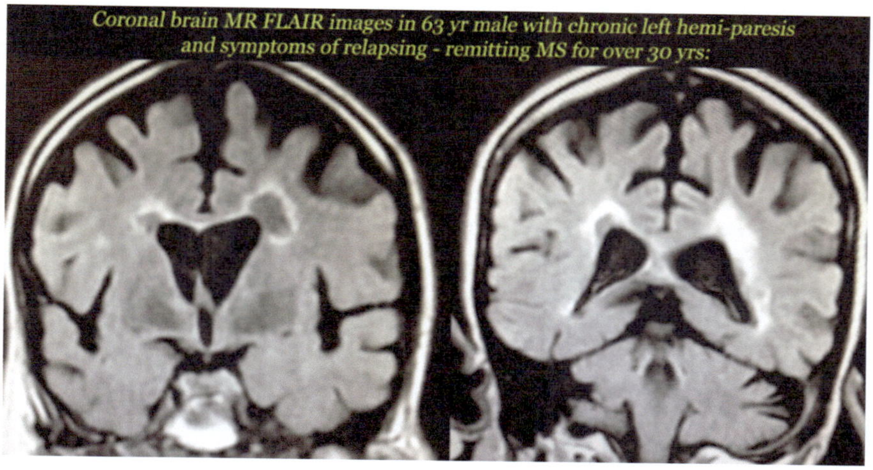

Fig. 5.14 Case example: periventricular predilection for demyelinating plaque

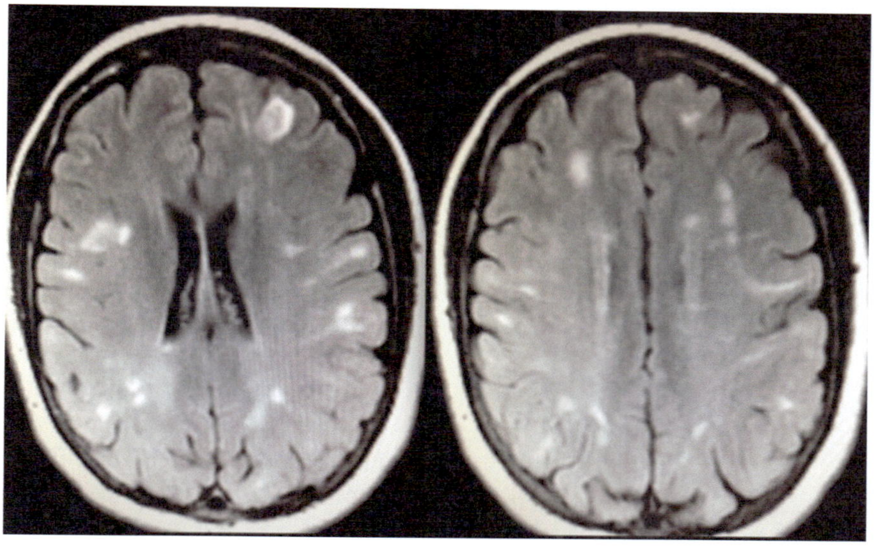

Fig. 5.15 Case example: juxta-cortical plaques; typical multiple sclerosis (MS) symptoms over 2 years in a 28-year-old female with atypical pattern of multi-focal juxta-cortical demyelinating lesions at *gray–white* juncture areas

both glatiramer acetate and the beta interferons reduce annual relapse rates by about 30%. Whereas glatiramer acetate is relatively free of major side effects, the interferons can induce transient flu-like symptoms after intramuscular injection. Glatiramer has an interesting design as a defined yet random assembly of the most frequent amino acid sequences found within the myelin basic protein.

Prior to the recent introduction of new oral agents discussed below, Natalizumab had been introduced as a therapeutic option. Designed as a humanized monoclonal antibody to the lymphocyte adhesion molecule alpha4–beta1 integrin, it blocks the normal binding that this integrin would have with vascular adhesion molecule VCAM-1 in the hope that this would reduce inflammatory lymphocyte entry across brain–blood vessels. Although Food and Drug Administration (FDA) approved for MS prophylaxis, Natalizumab has a black box warning about the risk for development of progressive multifocal leukoencephalopathy, which often can be fatal.

In the interest of enhancing convenience and compliance with treatment, multiple new oral agents have been developed, the first of which is known as fingolimod. Designed as a sphingosine-1 phosphate (S1P) receptor modulator to alter lymph node lymphocyte traffic, it can reduce peripheral blood lymphocyte counts by 70 % within 90 days. One study showed that once daily treatment reduced the annualized MS relapse rate by 54 % [15]. As S1P receptors are also expressed throughout the cardiovascular system, fingolimod can have a dose-dependent bradycardia effect, prompting the need for close monitoring upon starting this medication.

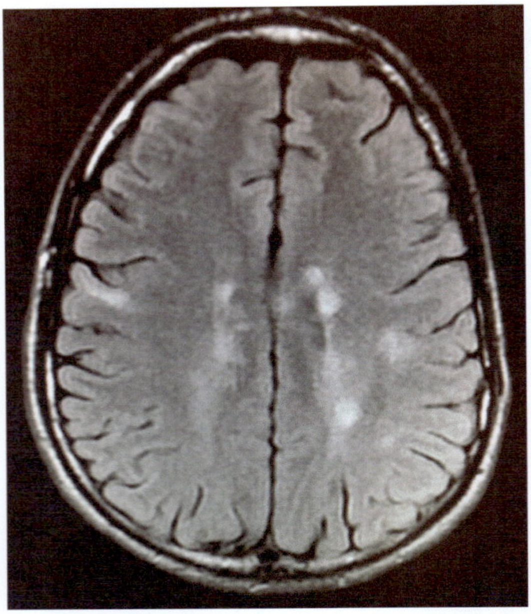

Fig. 5.16 Case example: mix of juxta-cortical with periventricular plaques

Teriflunomide is another oral MS medication and the active metabolite of the rheumatoid arthritis drug leflunomide; it inhibits dihydroorotate dehydrogenase, thereby inhibiting rapidly proliferating activated lymphocytes. Phase 3 studies have shown a annualized relapse rate reduction of 31.5 % compared to placebo. Like other oral agents, embryotoxicity and teratogenicity have been demonstrated in animal studies; a washout period of at least 8 months has been advised before contemplating pregnancy as the drug has a prolonged half-life.

Dimethyl fumarate is another new oral MS agent, and is chemically related to fumaric acid esters used in Germany for psoriasis treatment; for MS applications, treatment on a twice daily schedule reduced annualized relapse rate by 53 % compared to placebo. In addition to two psoriasis-treated patients developing PML, a fatal case of PML has been reported in a treated patient who had marked persistent lymphocytopenia [16].

Other new medications include alemtuzumab, which is a humanized monoclonal antibody against the CD52 lymphocyte antigen. The drug depletes the T and B lymphocyte population; although B cells can repopulate after treatment,

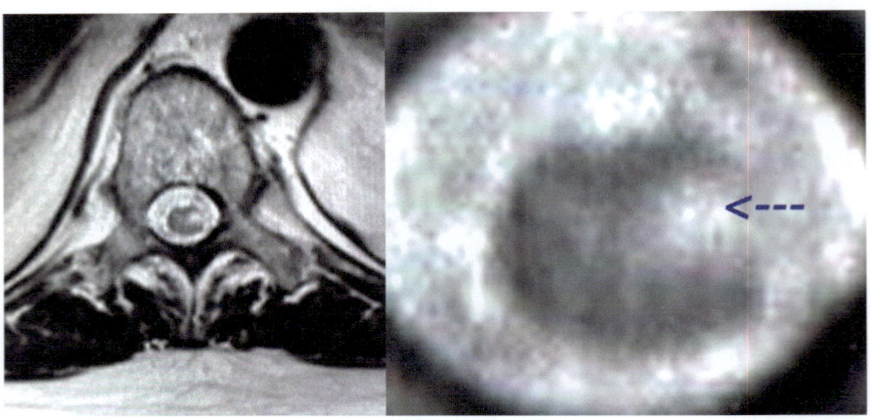

Fig. 5.17 Case example: demyelinating spinal cord plaque

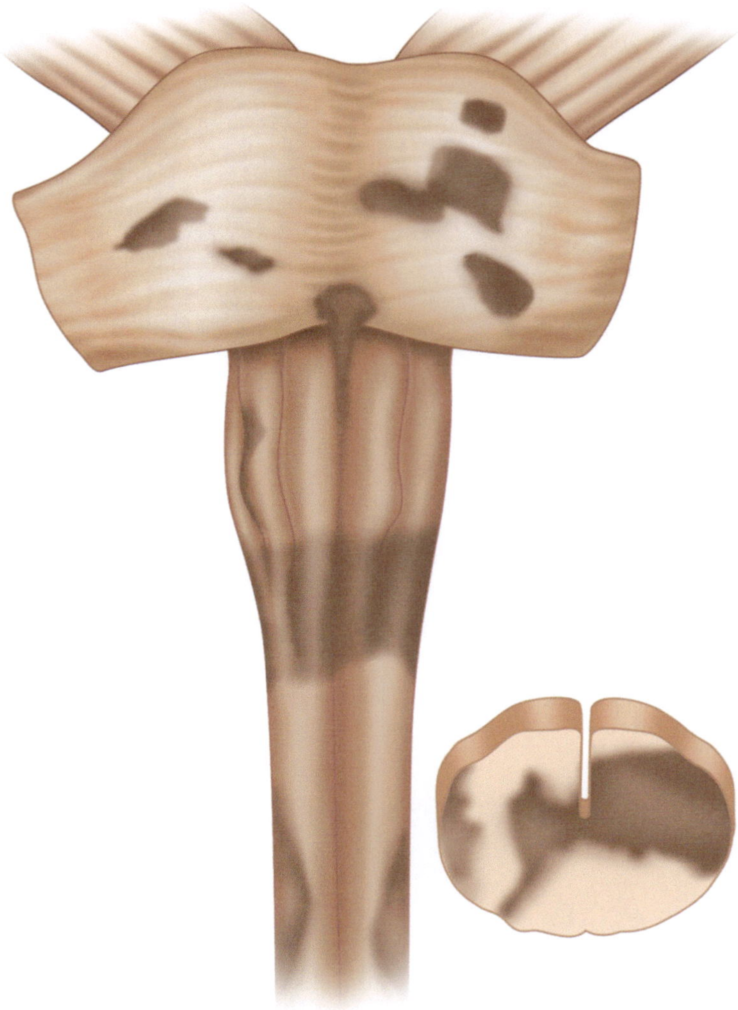

Fig. 5.18 The very first illustration of multiple sclerosis (MS) lesions, created in 1838 by the Scottish physician and artist, Dr Robert Carswell (adapted from the original drawing)

T cells are disproportionately affected. Although alemtuzumab reduced annualized relapse rate by 54.9 % at 2 years and 66 % at 5 years compared to interferon beta-1a, infusion reactions are very frequent and infections occur more frequently including cutaneous herpetic infections.

Another new humanized antibody therapy for MS is daclizumab which blocks the CD25 alpha sub-unit of the interleukin-2 receptor, which acts to restrict expansion of activated T cells. Monthly subcutaneous injections of 150 mg daclizumab reduced annualized relapse rate by 54 % compared to placebo [15].

From the first illustration of MS in 1838 (Fig. 5.18) to the current age of MRI, we now have gained the ability to go beyond standard imaging of demyelinating plaque in the subcortical white matter and can now look into the cortex with double inversion recovery MR sequences to reveal intra-cortical demyelination as an under-recognized phenomenon that may occur in the earliest stages of MS. Other new techniques include diffusion tensor imaging to reveal directionality and spatial orientation of white matter fiber tracts by color coding methods (Fig. 5.19) and three-dimensional tractography

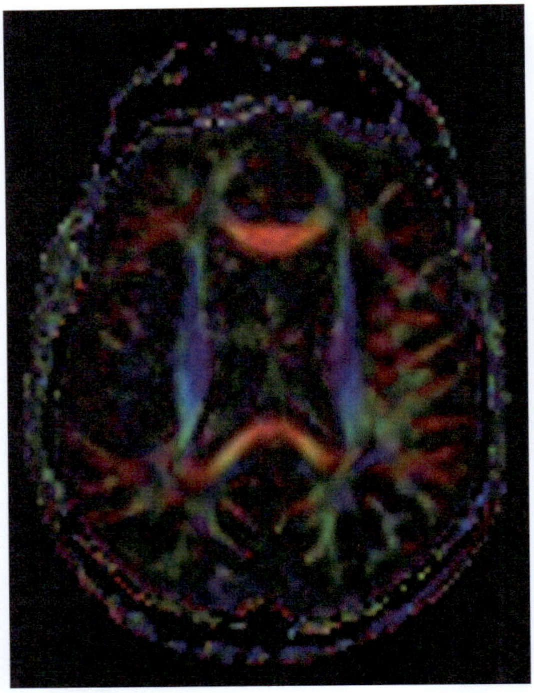

Fig. 5.19 Axial brain MR diffusion tensor image, with directionality to the fiber tracts color coded

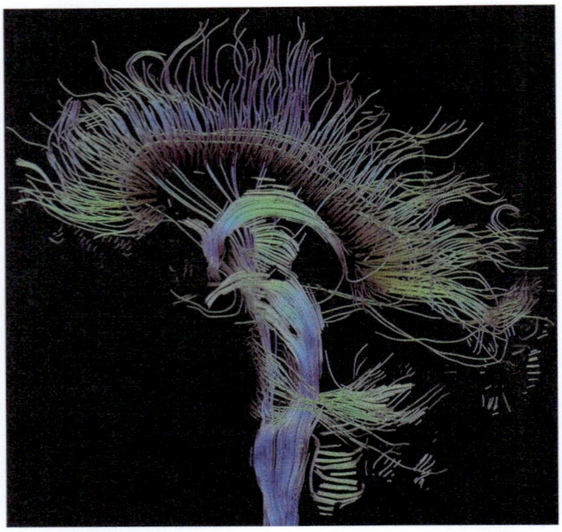

Fig. 5.20 3D rendering of MR tractography imaging (from Wikipedia)

(Fig. 5.20). New imaging modalities applicable to MS include imaging radiolabeled white cells (see Fig. 5.21). With these new advances in imaging coupled with amazing new development of a variety of immunomodulatory therapeutic agents, the outlook for patients with multiple sclerosis looks much brighter.

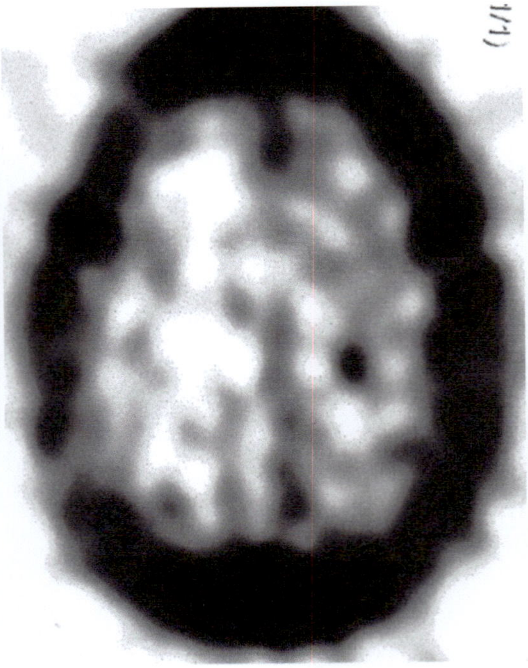

Fig. 5.21 A 24-year-old female with new onset of multiple sclerosis (MS) symptoms and active demyelinating plaques seen on MRI evaluated by SPECT imaging of 99mTc HMPAO radiolabeled autologous leukocytes: focally intense uptake is noted within the left semicentrum ovale white matter, reflecting localized infiltration into a newly forming demyelinating plaque

5.4 Leukodystrophies and Other Diseases of the White Matter

Leukodystrophies of childhood are tragic illnesses that stand in stark contrast to the normal pattern of development of myelination. Widespread degeneration of the subcortical white matter occurs in pediatric leukodystrophies and is often caused by defined genetic defects in the production of myelin-related sphigno-lipids, and include Krabbe's leukodystrophy or metachromatic leukodystrophy (Fig. 5.22). Other genetic defects resulting in white matter degeneration and secondary severe disability for affected children include Alexander's disease (Figs. 5.23 and 5.24), which

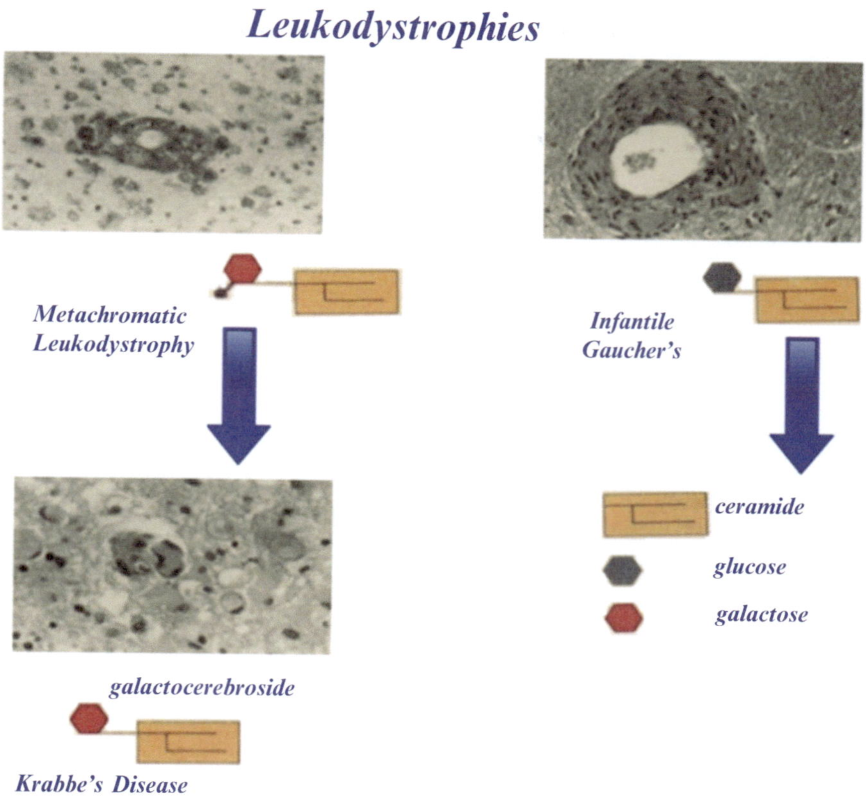

Fig. 5.22 Genetic metabolic defects in sphignolipid metabolism underlie metachromatic leukodystrophy, Krabbe's, and Gaucher's disease

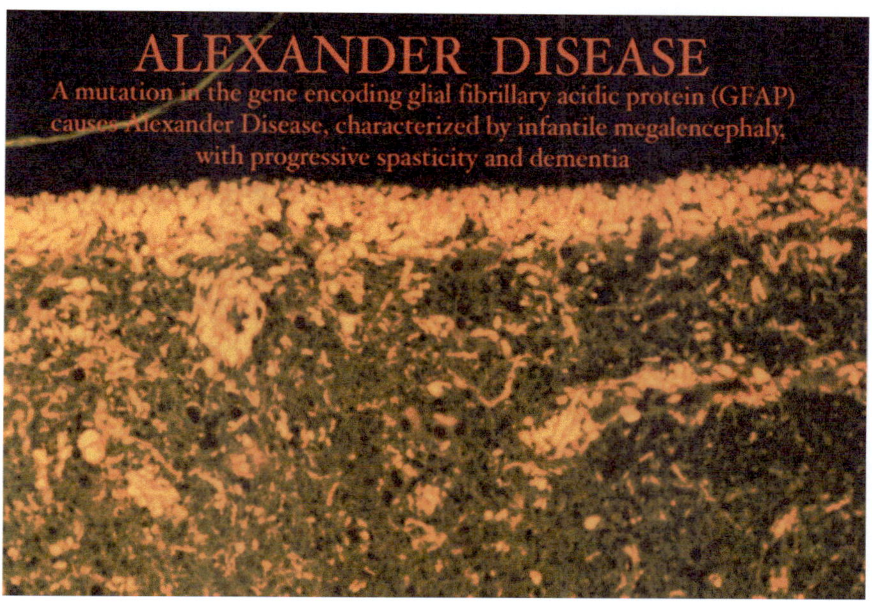

Fig. 5.23 Autofluorescent inclusions within the white matter in Alexander's disease

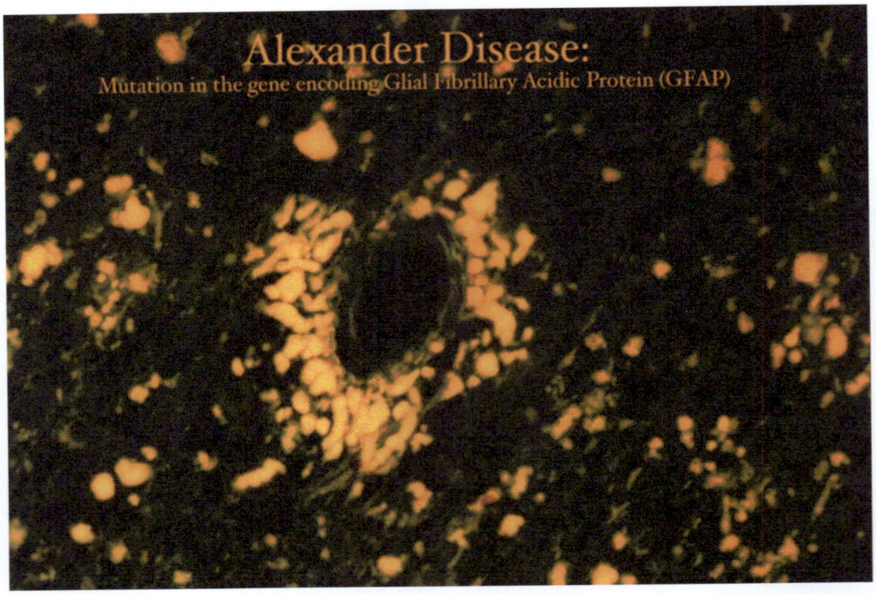

Fig. 5.24 Perivenular location of inclusions reflect the glial fibrillary acidic protein (GFAP) mutation-related pathology within astrocytic end-feet in Alexander's disease

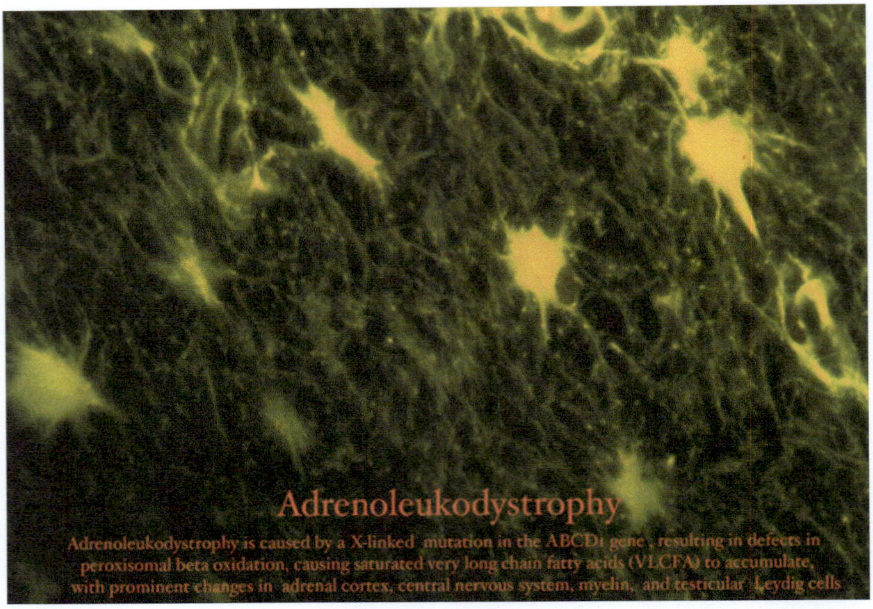

Fig. 5.25 Auto-fluorescent changes within degenerated white matter in adrenoleukodystrophy

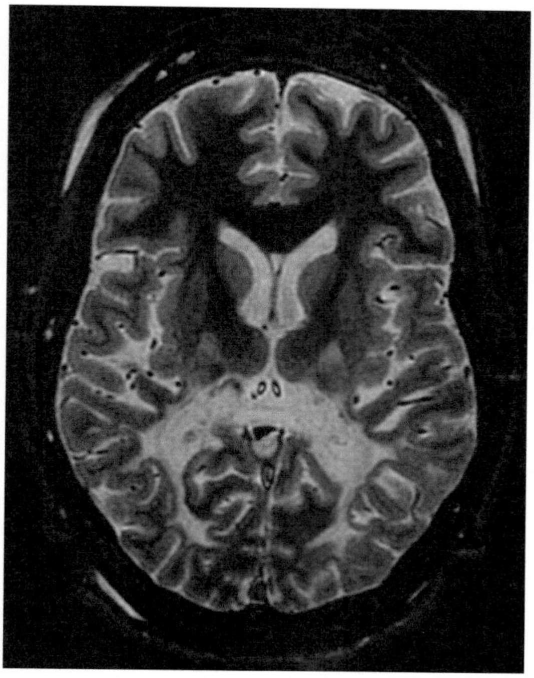

Fig. 5.26 Selective involvement of posterior white matter tracts in adrenoleukodystrophy (from Wikipedia)

relates to gene mutations in the gene encoding glial fibrillary acidic protein as a key astrocyte cytoskeletal component, and adrenoleukodystrophy (Figs. 5.25 and 5.26); a pathognomonic pattern for this disease is the striking selective involvement of the posterior half of the brain.

A variety of conditions show white matter pathology but are not primary leukodystrophies. Genetic conditions with white matter involvement that are not leukodystrophies include inherited vasculopathies such as CADASIL (cerebral autosomal dominant arteriopathy with subcortical infarcts and leukoencephalopathy). Similarly, it is important to note that some diseases have primary neuronal involvement yet generate secondary white matter changes and therefore are not true leukodystrophies; such disorders include but are not limited to GM1 and GM2 gangliosidosis, and neuronal lipofuscinosis. Genetic metabolic defects such as errors of amino acid metabolism can also induce secondary white matter abnormalities. Mitochondrial disorders such as MELAS can severely affect not only the gray matter but the white matter fiber tracts as well [17].

Other disorders with significant white matter involvement include multiple sclerosis and related autoimmune inflammatory central demyelinating disorders, such as post-infectious encephalomyelitis. Myelin injury can also relate to toxins, such as from drugs (e.g. heroin) or from pharmaceuticals (e.g. cyclosporine-related posterior reversible encephalopathy syndrome or PRES); with widespread access to MRI, PRES is an important white matter change that is recognized with increasing frequency (Fig. 5.27). External beam radiation can give rise to serious long-term myelin injury with delayed late radiation necrosis. Post-hypoxic injury, particularly in the perinatal period, can result in debilitating white matter alterations [18].

Figure 5.30 shows that electrolyte and fluid volume shifts such as with rapid correction of hyponatremia can induce osmotic demyelination within the white matter as in central pontine myelination (CPM) (Fig. 5.30). Small vessel ischemic vascular disease can be linked to multifocal white matter changes of ischemic demyelination.

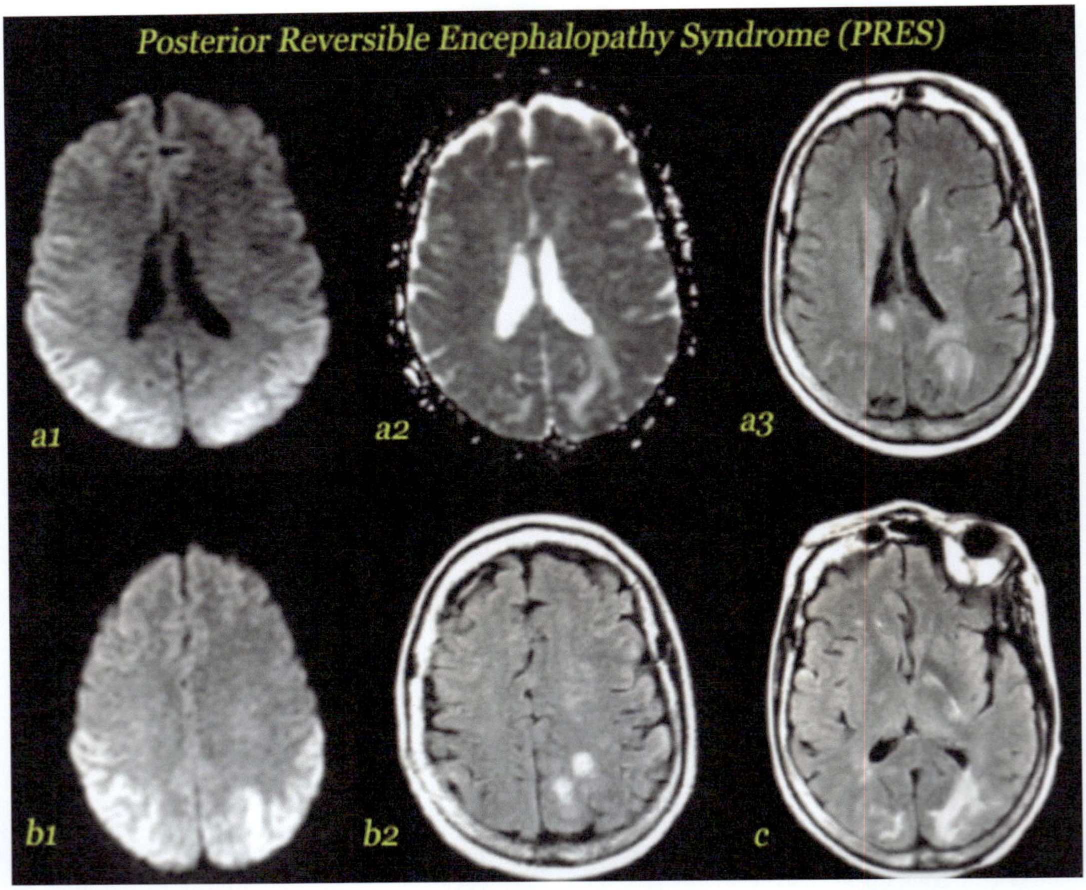

Fig. 5.27 Posterior reversible encephalopathy syndrome (PRES) in a 66-year-old female with acute transient visual loss and severe hypertension; al: positive axial diffusion scan; a2: ADC map

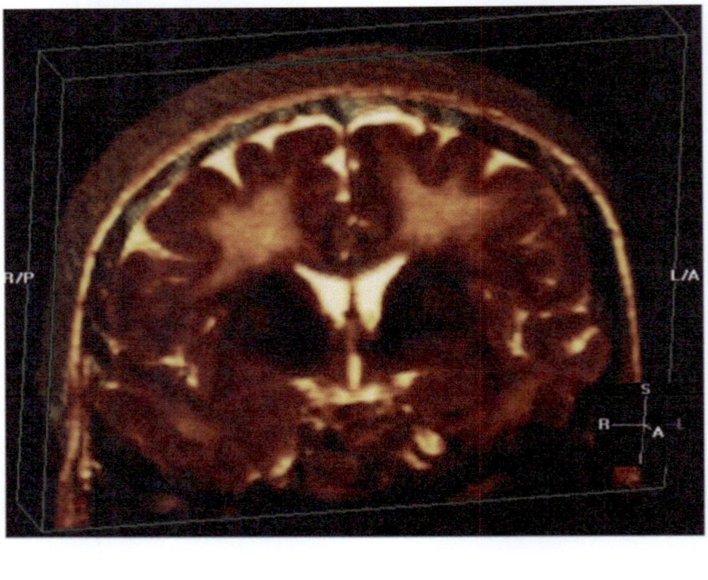

Fig. 5.28 Confluent bright signal within subcortical white matter in a case of delayed post-hypoxic leukoencephalopathy

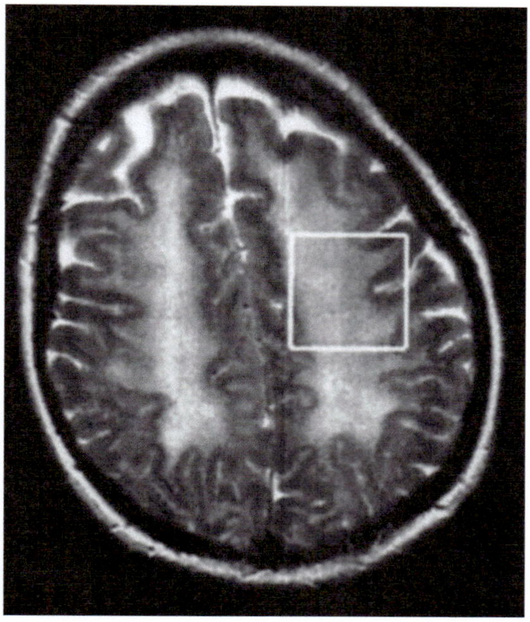

Fig. 5.29 As shown in Fig. 5.28, delayed post-hypoxic leukoencephalopathy: the patient who successfully recovered from a large overdose of diazepam and methadone, but then abruptly declined 3 weeks after the initial event. Magnetic resonance revealed confluent white matter hyperintensity on fluid-attenuated inversion recovery and T2-weighted sequences, and spectroscopy revealed elevated peaks in choline, creatinine, and lactate

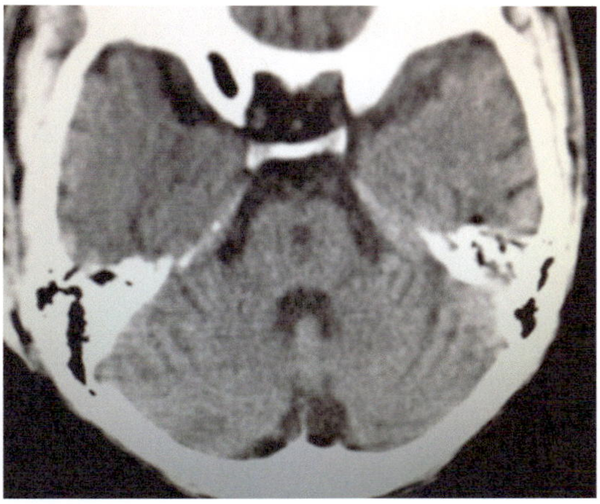

Fig. 5.30 CT revealing old central pontine myelinolysis in a young alcoholic

References

1. Fokke C, van den Berg B, Drenthen J, et al. Diagnosis of Guillain–Barré syndrome and validation of Brighton criteria. Brain. 2014;137(Pt 1):33–43.
2. Nyati KK. Role of campylobacter jejuni infection in the pathogenesis of Guillain–Barré syndrome: an update. Biomed Res Int. 2013;2013:852195.
3. Yuki N, Hartung HP. Guillain–Barré syndrome. N Engl J Med. 2012;366:2294–304.
4. van den Berg B, Bunschoten C, van Doorn PA. Mortality in Guillain–Barre syndrome. Neurology. 2013;80(18):1650–4.
5. Hughes RA, Swan AV, van Doorn PA. Intravenous immunoglobulin for Guillain–Barré syndrome. Cochrane Database Syst Rev. 2014;9:CD002063.
6. Bonnan M. Intrathecal IgG synthesis: a resistant and valuable target for future multiple sclerosis treatments. Mult Scler Int. 2015;2015:296184.
7. Magliozzi R, Howell O, Vora A, et al. Meningeal B-cell follicles in secondary progressive multiple sclerosis associate with early onset of disease and severe cortical pathology. Brain. 2007;130:1089–104.
8. Hansen T, Skytthe A, Stenager E, et al. Concordance for multiple sclerosis in Danish twins: an update of a nationwide study. Mult Scler. 2005;11:504–10.
9. Dodick DW, Silber MH, Noseworthy JH, et al. Acute disseminated encephalomyelitis after accidental injection of a hog vaccine: successful treatment with plasmapheresis. Mayo Clin Proc. 1998;73(12):1193–5.
10. Goldenberg MM. Multiple sclerosis review. P T. 2012;37(3):175–84.
11. Kamm CP, Uitdehaag BM, Polman CH. Multiple sclerosis: current knowledge and future outlook. Eur Neurol. 2014;72:132–41.
12. Polman CH, Reingold SC, Banwell B, et al. Diagnostic criteria for multiple sclerosis: 2010 revisions to the McDonald criteria (review). Ann Neurol. 2011;69: 292–302.
13. Balcer LJ. Optic neuritis. N Engl J Med. 2006;354:1273–80.
14. Frohman EM, Wingerchuk DM. Transverse myelitis. N Engl J Med. 2010;363:564–72.
15. Bridel C, Lalive PH. Update on multiple sclerosis treatments. Swiss Med Wkly. 2014;144:w14012.
16. Rosenkranz T, Novas M, Terborg C. PML in a patient with lymphocytopenia treated with dimethyl fumarate. N Engl J Med. 2015;372:1476–8.
17. Vanderver A, Tonduti D, Schiffmann R, et al. Leukodystrophy overview 2014. In: Pagon RA, Adam MP, Ardinger HH, et al., editors. GeneReviews® [Internet]. Seattle: University of Washington, Seattle; 2014. p. 1993–2015. http://www.ncbi.nlm.nih.gov/books/NBK184570/
18. Meyer MA. Delayed post-hypoxic leukoencephalopathy: case report with a review of disease pathophysiology. Neurol Int. 2013;5(3):e13.

6 The Hippocampus

6.1 Introduction

The hippocampus is a fundamentally important structure that is the key to understanding not only the biologic basis of memory, but other degenerative conditions such as Alzheimer's disease, where the first pathologic changes for the disease begins (Fig. 6.1). As the CA1 sector of the hippocampus is uniquely sensitive to any ischemic change, it is also the site for epileptogenic scarring that gives rise to a common form of epilepsy termed complex-partial seizures, otherwise known as temporal lobe epilepsy. The hippocampus and associated medial temporal lobe structures are the targets for infection by the herpes simplex virus; survivors of severe herpes simplex encephalitis are known to incur profound long-term memory deficits and suffer from recurrent complex-partial seizures. Basic science studies suggest that the hippocampus is important in spatial navigation and serves as a cognitive map of the environment; multiple clinical correlates have now been found to support this concept, including patients who suffer transient global amnesia on the basis of transient hippocampal ischemia and have transient loss in their frame of reference for space and time.

As revealed in this chapter, it is now well known since the famous 1953 surgical resection case of HM that the hippocampus is crucial for memory formation—this concept is well supported by not only countless subsequent clinical examples as in the case of herpes encephalitis survivors, but also extensively studied in animals. To refine the focus for memory formation further is the fascinating case of RB reported in 1986, nearly 30 years after HM [1]. This postmortem study confirms data also found in animals that the CA1 sector of the hippocampus plays a critical role in memory formation; however, the biologic mechanism remains elusive for this fundamental process of memory that helps define our existence.

The anatomy of the hippocampus is both fascinating and beautiful—the fine branches of dendritic trees, first evident in the 1890s by silver impregnation staining methods is truly dramatic when thinking that the fundamental yet elusive process of memory formation takes place in this area. The name Hippocampus derives from the Sea-Horse shape to the hippocampal folds from an outer six-layer entorhinal cortex that winds concentrically to form a single layer of pyramidal neurons, as shown in Fig. 6.1 in the coronal plane for the right temporal lobe (from the Greek word hippo for "horse", and kampos for "sea monster").

The hippocampal formation is located deep within the brain as an infolded structure along the bilateral medial aspects of the temporal lobes (Fig. 6.2). Best visualized in the coronal plane on MRI (Fig. 6.3), the hippocampus extends from the anterior medial aspects of the temporal lobe

M.A. Meyer, *Neurologic Disease*, DOI 10.1007/978-3-319-39581-4_6

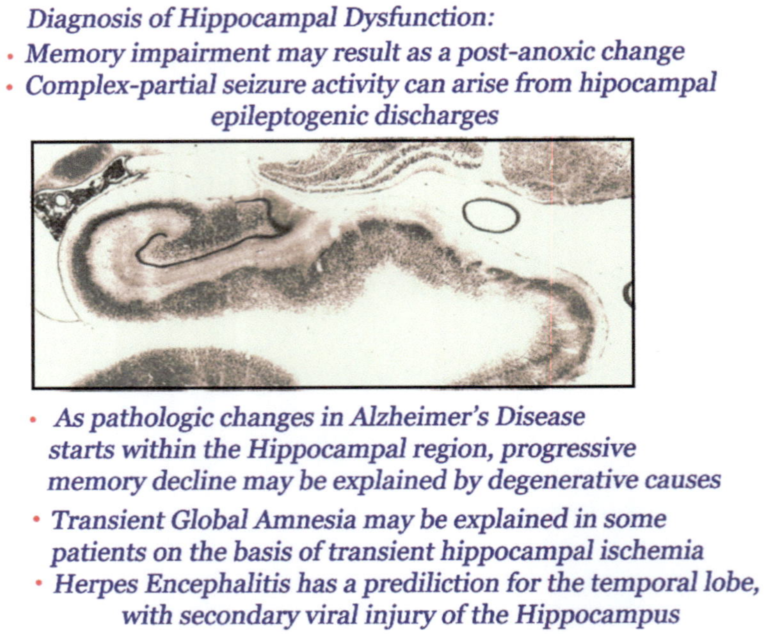

Fig. 6.1 Summary of major disease states affecting the hippocampus

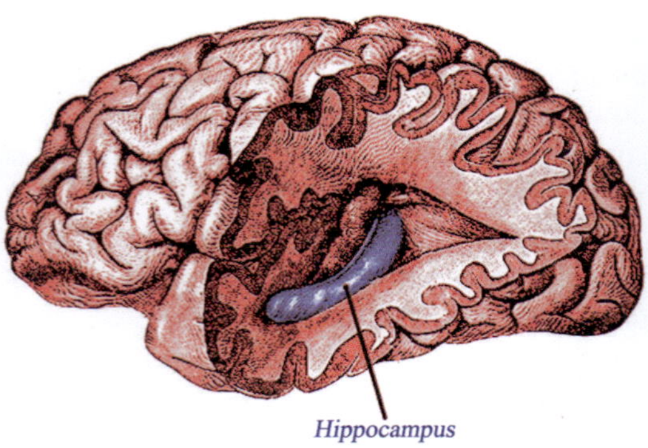

Fig. 6.2 The hippocampus is found within the medial aspects of the temporal lobe

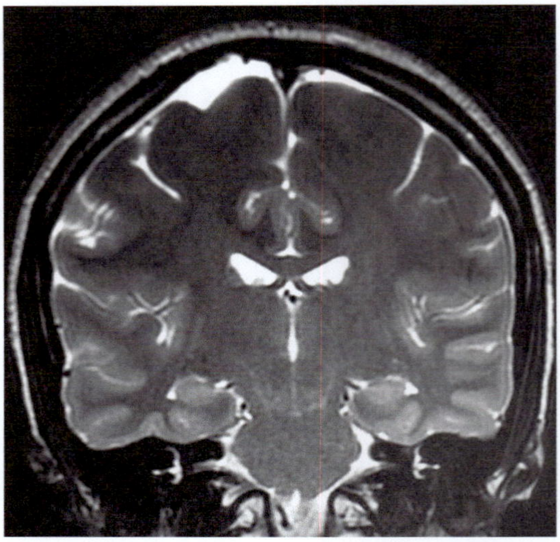

Fig. 6.3 Coronal T2-weighted MR exam revealing the bilateral hippocampal formations

back toward the ventricles, and sits just above the inter-connected entorhinal cortex; in horizontal cross section at eye level it can be seen as a highly infolded structure (Figs. 6.4 and 6.5).

As shown in Fig. 6.6, the hippocampus is comprised of two interlocking "C" shaped structures with one being the dentate gyrus, and the other being a pyramidal cell monolayer, which is further subdivided into regions CA1 through CA4 (CA being the abbreviation of Cornu Ammonis, named by early anatomists in Latin for the hippocampal curled shape resembling a Ram's Horn). As shown in Figs. 6.7 and 6.8, the dentate gyrus is densely packed with a single layer of granule cells which project their output as a bundle of axonal fibers (termed mossy fibers) that terminate upon the proximal aspects of relatively taller dendritic trees of CA3 pyramidal neurons within the complementary interlocking pyramidal cell monolayer. The CA3 neurons not

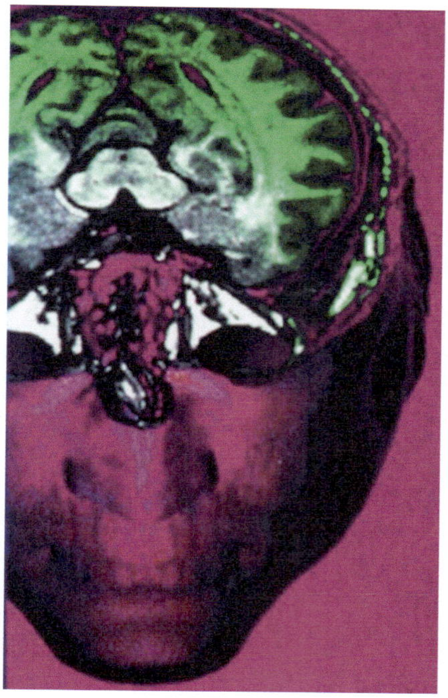

Fig. 6.4 Axial T1 view by MRI sectioning through the hippocampus at eye level

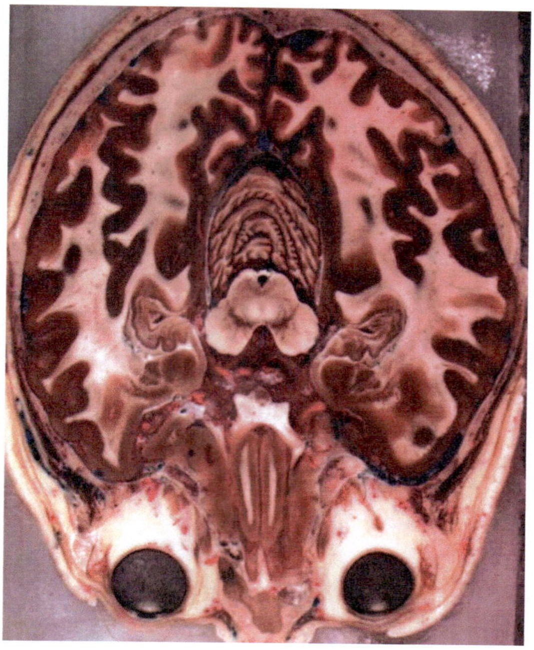

Fig. 6.5 Axial postmortem section through the temporal lobes

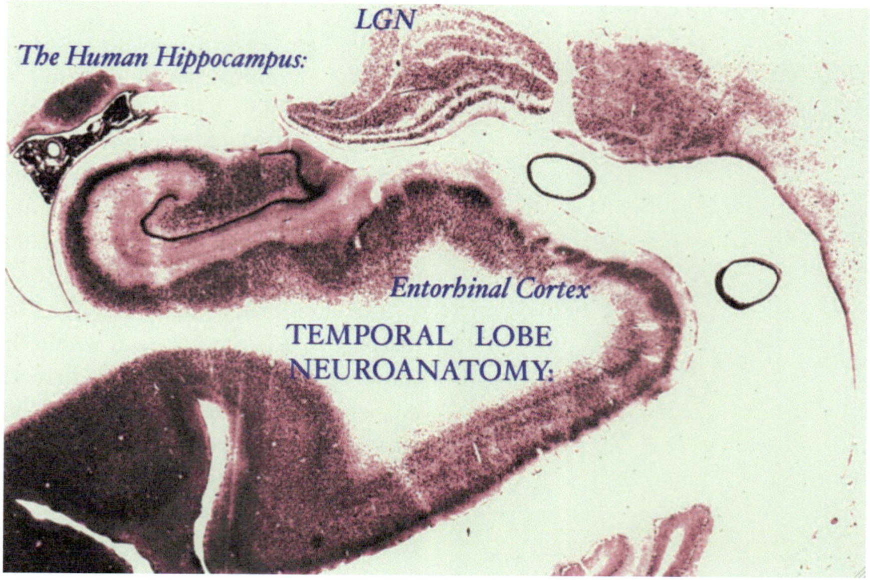

Fig. 6.6 Coronal histologic section through the hippocampus at the level of the lateral geniculate (LGN), revealing the dentate gyrus and entorhinal cortex

only project their output to other limbic structures but also pass collateral fibers (known as Schaffer collaterals) to the nearby CA1 dendrites within the stratum radiatum. Major inputs to the hippocampus arise from the nearby entorhinal cortex with layer 2 neurons projecting to the dentate gyrus versus layer 3 projecting to the outer apical dendrites of the CA1 neurons; as the innervating fiber tracts

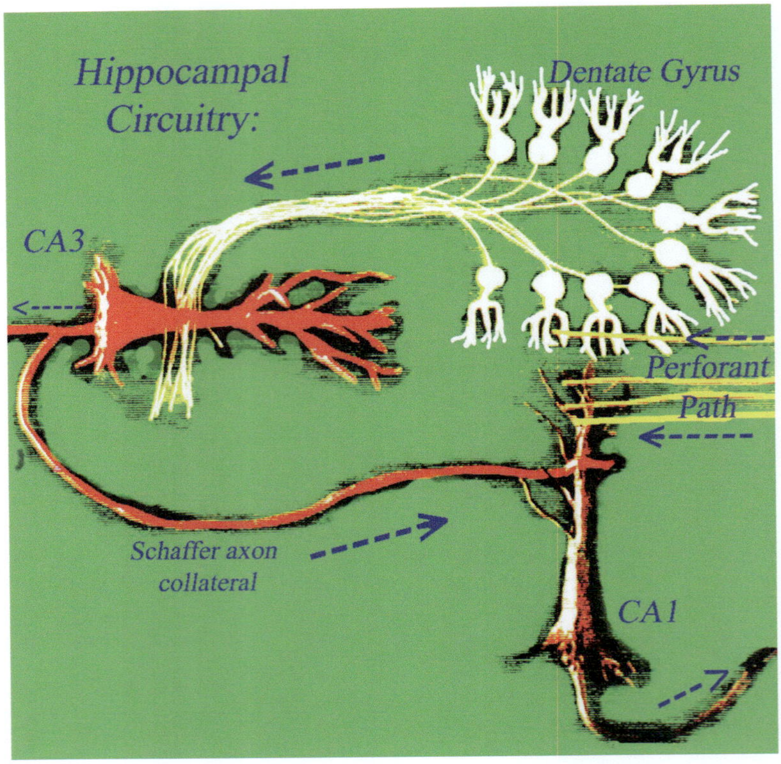

Fig. 6.7 Hippocampal interconnectivity: afferent activation of CA1 dendrites via the perforant path

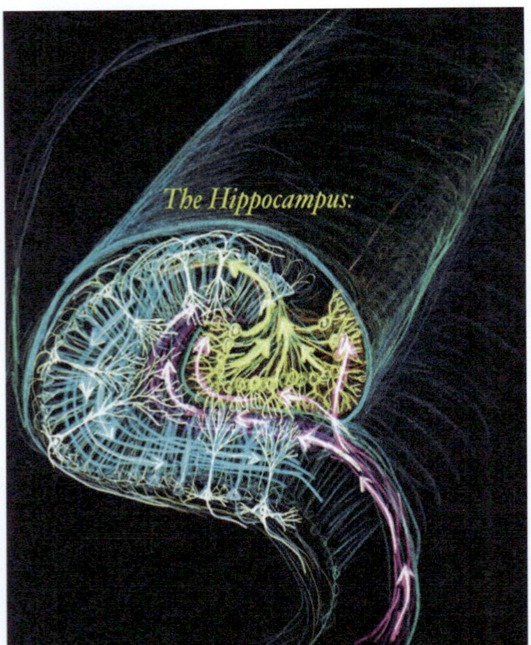

Fig. 6.8 Hippocampal circuitry: *arrows* depict the path for flow of information within the medial temporal lobe

from the entorhinal cortex perforate the hippocampal formation, it is termed the perforant pathway. Despite detailed knowledge about the anatomical circuitry for the flow of information within the hippocampus, how this translates into the phenomenon of memory formation remains an enigma.

The entorhinal cortex is important for multiple reasons, as it is the first area within the brain to show pathologic changes characteristic to Alzheimer's disease; both animal and human clinical studies confirm that this region plays a role in spatial navigation and forms a cognitive map of the spatial environment through the interconnection of grid cells that fire according to position and direction of the head within the environment. In this regard, a clinical preoperative electrophysiologic study on epileptic patients found that entorhinal cortex electrical stimulation can enhance spatial learning abilities. The hippocampus is also believed to play important roles in spatial navigation; although well described in

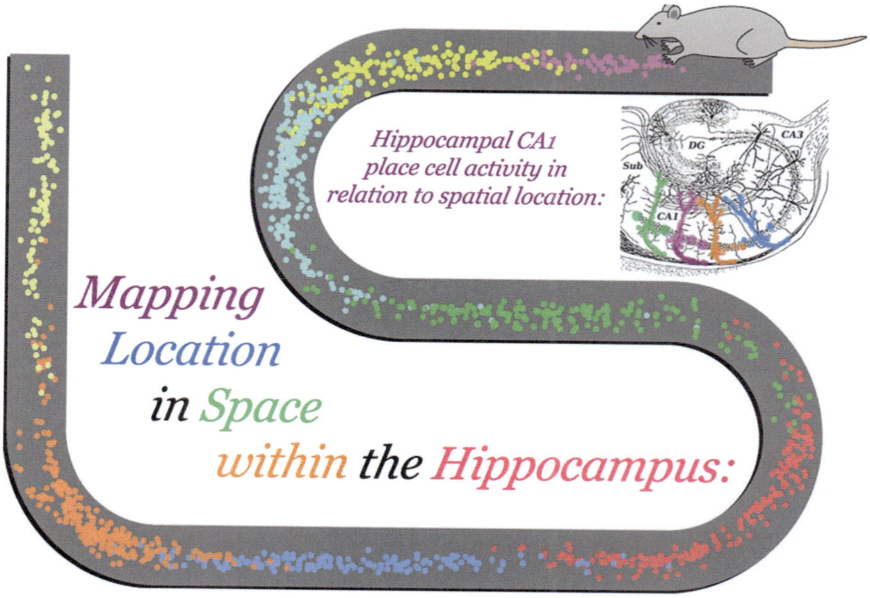

Fig. 6.9 The hippocampus as a spatial frame of reference: selective activation of hippocampal neurons according to spatial location of the head (adapted from Wikipedia)

animals where hippocampal neurons selectively fire in specific spatial locations during free range roaming (Fig. 6.9), analogous human hippocampal neuronal activity has been recorded while exploring and navigating a virtual town [2, 3].

Other important disease states linked to hippocampal and entorhinal cortex dysfunction include schizophrenia, where neuropathologic autopsy studies reveal developmental anomalies of neuronal organization including aberrant invaginations of the cortical surface, disruption of cortical layers, heterotopic displacement of neurons, and paucity of neurons in superficial layers [4–7]. Collectively, these changes suggest altered development of these important limbic system structures in schizophrenia and may play a role in the pathophysiology of the disease. In contrast, the normal postnatal pattern of development for the hippocampus is shown in Fig. 6.10.

As shown in Figs. 6.11 and 6.12, the hippocampus has a fairly well protected blood supply pattern that relies upon the interconnection of the anterior choroidal artery as the last branch from the distal terminal aspect of the internal carotid, with the hippocampal artery that arises from the posterior cerebral artery. Despite this protected pattern for a dual blood supply arising from both the anterior and posterior circulations, occasional ischemic events occur that are now known to be linked to the phenomenon of transient global amnesia (TGA); in many patients, this remarkably alarming transient state of confusion is increasingly more recognized as a TIA equivalent affecting the hippocampus that often resolves spontaneously. A study of 41 patients with TGA revealed that most cases had associated diffusion MR abnormalities, with 94 % being within the CA1 region, further emphasizing the metabolic vulnerability of this important area [8, 9].

A key concept in understanding the hippocampus lies appreciating its interconnections with other structures, collectively termed the limbic system. Limbic areas include the mammillary bodies that project to the anterior thalamic nucleus; damage to either of these structures can result in severe memory impairments. Limbic structures also include the fornix, which is a major white matter fiber tract exiting the tail of the hippocampus and readily identified in the midline on coronal MR images (Fig. 6.3). Anterograde amnesia can result from selective damage to the fornix, which interconnects the

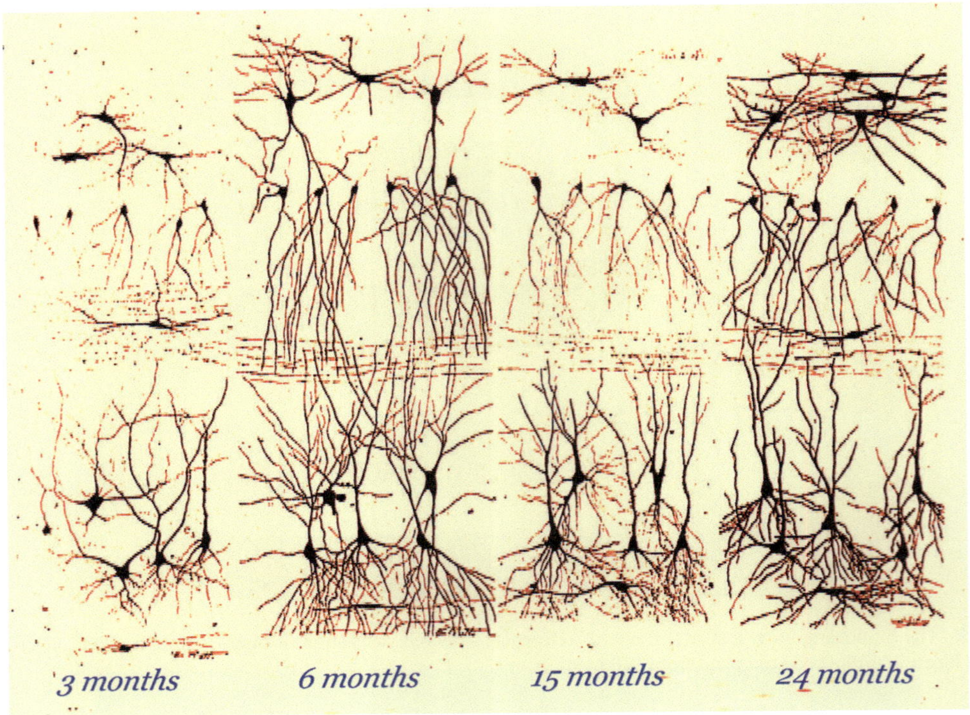

Fig. 6.10 Human cytologic development of the hippocampus (age in months)

Fig. 6.11 Dual blood supply to the hippocampus via branches of the internal carotid (anterior choroidal artery) and posterior cerebral (hippocampal artery)

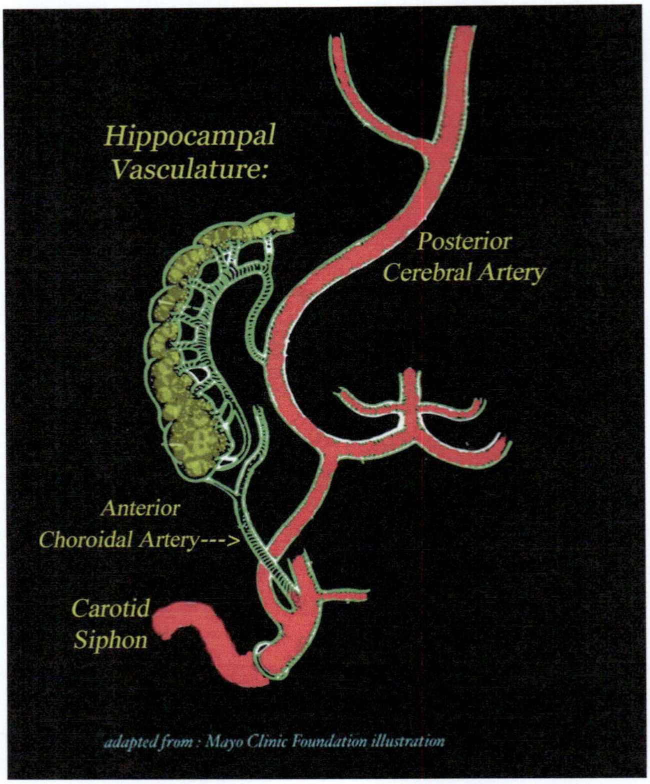

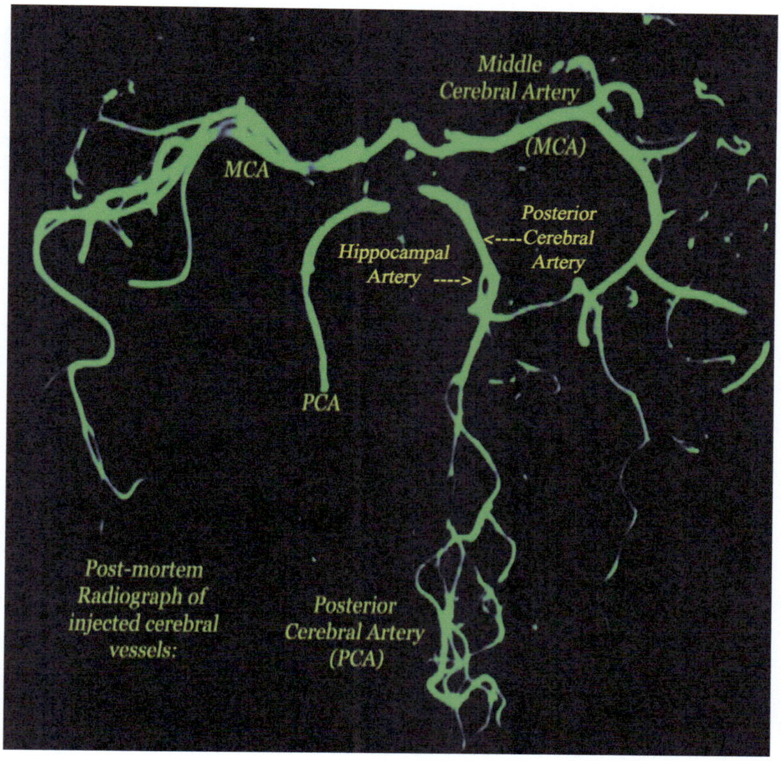

Fig. 6.12 Human hippocampal vasculature

hippocampus with the mammillary bodies; clinical examples include a fascinating case report of an individual who had selective infarction of the anterior fornix and genu of the corpus callosum and had developed sudden apathy and anterograde amnesia [10].

Where does the hippocampus project to? This was well delineated for monkey cerebral cortex with amino acid injections by Goldman-Rakic [11] to trace anterograde versus retrograde labeling, confirming that the posterior parietal cortex is an inter-connected region (amongst other cortical projection targets) and serves as a complex association area and correlates well to the consistent PET findings seen in Alzheimer's disease that reveal functional and therefore metabolic defects within the posterior parietal cortex.

The key role that the hippocampus has in memory formation is best illustrated by the unfortunate case of Mr. Henry Molaison, referred to in the medical literature as HM (Fig. 6.13). This individual suffered from intractable post-traumatic epilepsy localized to the medial temporal lobes. At age 27, at the Hartford Hospital in Hartford, Connecticut, he underwent surgical resection of the bilateral hippocampal formations and adjacent structures, including most of the amygdala and entorhinal cortex. His neurosurgeon Dr. William Scoville noted that although his epilepsy was remarkably improved, it came at the expense of a profound memory deficit: although distant memories were intact, he had difficulty in recalling the last 3 years (partial retrograde amnesia) but more importantly could not form new memories (profoundly severe anterograde amnesia). He was subsequently referred to Neuropsychologist Dr. Brenda Milner at the Montreal Neurologic Institute for further evaluation; her subsequent work with HM opened the door to new insights into the anatomical basis for memory; a remarkable postmortem study was carried out that involved serial sectioning of the entire brain [12].

Dr Milner observed over the years that his anterograde amnesia was persistently severe and apparently permanent: "After operation this

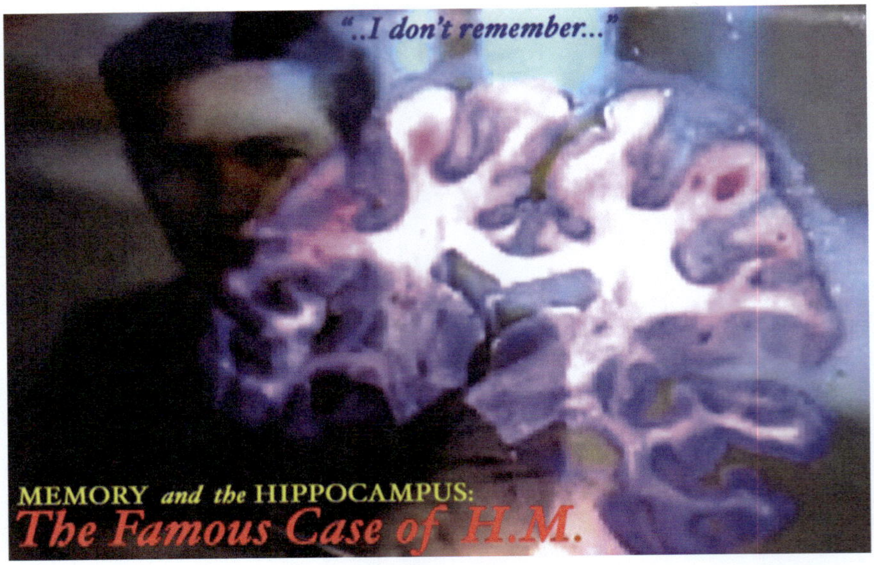
"..I don't remember..."
MEMORY and the HIPPOCAMPUS:
The Famous Case of H.M.

Fig. 6.13 Histologic section of the brain of patient HM illustrating the large postsurgical bilateral hippocampal defects

young man could no longer recognize the hospital staff nor find his way to the bathroom, and he seemed to recall nothing of the day-to-day events of his hospital life. There was also a partial retrograde amnesia, in as much as he did not remember the death of a favourite uncle 3 years previously……. His early memories were apparently vivid and intact. In conversation, the reverted constantly to boyhood events and seemed scarcely to realize that he had undergone an operation…….. In summary, this patient appears to have a complete loss of memory for events subsequent to bilateral medial temporal-lobe resection 19 months before, together with a partial retrograde amnesia for the 3 years leading up to his operation; but early memories are seemingly normal and there is no impairment of personality or general intelligence." [13]. Dr Milner reported that he likened his problem to, "like waking from a dream … every day is alone in itself…" [14]. Detailed neuropsychological testing revealed he could in fact learn new motor skills, such as accurately tracing patterns that had been reversed by mirrors, but had no recollection learning these skills.

Almost 30 years after the seminal 1957 publication of the HM case by Scoville and Milner came an even more remarkable case report of patient RB who suffered selective ischemic damage to the CA1 sector of the hippocampus (Fig. 6.14). Although displaying little if any retrograde amnesia, the authors of the landmark 1986 paper noted he "exhibited marked anterograde amnesia,….and showed no signs of cognitive impairment other than memory. Thorough histological examination revealed a circumscribed bilateral lesion involving the entire CA1 field of the hippocampus………To our knowledge, this is the first reported case of amnesia following a lesion limited to the hippocampus in which extensive neuropsychological and neuropathological analyses have been carried out" [1].

Since that time, other clinical and basic science studies have been published that add support to the concept that the CA1 sector of the hippocampus is critically important, as exemplified by a study on 14 individuals with selective focal lesions in the CA1 sector and displayed profound impairments in place learning. An outstanding basic science study on the importance of CA1 hippocampal neurons in memory formation by turning cells on and off with elegant optogenetic technologies that relies on transfection-induced expression of a light-sensitive neuronal membrane protein that can change its conformation and alter channel conductivity. This study by

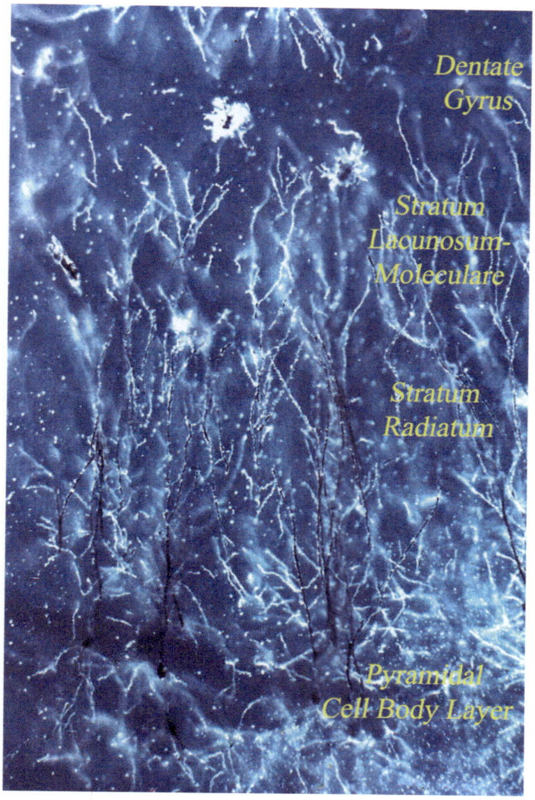

Fig. 6.14 Dark field view of Golgi impregnated silver-stained CA1 sector

Goshen et al. [15] found "….that contextual fear memory recall, even weeks after training, can be reversibly abolished by temporally precise optogenetic inhibition of CA1. When this inhibition is extended to match the typical time course of pharmacological inhibition, remote hippocampus dependence converts to hippocampus independence, suggesting that long-term memory retrieval normally depends on the hippocampus but can adaptively shift to alternate structures".

The molecular mechanism of memory still remains elusive, although reflected by structural alterations with the formation of dendritic spine synapses and physiologically by the phenomenon of long-term potentiation with prolonged strengthening of synaptic transmission; the neurochemistry of how this happens within CA1 hippocampal neurons remains a mystery (Fig. 6.15). To further explore this, the author conducted a study on a data base of 1013 genes [16], where 16 were identified that had selective localization of gene expression within the CA1 region, and included Angpt2, ARHGEF6, CCK, Cntnap1, DRD3, EMP1, Epha2, Itm2b, Lrrtm2, Mdk, PNMT, Ppm1e, Ppp2r2d, RASGRP1, Slitrk5, and Sstr4 (Fig. 6.16). Of the 16 identified, the most selective and intense localization for both adult and postnatal day 7 was noted for ARHGEF6 (Fig. 6.17), which is known to be linked to non-syndromic mental retardation, and has also been localized to dendritic spines. Gene expression atlases are particularly useful in unraveling the mystery of hippocampal physiology; it is remarkable to find some genes expressed in very selective locations that range from only the dentate gyrus to other patterns that are CA1-selective (Figs. 6.18, 6.19, and 6.20).

Another mystery about the hippocampus that has clinical implications centers on the extreme sensitivity and vulnerability that CA1 neurons have with transient ischemia. Whereas most other brain regions can tolerate brief periods of reduced cerebral blood flow, the neurons within the CA1 region cannot and undergo apoptotic programmed cell death over a period of a few days should this occur, leaving the patient with long-term memory deficits. Insight into this phenomenon of metabolic vulnerability is gained from a review of mitochondrial cytochrome oxidase staining (Fig. 6.21) and glucose uptake as assessed by radiolabeled deoxyglucose autoradiography (Fig. 6.22). Unlike other areas of the brain, the distal dendrites within the stratum lacunosum-moleculare of the CA1 neurons have high rates of metabolic activity; any significantly prolonged interruption in blood flow to this area can easily trigger the release of highly concentrated mitochondrial cytochrome to initiate the cascade of programmed cell death neuronal apoptosis.

Another important feature to this outer dendritic layer known as the lacunosum-moleculare (SLM) of the CA1 neurons is the innervation by myelinated afferents of the perforant pathway originating from the entorhinal cortex (Fig. 6.23). Recent studies have now shown that inhibitory neurons within the SLM modulate this excitatory input from the perforant pathway [17], raising speculation about their potential role in

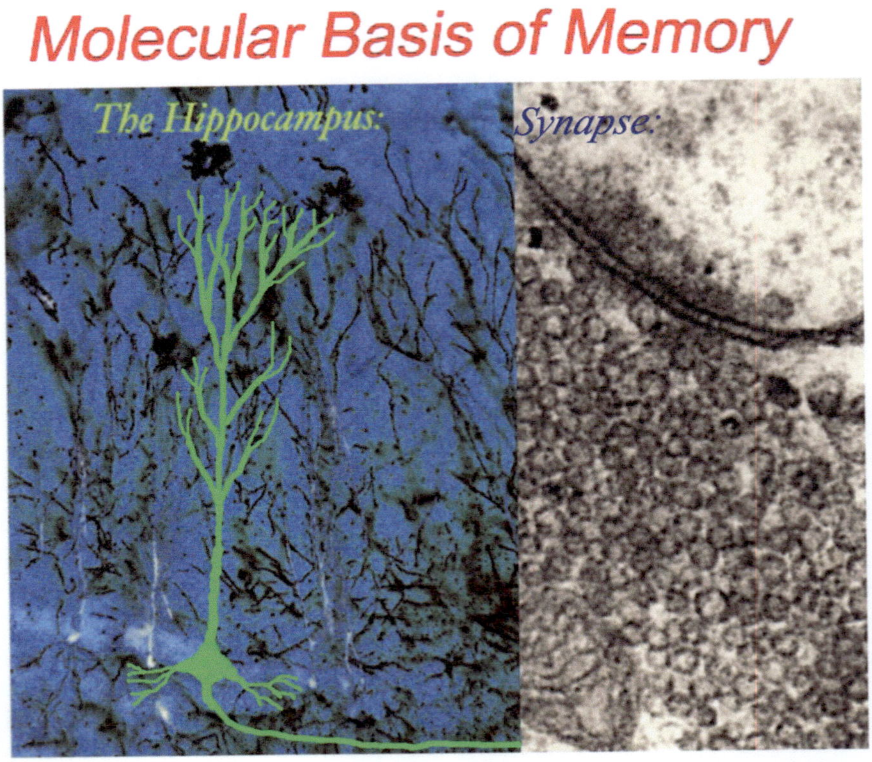

Fig. 6.15 Investigating the molecular mechanisms of memory at two different levels of resolution: by light microscopy at *left* versus the ultra-structural synaptic level at *right*

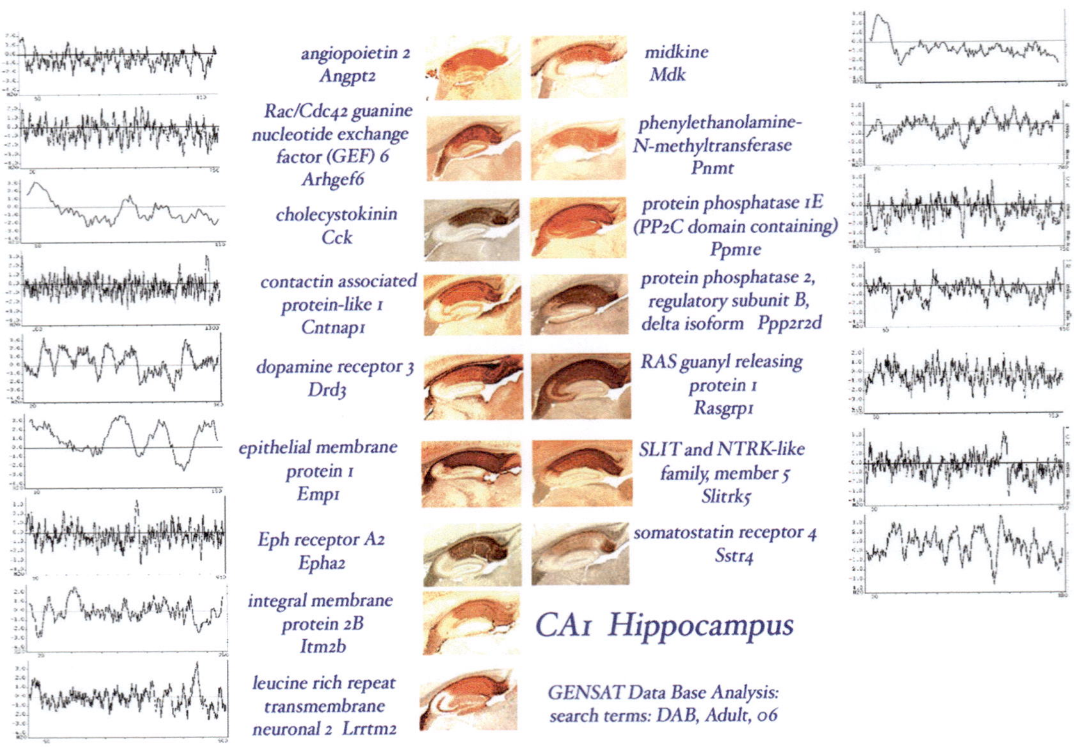

Fig. 6.16 Investigating the molecular mechanism of memory using a gene expression on-line atlas to identify genes that are strongly expressed within the CA1 region

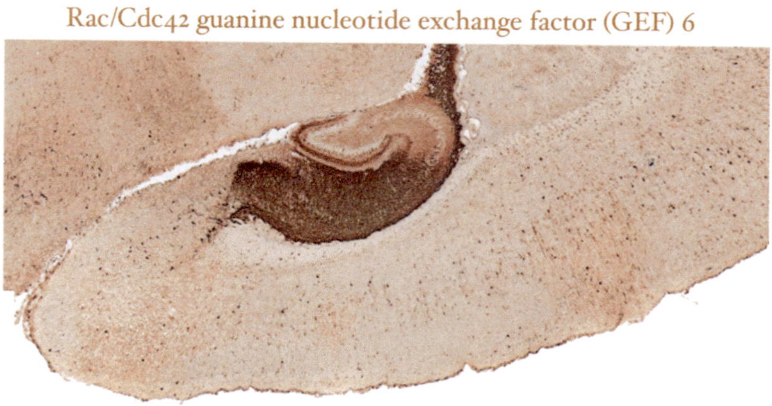

Fig. 6.17 ARHGEF6 gene mutations underlie some non-syndromic forms of mental retardation; the normal gene product of Arhgef6 is linked to dendritic spine formation and appears selectively expressed within the CA1 region

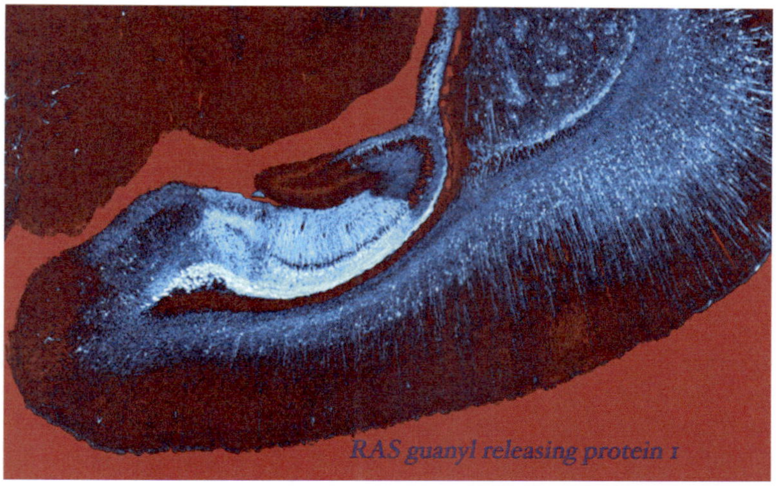

Fig. 6.18 As an example of CA1-selective gene expression, Ras guanyl releasing protein 1 is illustrated to stand in contrast to other genes that are selectively expressed within the dentate gyrus

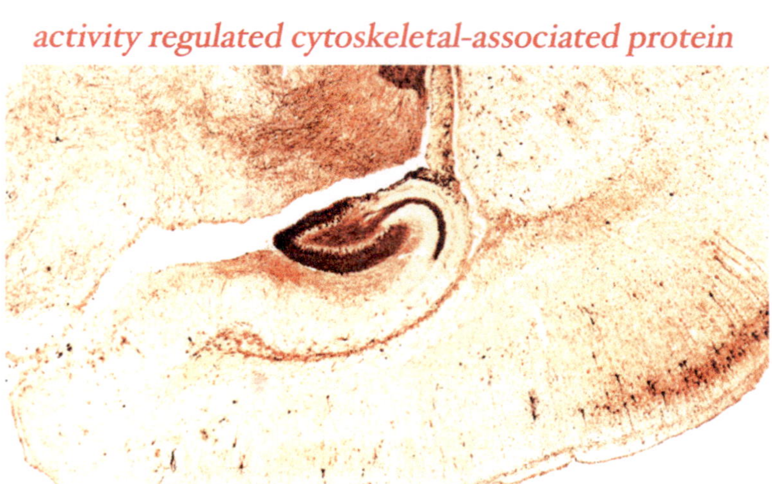

Fig. 6.19 Activity regulated cytoskeletal associated protein is an example of another gene that is selectively expressed within the dentate gyrus

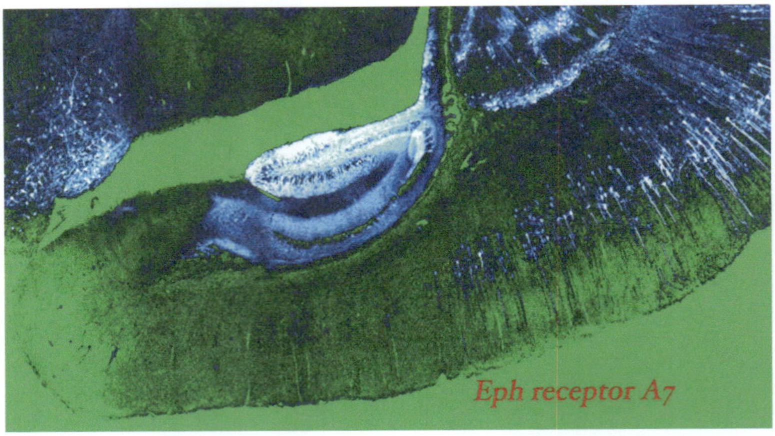

Fig. 6.20 Eph receptor a7 shows predominantly dentate gyrus expression and belongs to the ephrin receptor subfamily of the protein-tyrosine kinase family that helps mediate brain development

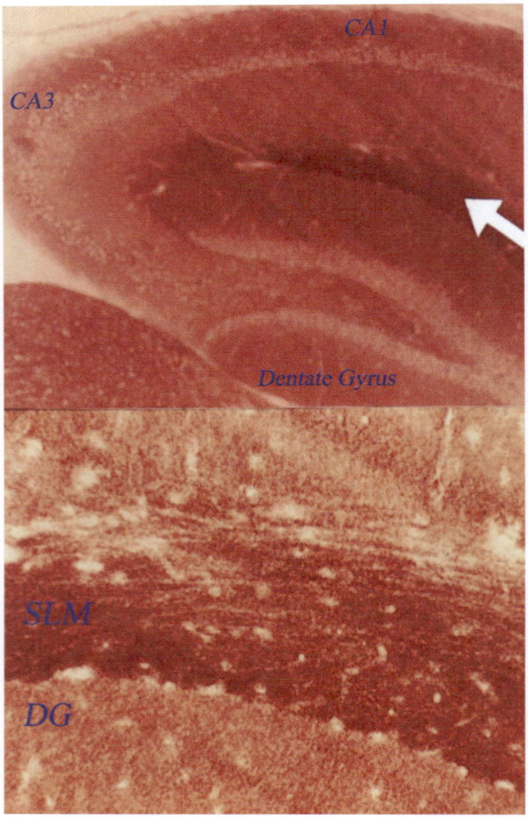

Fig. 6.21 Cytochrome oxidase histochemical staining for the mouse hippocampus, demonstrating intense activity within the neuropil of outer dendritic trees of CA1 neurons

CA1-mediated memory formation. Known as neurogliaform cells, these interneurons mediate feedforward inhibition of CA1 pyramidal cells via chemical and electrical synapses, and evoke GABA-mediated slow inhibitory synaptic currents.

6.1.1 Clinical Case Examples

To further illustrate the key role that the hippocampus plays in memory formation, the case of a 75-year-old with acute sudden loss of memory is illustrated in Fig. 6.24. The patient returned from driving her granddaughter one morning and suddenly developed disorientation where her frame of reference was transiently lost and kept asking the same question of what had happened and where she was. Despite multiple attempts by family to reassure her, she could not retain any new information over the next 12 h. She was brought to the local emergency room where intermittent paroxysmal atrial fibrillation was noted. Although speech was intact, and distant long-term recall was intact, she could not recall events of the preceding 3 weeks nor recall any of four simple words that were given to her on neurologic exam in the emergency room. By the next day, she improved but had never been able to recall the personal experience of how she wound up in the hospital; MR imaging disclosed a focal ischemic change within the left fornix (see Fig. 6.24 illustrating this important fiber tract that transmits the output of the hippocampus to the mammillary bodies).

An unusual case of paraneoplastic limbic encephalitis affecting the right hippocampus is shown in Fig. 6.25. Shortly after Thanksgiving in late November, a 45-year-old smoker developed a profoundly severe short-term memory deficit that became progressively worse over a

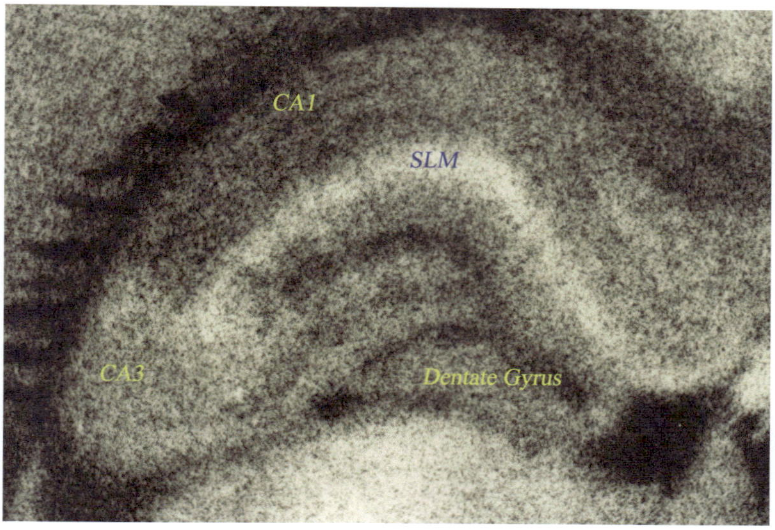

Fig. 6.22 14C-2-deoxyglucose autoradiogram of the rat hippocampus, demonstrating intense metabolic activity within the same area that has intense mitochondrial cytochrome oxidase activity

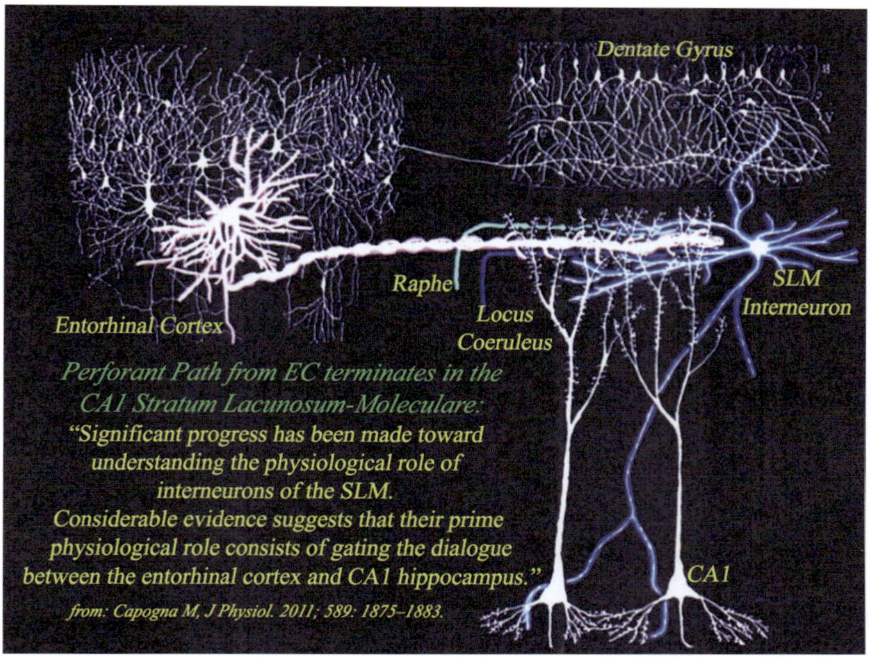

Fig. 6.23 Summary diagram showing innervation of the outer dendritic region of CA1 neurons, including inhibitory input from interneurons within the stratum lacunosum-moleculare

period of 2 weeks that prompted in-patient hospital evaluation, where small cell lung carcinoma was discovered. An abnormal bright T2 signal abnormality was seen in the right hippocampus that corresponded to a mild to moderate increase in hippocampal cerebral perfusion as assessed by brain SPECT; CSF exam and repeat imaging studies failed to demonstrate metastatic disease, leading to the diagnosis of a remote paraneoplastic effect upon hippocampal-mediated memory formation. Clinical improvements in memory and cognition was coincident with an objective positive response of the lung neoplasm to chemotherapy.

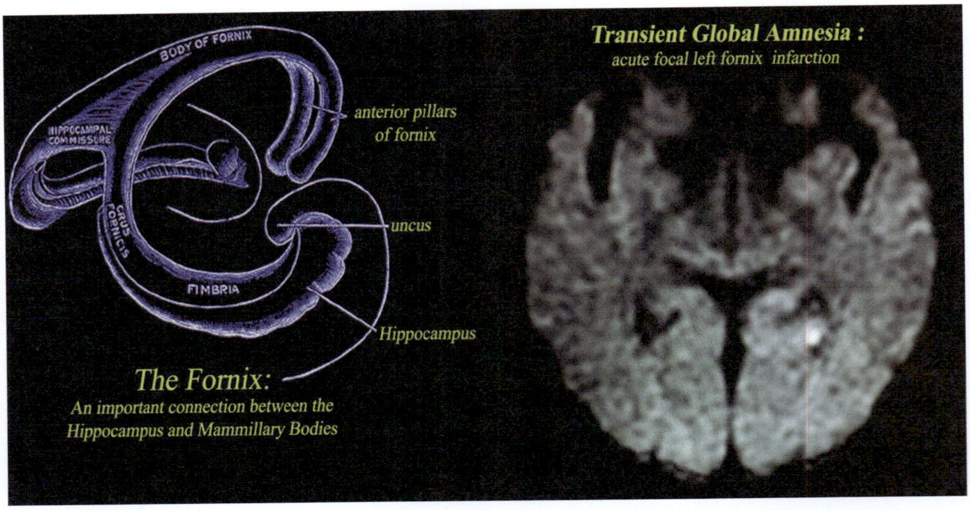

Fig. 6.24 Clinical example of hippocampal dysfunction due to a highly focal left fornix infarct producing a state of transient global amnesia

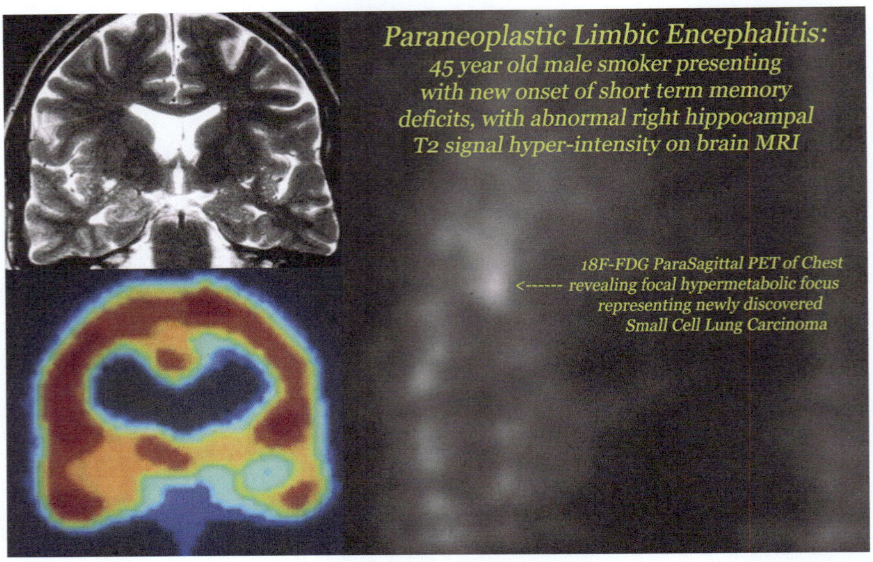

Fig. 6.25 Clinical example of right hippocampal dysfunction due to a remote paraneoplastic effect from small cell lung cancer

References

1. Zola-Morgan S, Squire LR, Amaral DG. Human amnesia and the medial temporal region: enduring memory impairment following a bilateral lesion limited to field CA1 of the hippocampus. J Neurosci. 1986;6:2950–67.
2. Suthana N, Haneef Z, Stern J, et al. Memory enhancement and deep-brain. Stimulation of the entorhinal area. N Engl J Med. 2012;366:502–10.
3. Ekstrom AD, Kahana MJ, Caplan JB, et al. Cellular networks underlying human spatial navigation. Nature. 2003;425:184–7.
4. Honer WG, Bassett AS, Falkai P, et al. A case study of temporal lobe development in familial schizophrenia. Psychol Med. 1996;26:191–5.
5. Falkai P, Bogerts B, Rozumek M. Limbic pathology in schizophrenia: the entorhinal region—a morphometric study. Biol Psychiatry. 1988;24:515–21.
6. Arnold SE, Hyman BT, Van Hoesen GW, Damasio AR. Some cytoarchitectural abnormalities of the ento-

rhinal cortex in schizophrenia. Arch Gen Psychiatry. 1991;48:625–32.
7. Conrad AJ, Abebe T, Austin R, Forsythe S, Scheibel AB. Hippocampal pyramidal cell disarray in schizophrenia as a bilateral phenomenon. Arch Gen Psychiatry. 1991;48:413–7.
8. Bartsch T, Alfke K, Stingele R, et al. Selective affection of hippocampal CA-1 neurons in patients with transient global amnesia without long-term sequelae. Brain. 2006;129(Pt 11):2874–84.
9. Bartsch T, Schönfeld R, Müller FJ, et al. Focal lesions of human hippocampal CA1 neurons in transient global amnesia impair place memory. Science. 2010; 328(5984):1412–5.
10. Saito Y, Matsumura K, Shimizu T. Anterograde amnesia associated with infarction of the anterior fornix and genu of the corpus callosum. J Stroke Cerebrovasc Dis. 2006;15(4):176–7.
11. Cavada C, Goldman-Rakic PS. Posterior parietal cortex in rhesus monkey: I. Parcellation of areas based on distinctive limbic and sensory corticocortical connections. J Comp Neurol. 1989;287:393–421.
12. Annese J, Schenker-Ahmed NM, Bartsch H. Postmortem examination of patient H.M.'s brain based on histological sectioning and digital 3D reconstruction. Nat Commun. 2014;5:3122.
13. Scoville WB, Milner B. Loss of recent memory after bilateral hippocampal lesions. J Neurol Neurosurg Psychiatry. 1957;20:11.
14. Squire LR. The legacy of patient H.M. for neuroscience. Neuron. 2009;61:6–9.
15. Goshen I, Brodsky M, Prakash R, et al. Dynamics of retrieval strategies for remote memories. Cell. 2011; 147:678–89.
16. Meyer MA. Highly expressed genes within hippocampal sector CA1: implications for the physiology of memory. Neurol Int. 2014;6:5388.
17. Capogna M. Neurogliaform cells and other interneurons of stratum lacunosum-moleculare gate entorhinal-hippocampal dialogue. J Physiol. 2011; 589(Pt 8):1875–83.

7 Alzheimer's Disease

Alzheimer's disease (AD) is a tragic illness that robs the affected individual of their cognitive skills, leading from an initial stage of mild cognitive impairment to progressively severe dementia. Despite being highly prevalent in the geriatric population, there still is no effective treatment that halts the progression of the disease; despite detailed knowledge about the pathophysiology of neurotoxic neurofibrillary plaque and tangle formation, AD remains a major cause of dementia that still has no effective treatment. Although medications such as cholinesterase inhibitors can be of mild to moderate help with some of the symptomatic impairments in memory, there is no treatment yet available that addresses the core problem of progressive neuronal dysfunction and cell death. The numbers of affected patients are staggering with more than 35 million worldwide suffering with AD and other dementias; the incidence also doubles for every 5 years after 65 years of age; economic costs of the disease are substantial, and anticipated to exceed $1 trillion by 2050.

Many neurodegenerative disorders, such as Alzheimer's have no effective treatments currently available despite knowing a great amount of detail on disease pathophysiology. A key common mechanism of disease relates to misfolding of proteins that normally play key roles in neuronal functioning—in multiple disease states, focal gene mutations have been found to give rise to abnormal protein products that misfold rendering them dysfunctional and in some cases cause the proteins to self-aggregate producing insoluble cellular debris that accumulate within the neuron causing further dysfunction.

With regards to AD, a key pathophysiologic link to keep in mind when reviewing information on the disease is the neuronal cytoskeleton, which must remain intact for proper neuronal health and to maintain axonal transport. For AD, there is a prominent disruption of the neuronal cytoskeleton, with dissolution of the supportive framework for axonal transport being a primary event in this illness as well as other degenerative illnesses such as amyotrophic lateral sclerosis (ALS), which is known to be caused by a variety of mutations, including the gene for heavy neurofilament production (NFH).

The most common form of dementia in the elderly is attributable to AD, comprising about half of all cases of dementia with an additional 15–25 % of dementia cases accounted by Lewy body dementia and frontotemporal dementia (FTD); vascular multi-infarct states may be a superimposed factor in up to 25 % of cases. Although AD is a distinct neurodegenerative process with a characteristic neuropathologic change with plaques and tangles, the clinical features of progressive memory and cognitive impairment are nonspecific and seen with the early clinical stages of other forms of dementia. However, age of onset can be a clear factor that may separate genetic causations in the form of familial early-

M.A. Meyer, *Neurologic Disease*, DOI 10.1007/978-3-319-39581-4_7

onset AD (EOAD) versus the far more common multi-factorial sporadic late-onset AD (LOAD). Although LOAD shares some of the same pathogenetic factors linked to amyloid production seen in EOAD, it is likely a more complex process that may be further complicated by other yet to be determined genetic factors as well as a multitude of acquired factors including cerebrovascular disease. Genetic factors have been identified that involve mutations that cause alterations in the processing of amyloid precursor protein (APP) that induce production of abnormal beta amyloid fragments which can then clump together to form toxic aggregates of amyloid in the extracellular space.

Dramatic individual patient cases have been known to inspire physician-scientists to explore their illness in great detail that have lead to important medical advances. This was certainly the case for Dr. Alois Alzheimer who encountered a 51-year-old female named Auguste Deiter at a mental hospital in Frankfurt, Germany (Fig. 7.1); he was struck by the premature nature of her illness and dramatic symptoms noted by her husband in addition to cognitive decline starting in her late 40s, she would have trouble sleeping with dragging of bed sheets and scream repeatedly throughout the night. Progressive sleep and memory disturbance, aggression, and confusion, with paranoia was noted. During his November, 1901 examination of the patient, he noted her writing her name repeatedly while muttering "I have lost myself"; her dramatic unfortunate case of progressive presenile early-onset of dementia captured his long-term interest from that point onward; despite relocating to Munich, he followed her progressive cognitive decline at a distance to the point where she was bedridden and at age 56, had fatal sepsis due to infected bed sores. Her medical records and autopsy brain specimen were sent to him in Munich, where he collaborated with Dr. Emil Kraepelin to prepare and study histologic sections using silver staining techniques to discover the presence of very numerous extracellular amyloid plaques within her brain in conjunction with numerous intraneuronal neurofibrillary tangles, leading Kraepelin and colleagues to refer to these findings as "Alzheimer's Disease". Modern day mutational analysis of the preserved brain tissue from this first case [1] identified the presence of a T→C substitution at position 526 within exon 6 of gene on chromosome 14 that encodes for a key protein that complexes with 3 other proteins to form the gamma secretase complex (see follow-up studies [2]). Known as the presenilin 1 gene (PSEN1), mutations have now been linked as a causative agent in many cases of familial EOAD (early-onset Alzheimer's disease); early-onset cases comprises only 5–10% of all cases, with familial forms being even less frequent at only 13% of the EOAD group. PSEN1 gene mutations are also implicated in extremely rare cases of very early-onset Alzheimer's disease (VEOAD), as shown for the case of an affected 32-year-old with dementia, with the very youngest known case to be 24 years old [3].

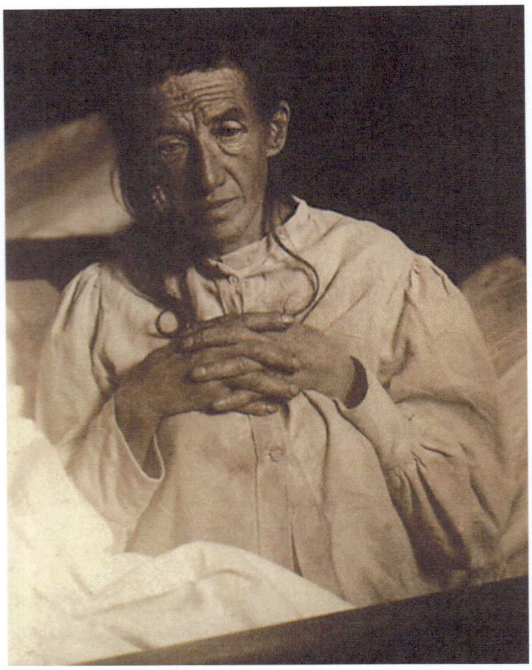

Fig. 7.1 Alzheimer's initial patient: Auguste Deiter (from Wikipedia)

Modern-day analysis of the remaining original tissue sections from the famous case of Auguste confirmed "...there were numerous neurofibrillary tangles and many amyloid plaques, especially in the upper cortical layers of this patient. Yet, there was no microscopic evidence for vascular, i.e., arteriosclerotic, lesions…" [4]. The APOE (apolipoprotein E) genotype of this patient was also shown to be homozygous for epsilon3, which is a neutral factor with respect to risk for AD, in contrast to Apolipoprotein E epsilon 4 (ε4) is considered to be a significant genetic risk factor for late-onset Alzheimer's Disease (LOAD); APOE epsilon 4 homozygosity can be found amongst Northern European Alzheimer patients at a high prevalence rate of 15.7 % for Sweden versus lower prevalence rates for AD patients from South Korea at 2.24 % [5]. In this regard, it is also noted that global geographic variations for the prevalence of dementia in the over 60-year-old population, with a low of 1.6 % for Africa versus 6.4 % for North America [6].

It is important to note that other case material originally studied by Alzheimer survive today for modern genetic analysis. In fact, his second case of early-onset dementia was a 56-year-old male named Johann F. who came to autopsy examination that curiously revealed only numerous amyloid plaques yet no neurofibrillary tangles in the cerebral cortex; subsequent 1997 analysis of this case from 1911 was also shown to be homozygous for apolipoprotein allele epsilon3 genotype and lacked mutations in the amyloid precursor protein gene at codons 692, 693, 713, and 717 [7].

Since the original 1906 and 1911 cases described by Alzheimer, worldwide recognition and concern for this disease continues to grow as there currently are now over 25 million affected individuals worldwide; in the US alone, economic costs of the disease are substantial, and anticipated to exceed $1 trillion by 2050 [8]. Most importantly, AD limits lifespan, as the median survival time for those newly diagnosed with disease ranges from 3 to 6 years [9]. Despite the alarming implications for limiting survival and despite the high prevalence and cost, there remains little in the way of inexpensive and easy accessible biomarker testing to accurately diagnose Alzheimer's disease and grade disease activity. With regards to AD biomarkers, diagnostic testing of spinal fluid may include checking for the proteolytic fragment of the amyloid precursor protein, Aβ1-42, in addition to total tau (t-tau) and phosphorylated tau 181 protein (p-tau) levels; imaging studies include structural MRI to assess hippocampal volume as well as experimental approaches with functional MRI. Although brain SPECT is relatively inexpensive, brain PET imaging of glucose metabolism with 18F-FDG is a more accurate and sensitive test for AD-associated posterior parietal hypometabolism; brain PET imaging of amyloid avid tracers is a new emerging option to evaluate differential diagnostic possibilities.

A basic clinical approach to the diagnostic evaluation of suspected Alzheimer's dementia is outlined in Fig. 7.2. Lab tests are needed to

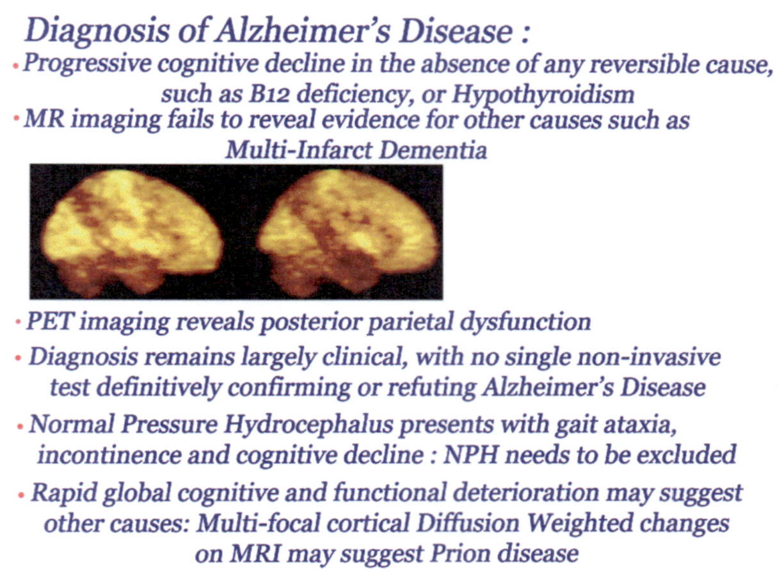

Fig. 7.2 Differential diagnosis of Alzheimer's disease (AD) and general clinical approach

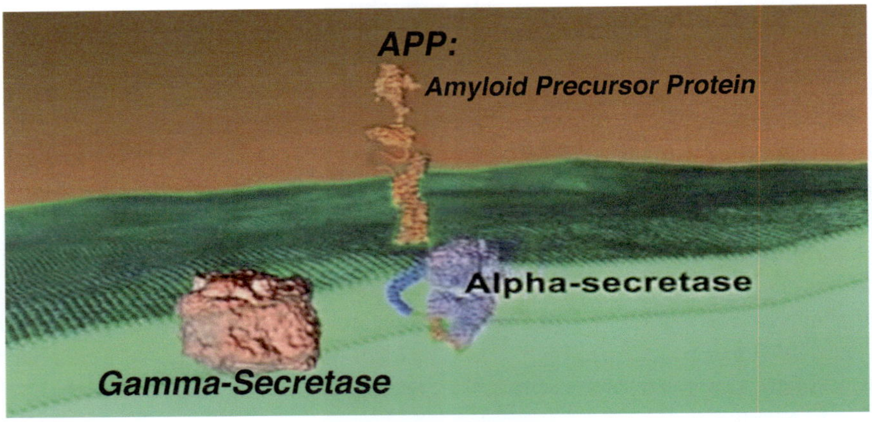

Fig. 7.3 Intramembranous nature of amyloid precursor protein (APP)

exclude vitamin B12 deficiency and hypothyroidism; CT and/or MRI are helpful in excluding multi-infarct dementia as well as normal pressure hydrocephalus, with MRI diffusion sequences being critically important for evaluating rapidly progressive severe dementia, as patchy segmental diffusion restriction within the cerebral cortex may identify patients with the rarely encountered Creutzfeldt–Jacob disease. PET and/or SPECT imaging of the brain can help give clues to the diagnosis of AD if posterior parietal defects in metabolism or perfusion are present.

An interesting story regarding the important role of amyloid formation in the development of Alzheimer's disease begins with an understanding about the normal functions for the amyloid precursor protein (APP; see Fig. 7.1). Known to be an ancient and highly conserved protein, it is encoded by a gene within chromosome 21, which likely interrelates to the high incidence of Alzheimer type neuropathologic changes seen in trisomy 21 (Down's syndrome). APP is an integral membrane protein found in many types of tissue but highly concentrated within neurons and especially at synapses, where it plays a role in synapse formation and repair, as well as in brain development, memory, and synaptic plasticity [10]. As shown in Fig. 7.3, most of the molecules are extracellular; after enzymatic processing, extracellular fragments are released that are felt to be neuroprotective. APP also seems to play a role in fast anterograde axonal transport, where a 15 amino acid peptide sequence from the cytoplasmic C terminus of APP mediates the interaction of kinesin with cargo needed to transport material down the axon [11], suggesting APP normally activates axonal mechanisms for fast transport to take place.

The amyloid hypothesis for the pathogenesis of AD focuses on how APP is processed by cellular enzymes (Fig. 7.4), which normally occurs by the action of alpha secretase followed by that of beta secretase. In AD, amyloidogenic fragments can be generated by the sequential action of beta secretase upon the intramembranous APP molecule, followed by the action of the gamma secretase enzyme complex (Fig. 7.5). The complex is comprised of four different proteins: Nicastrin, anterior pharynx-defective 1 (APH-1), presenilin enhancer 2 (PEN-2), as well as Presenilin (Fig. 7.6). Aside from being able to cleave the membrane-spanning domain of APP, it can act upon other signaling proteins, including the very important Notch signaling pathway for cell-to-cell communication. Notch is a cell-surface receptor that interacts with transmembrane ligands on neighboring cells; cleavage by gamma secretase releases the Notch intracellular domain fragment (NICD), which then enter the cell nucleus to regulate gene transcription.

Gamma secretase will cleave APP in multiple ways to liberate a variety of peptide fragments varying from 39 to 42 amino acids in length (Fig. 7.7), with Aβ40 being the most common

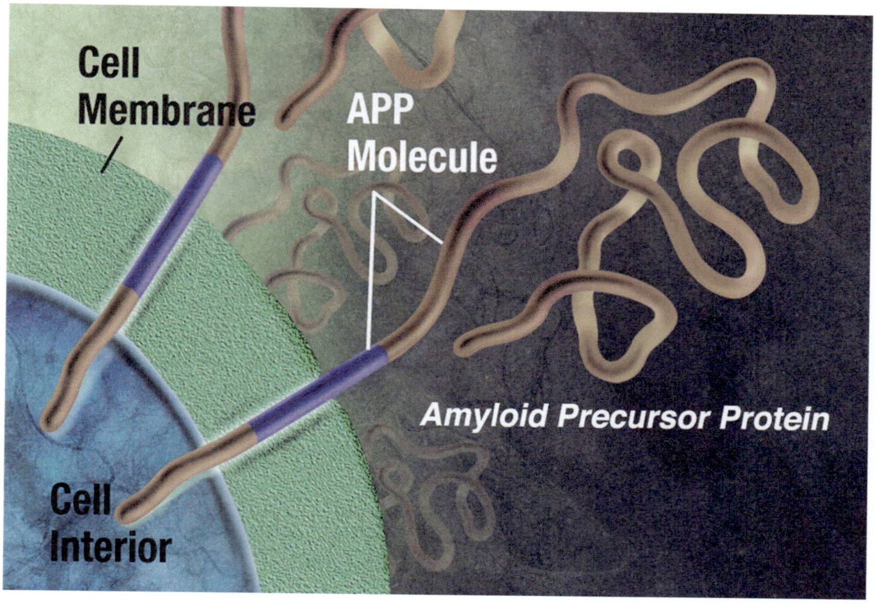

Fig. 7.4 Amyloid precursor protein (APP) has a large extracellular domain

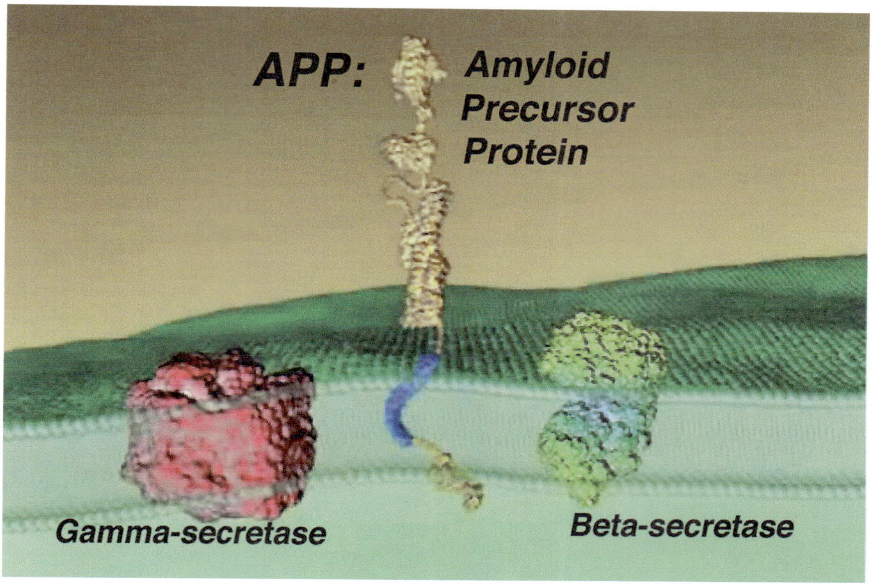

Fig. 7.5 Beta and gamma secretase can cleave APP to generate amyloidogenic fragments

type yet Aβ42 is a dangerous form that can lead to self-aggregation, forming toxic clumps of amyloid (Figs. 7.8 and 7.9). Mutations within the APP and presenilin genes are associated with increased Aβ42 production, thereby causing early-onset form of familial AD. The histologic changes characteristically show extracellular clumped collections of beta-amyloid within senile plaques in the late-onset form of the disease (LOAD), as shown in Fig. 7.10. As shown in Fig. 7.11, the neuropathologic changes for AD show not only large extracellular amyloid

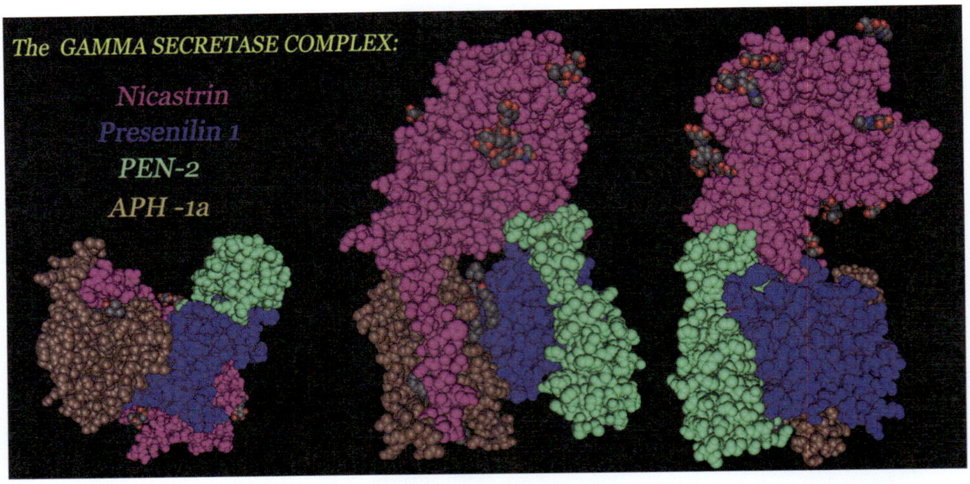

Fig. 7.6 The gamma secretase complex

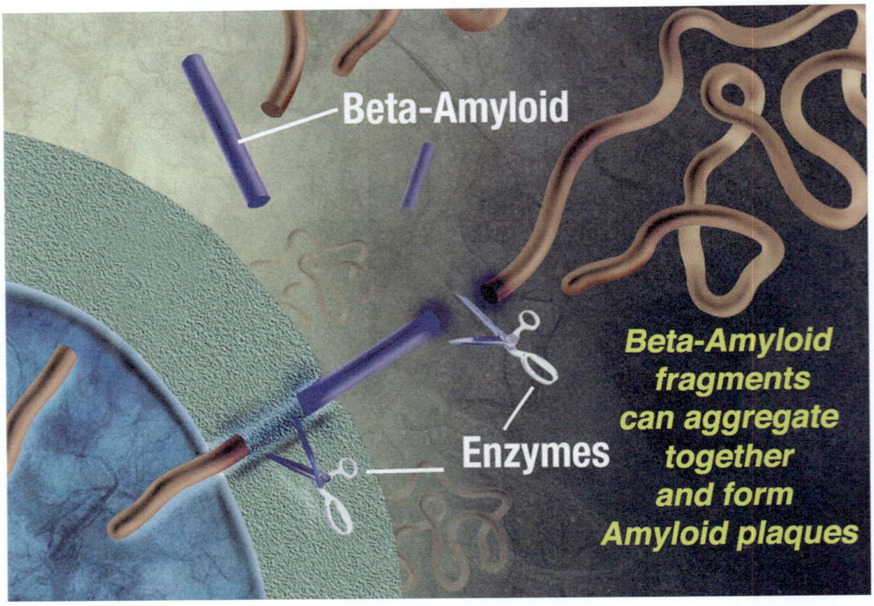

Fig. 7.7 Beta amyloid fragments arise from amyloid precursor protein (APP) cleavage

plaques but also reveal intraneuronal neurofibrillary tangles.

To understand the pathologic changes that occur within the microtubule system in AD, it is important to appreciate the normal structure and function of tau (Fig. 7.12). By binding to microtubules, tau has a stabilizing effect and keeps the microtubule-based system of axonal transport intact and preserves the integrity of the neuronal cytoskeleton. As noted by Zhou et al. [12], the human tau gene is encoded by a gene on chromosome 17q21 that contains 16 exons with exons 2, 3, and 10 undergoing alternative splicing, producing six isoforms of the tau protein; in contrast to the fetal tau isoform that excludes exons 2, 3, and 10, adults express all six tau isoforms of tau that range from 352 to 441 amino acids in length, depending on the presence or absence of exons 2, 3, and 10.

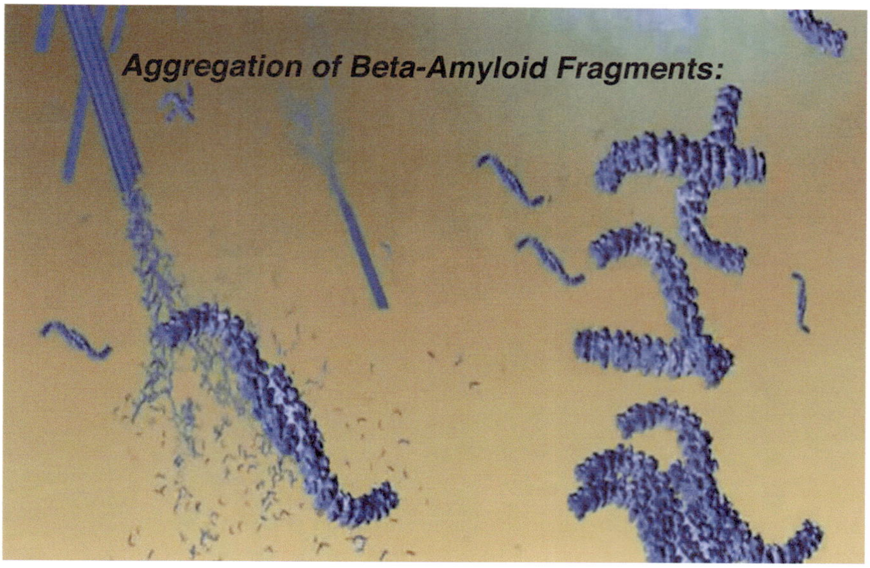

Fig. 7.8 Beta amyloid fragments can self-associate and aggregate together

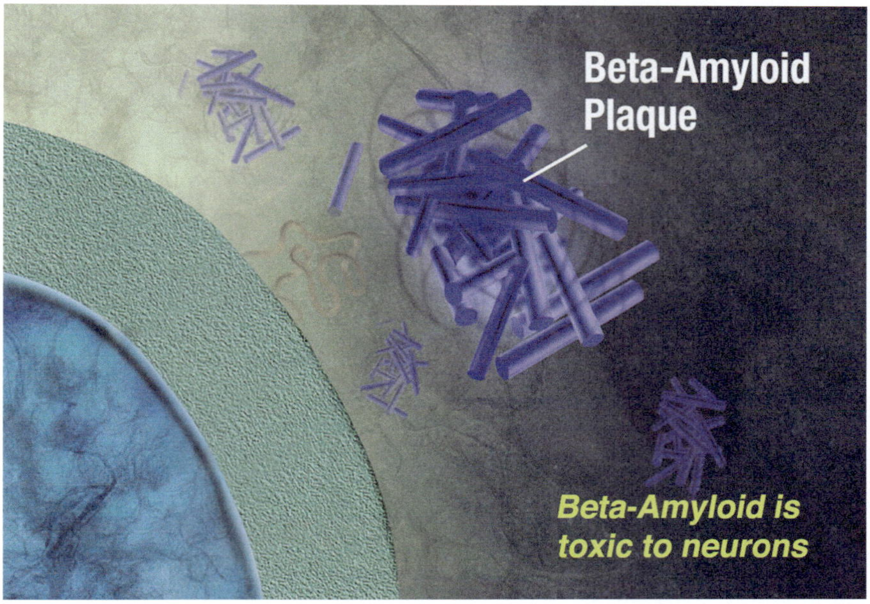

Fig. 7.9 Amyloid plaque formation

Tangles form within the brain tissue of AD patients when tau dissociates from the microtubules (Figs. 7.13 and 7.14). Comprised of hyperphosphorylated insoluble aggregates of disassembled microtubule-associated tau protein, the intraneuronal tangles actually appear to be paired helical filaments when examined by electron microscopy (Fig. 7.15). A summary illustration of the AD neuronal landscape is shown in Fig. 7.16 in contrast to the normal cellular architecture; after the affected neurons degenerate and die off, dense tangles may remain behind as well

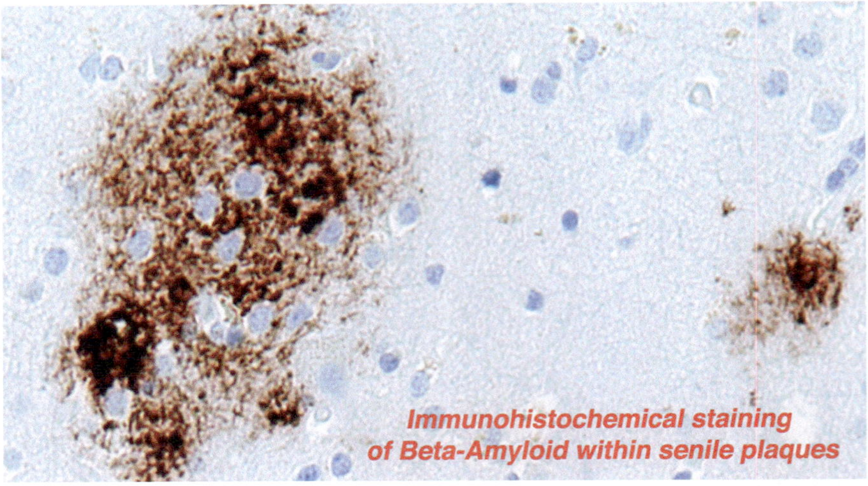

Fig. 7.10 Histochemical stains reveal the extracellular nature to beta amyloid (from Wikipedia)

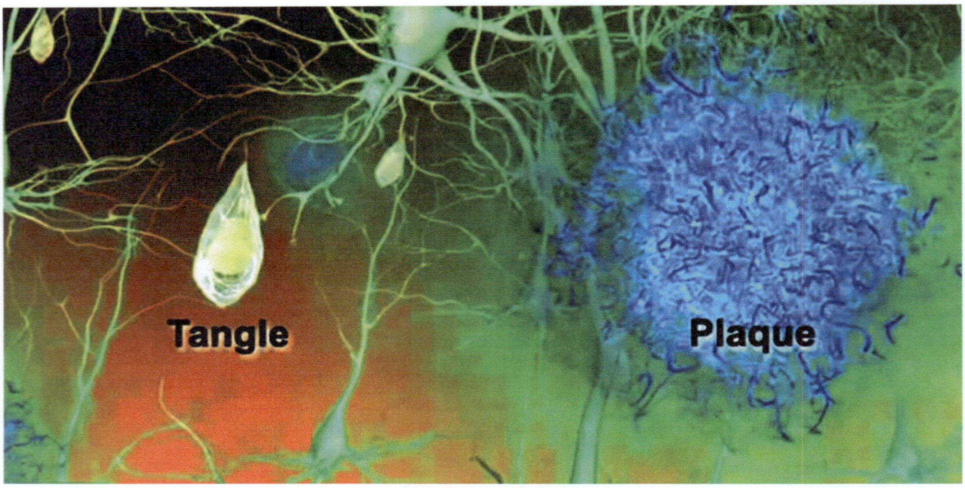

Fig. 7.11 Intracellular localization of tangles versus extracellular location of amyloid plaque material

("ghost tangle"). It should be noted that some forms of AD turn out at autopsy to predominantly show tangles with little in the way of plaque formation; one study estimated the incidence of tangle-only dementia at 3.9 % of all dementia cases examined with onset age averaging 84 years and death at age 88 years [13]. In general, the presence of tangles reflect the end stage of a progressive symptomatic and ultimately fatal paralysis of the microtubule-based system of axonal transport; however, an alternate view taken by other researchers is that this collapse of the axonal transport system reflects a secondary downstream effect of a more primary and devastating toxic effect elsewhere, such as from amyloid plaque. However, multiple types of gene mutations within the gene encoding the tau protein have been identified in not only AD, but also in fronto-temporal dementia as well as in progressive supranuclear palsy [12].

Regarding acquired factors that also produce neurofibrillary tangles and interrelate to AD

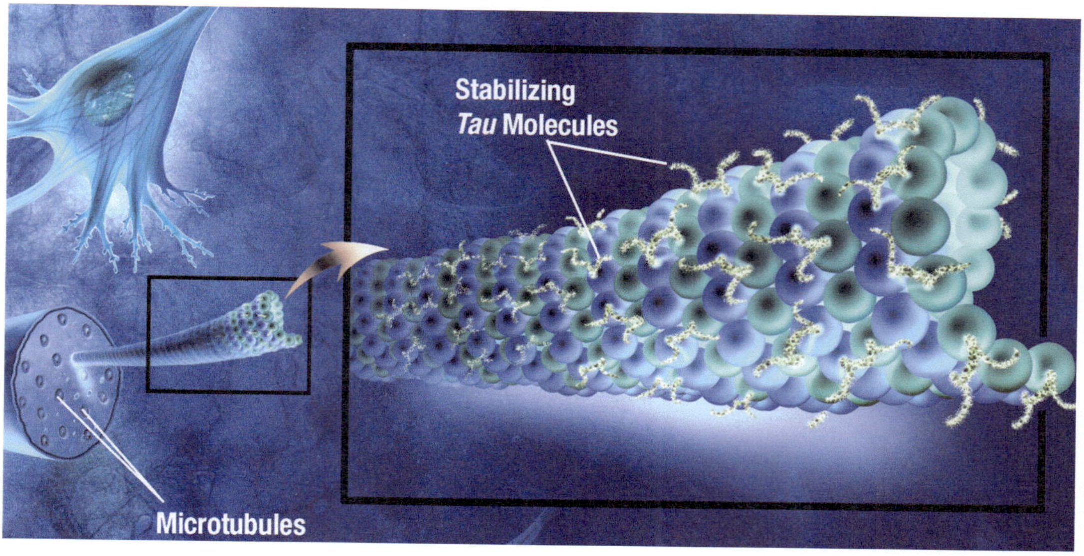

Fig. 7.12 Normal pattern of tau association with axonal microtubules

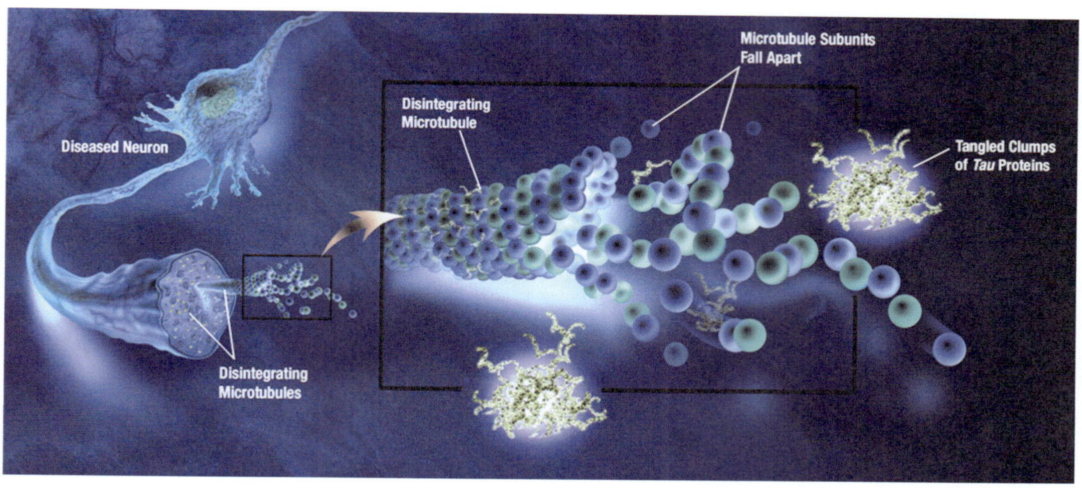

Fig. 7.13 Dissociated tau in Alzheimer's disease (AD)

pathogenesis, it is important to note that about 17 % of cases of repetitive concussion or mild traumatic brain injury may be at risk for developing chronic traumatic encephalopathy (CTE), as seen in Fig. 7.14. As noted by McKee et al. [14], although CTE shares many features of other neurodegenerative disorders, it is a distinct, progressive tauopathy with a clear posttraumatic etiology; in terms of the distinct neuropathologic findings, "….there are extensive tau-immunoreactive neurofibrillary tangles, astrocytic tangles, and spindle-shaped and threadlike neurites throughout the brain. The neurofibrillary degeneration of CTE is distinguished from other tauopathies by preferential involvement of the superficial cortical layers, irregular, patchy distribution in the frontal and temporal cortices, propensity for sulcal depths, prominent perivascular, periventricular and subpial distribution, and marked accumulation of tau-immunoreactive astrocytes".

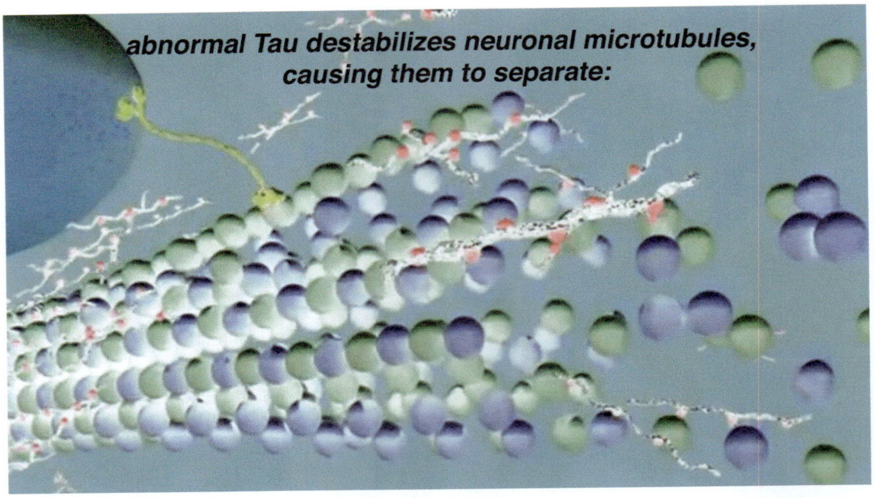

Fig. 7.14 Disassembly of microtubules in Alzheimer's disease (AD)

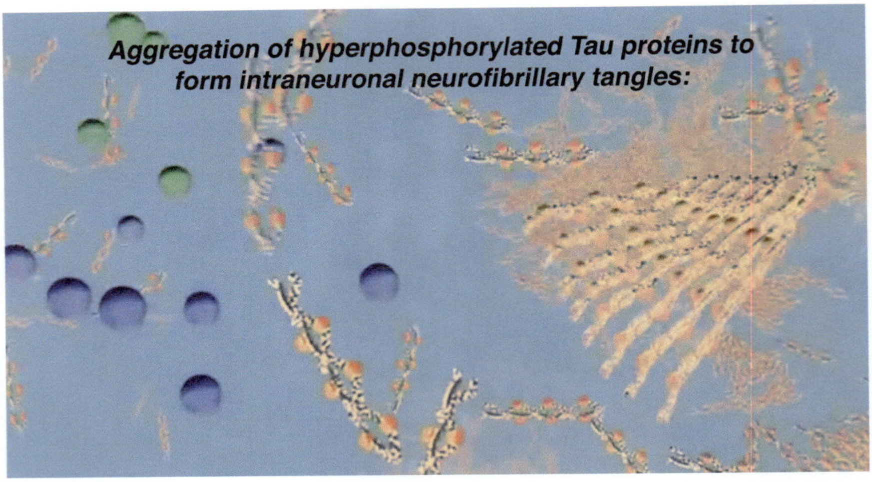

Fig. 7.15 Paired helical filament formation by phosphorylated tau

7.1 Clinical and Radiographic Aspects of Alzheimer's Disease

As illustrated in Fig. 7.17, brain SPECT can be very useful to reveal bilateral perfusion defects within the posterior parietal cortices consistent with the clinical impression of probable Alzheimer's disease for this 65-year-old female. As shown in Fig. 7.17, these bilateral functional defects are found in the absence of any structural lesion as shown by the negative brain MRI examination (see T2 axial section in the left-hand panel of Fig. 7.17). Despite having a lower resolution than PET, brain SPECT has certain advantages of accessibility and a relatively lower cost.

In contrast to brain SPECT, brain PET is a higher resolution test with greater sensitivity, and able to capture subtle yet definite patterns of progressive change over time; as shown Fig. 7.18, a clear and definite new reduction in glucose metabolism within the left posterior parietal cortex is evident 27 months after an initial

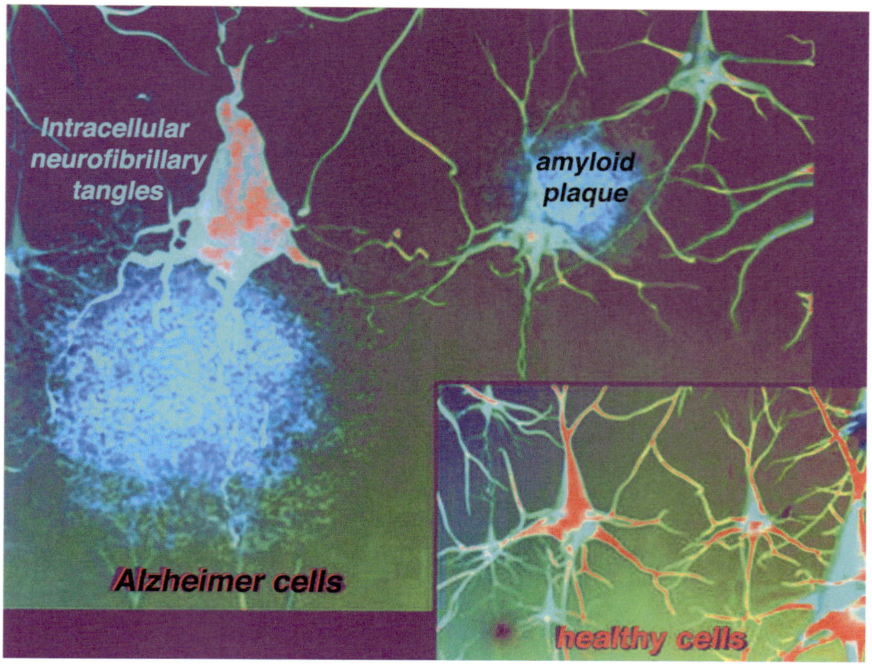

Fig. 7.16 Normal versus Alzheimer's disease (AD) neuronal landscape with numerous plaques and tangles

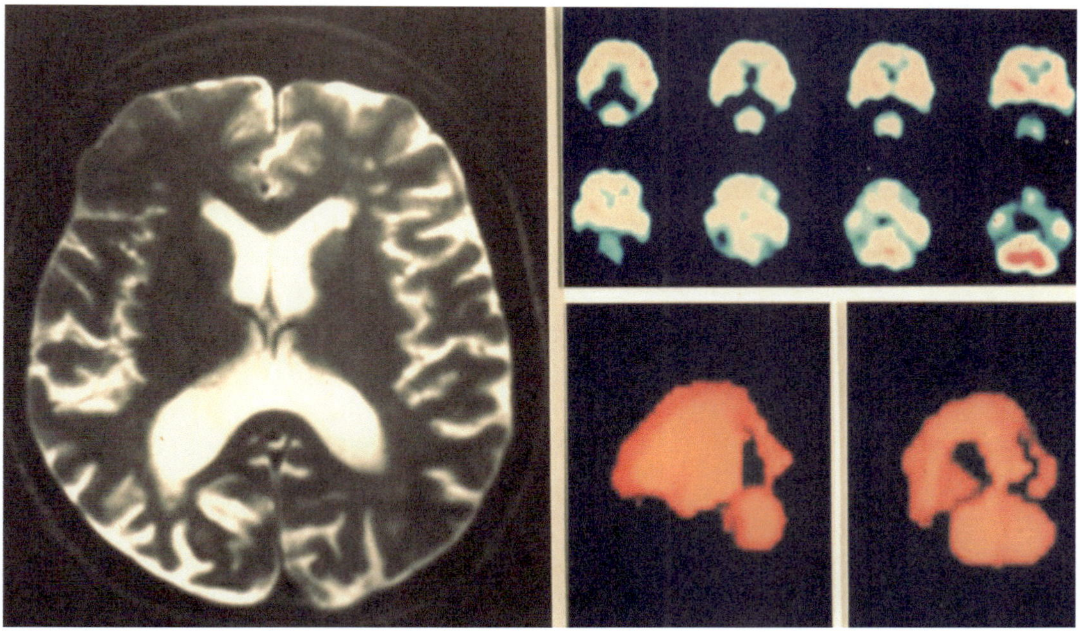

Fig. 7.17 Brain SPECT in Alzheimer's disease (AD)

PET scan revealed unilateral right posterior parietal hypometabolism that confirmed the clinical suspicion for Alzheimer's disease. The PET tracer used was the standard radiolabeled glucose analogue, 18F-FDG. Published studies have demonstrated the pre-mortem accuracy of FDG PET imaging in predicting the post-mortem neuropathologic diagnosis. As noted by Mosconi

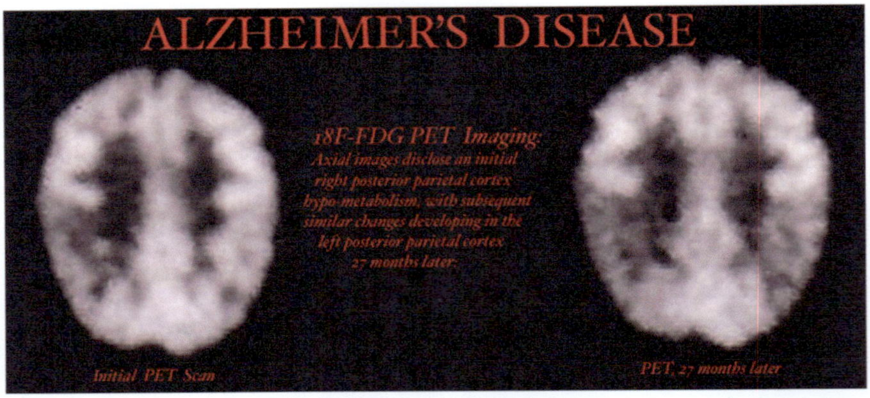

Fig. 7.18 PET can reveal subtle yet definite cortical metabolic changes over time in AD

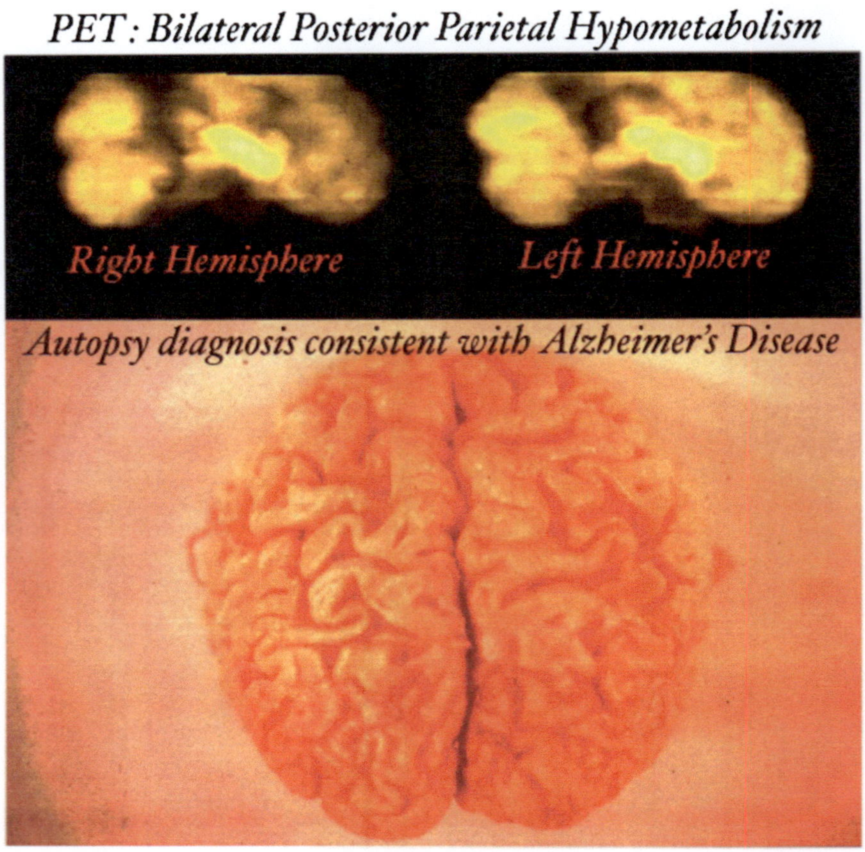

Fig. 7.19 Histologic examination post-mortem confirmed pre-mortem PET findings consistent with Alzheimer's disease (AD); note lack of focal posterior parietal atrophy on gross examination

et al. progressive metabolic reductions on FDG-PET brain imaging occur years in advance of clinical Alzheimer's disease symptoms in patients with pathologic verification of the disease at autopsy [15]. As shown in Fig. 7.19, bilateral posterior parietal defects on FDG PET imaging

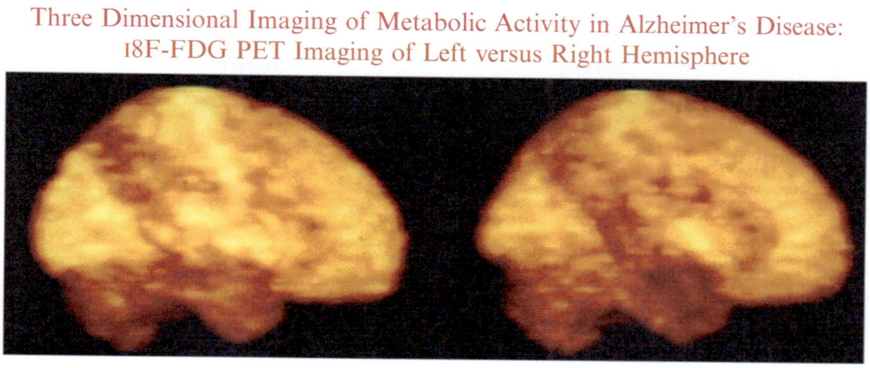

Fig. 7.20 3D reconstructions of hemispheric fluorodeoxyglucose (FDG) uptake in Alzheimer's disease (AD)

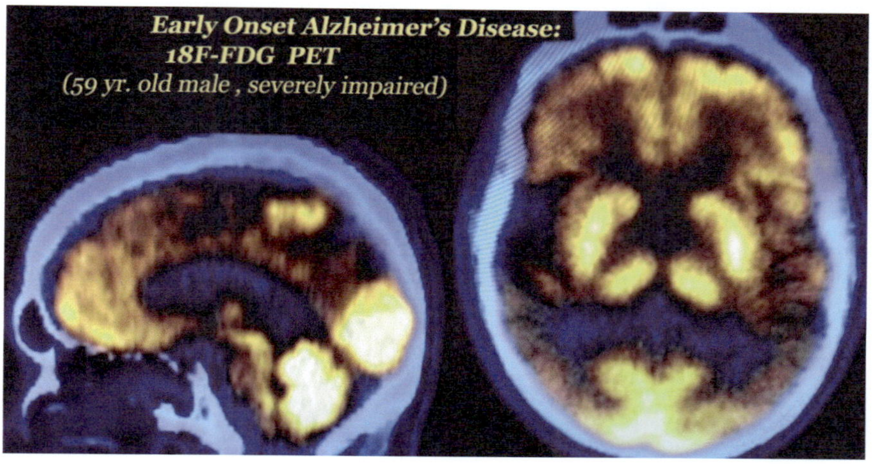

Fig. 7.21 PET findings in EOAD (59-year-old patient with progressive dementia)

in a patient with progressive dementia suggested a diagnosis of Alzheimer's disease, which was clearly confirmed at autopsy by histologic confirmation of numerous plaques and tangles; note that gross examination fails to reveal focal posterior parietal atrophy despite prominent bilateral metabolic and functional deficits seen during life by PET; bilateral posterior parietal deficits are shown for another AD case in Fig. 7.20, which uses three-dimensional reconstruction techniques to form minimal intensity projection images of hemispheric activity.

PET is particularly helpful in the assessment of younger individuals who require the most aggressive and comprehensive evaluation possible when early-onset Alzheimer's disease (EOAD) is suspected. As shown in Fig. 7.21, PET can be very helpful in identifying the characteristic posterior parietal defects that typically signify underling AD. As shown in Fig. 7.22 for another EOAD case, the original PET data can be transformed into a standardized format as statistical parametric map (SPM) that normalizes the data to a normative group of neurologically intact normal individuals; departures from normal are color coded as shown in the lateral hemispheric projections that support the EOAD diagnosis with noting posterior parietal metabolic defects.

What is the significance of the posterior parietal defects in AD? Does this reflect loss of small intrinsic GABAergic neurons within the posterior parietal cortex? To investigate the cause of

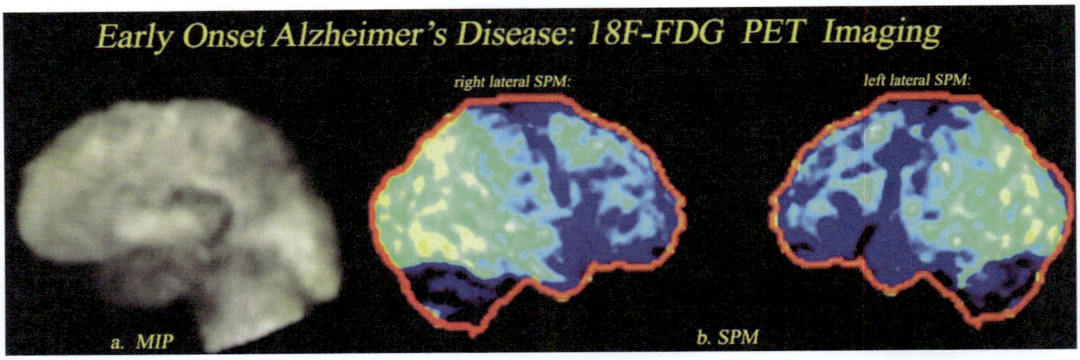

Fig. 7.22 Statistical parametric maps illustrate departures from normal control values

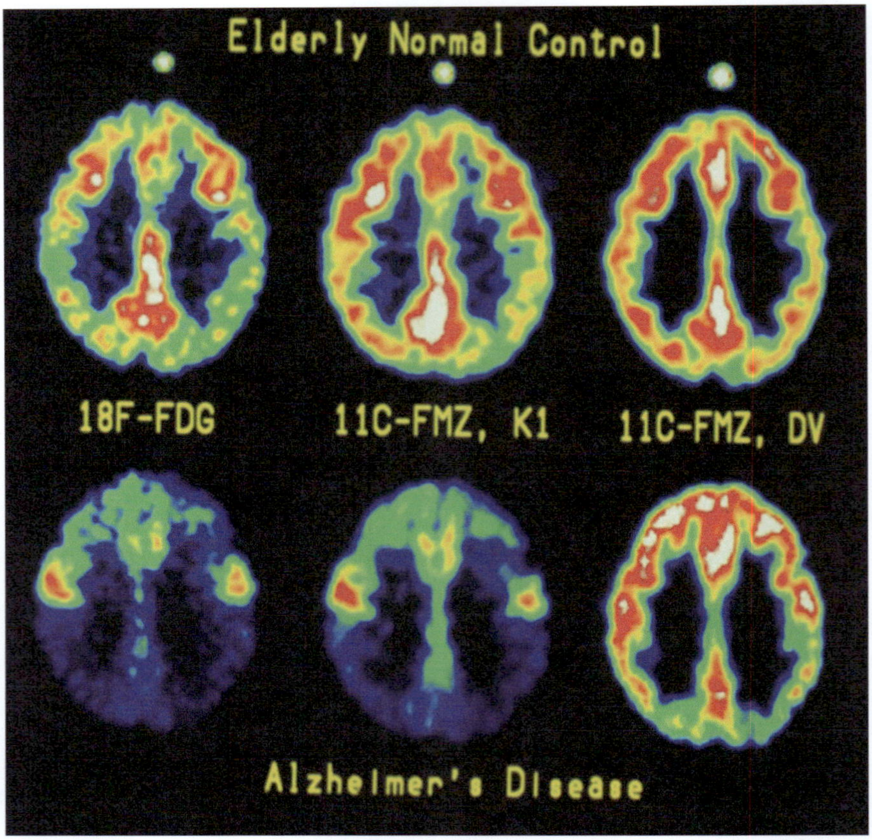

Fig. 7.23 11C-flumazenil binding in Alzheimer's disease (AD) to illustrate preservation of GABAergic synapses

these characteristic changes seen in AD, investigators at the University of Michigan used a radiolabeled ligand to reveal GABAergic synaptic receptors with 11C-flumazenil [16]. As shown in Fig. 7.23, flumazenil binding was intact within dysfunctional hypometabolic areas of posterior parietal cortex in AD, suggesting that the intrinsic cortical neuropil is intact but suffers from lack of activating input from the hippocampus and elsewhere.

An emerging technology in evaluating patients for developing possible AD is the use of PET to image radiolabeled ligands that bind amyloid, such as 11C-PiB (Fig. 7.24). One recent study from China has reviewed the literature and formed a collective analysis of 352 mild cognitive impairment cases reported from 11 studies [17]. The investigators found that pooled estimates of the sensitivity and specificity of PIB PET imaging for predicting conversion to AD was 94.7 % and 57.2 % respectively. Despite this suboptimal specificity of 57 %, one recent study found a good correlation between uptake of the amyloid PET imaging agents 11C-PiB and 18F-flutemetamol and amyloid-β measured by histochemical staining in frontal cortical biopsy specimens from normal pressure hydrocephalus (NPH) patients [18]. Of additional note, another recent study found 11C-PIB retention was limited to the high-convexity parasagittal areas in idiopathic NPH, versus the AD pattern of frontal and parietotemporal localization of the amyloid avid tracer [19].

It is important to note that many elderly patients with NPH may have co-existent AD, and may fail to improve after surgical procedures to shunt dilated ventricles. This was formally studied by investigators at the University of Pennsylvania who examined cortical biopsies obtained during shunt insertion and found that patients with little to no tau and Aβ pathology showed significant improvements after surgery yet those with moderate-to-severe AD pathology did not show improvement on any study measure of gait and overall clinical improvement [20]. Although some cases of NPH are of an extreme nature and require at the very least an attempt at shunting as shown for the case illustrated in Fig. 7.24, other more subtle presentations of NPH in elderly individuals may benefit from further investigation to insure the unlikelihood of co-existent AD; however, to complicate matters further, Alzheimer spinal fluid biomarkers may be misleading in normal-pressure hydrocephalus [21].

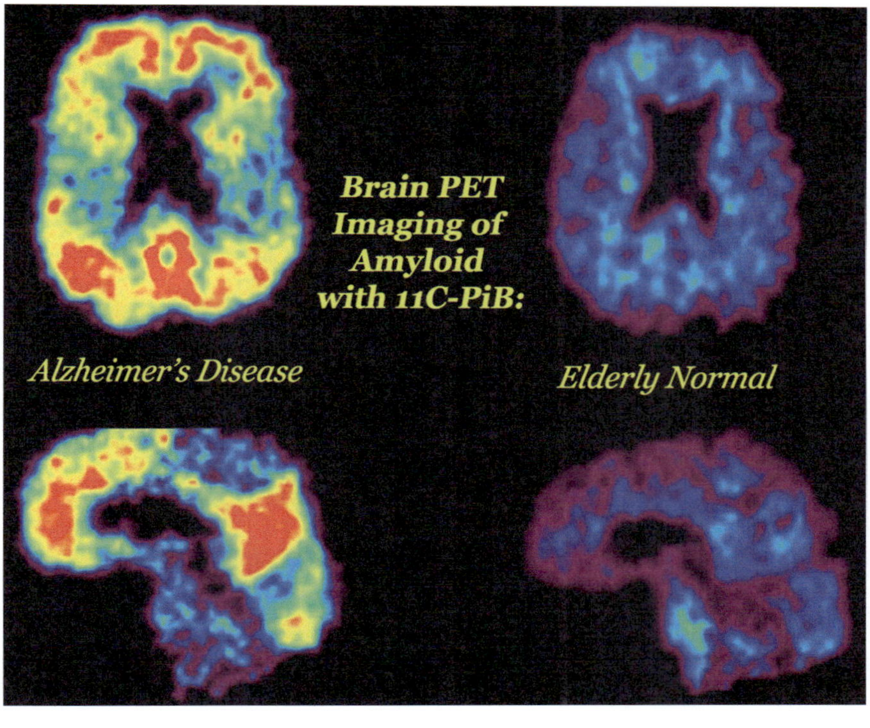

Fig. 7.24 11C-PiB PET imaging of brain amyloid deposits (from Wikipedia)

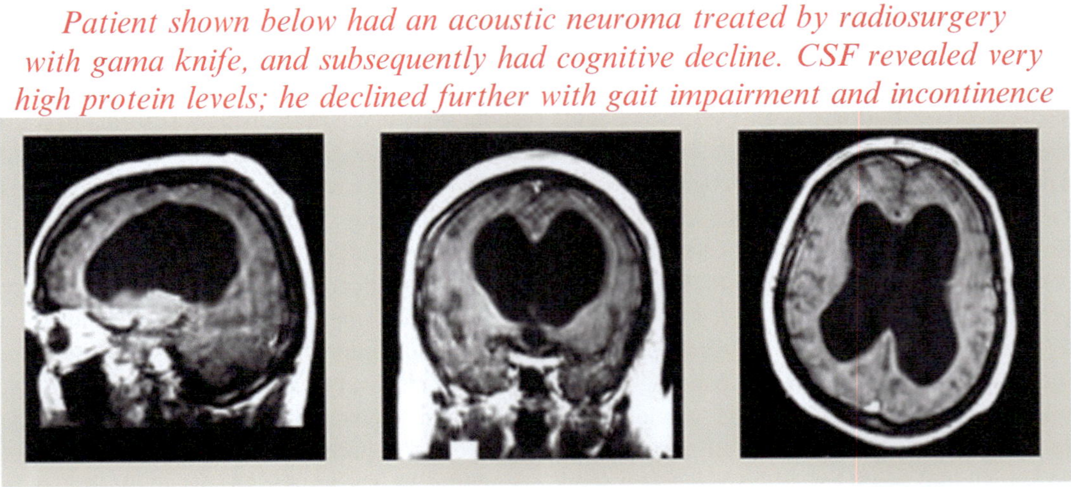

Fig. 7.25 Normal pressure hydrocephalus: an extreme example with very large ventricles

References

1. Müller U, Winter P, Graeber MB. A presenilin 1 mutation in the first case of Alzheimer's disease. Lancet Neurol. 2013;12:129–30.
2. Rupp C, Beyreuther K, Maurer K, Kins S. A presenilin 1 mutation in the first case of Alzheimer's disease: revisited. Alzheimers Dement. 2014;10:869–72.
3. Filley CM, Rollins YD, Anderson CA, et al. The genetics of very early onset Alzheimer disease. Cogn Behav Neurol. 2007;20:149–56.
4. Graeber MB, Kösel S, Grasbon-Frodl E, et al. Histopathology and APOE genotype of the first Alzheimer disease patient, Auguste D. Neurogenetics. 1998;1:223–8.
5. Ward A, Crean S, Mercaldi CJ, et al. Prevalence of apolipoprotein E4 genotype and homozygotes (APOE e4/4) among patients diagnosed with Alzheimer's disease: a systematic review and meta-analysis. Neuroepidemiology. 2012;38(1):1–17.
6. Ferri CP, Prince M, Brayne C, et al. Global prevalence of dementia: a Delphi consensus study. Lancet. 2005;366(9503):2112–7.
7. Graeber MB, Kösel S, Egensperger R, et al. Rediscovery of the case described by Alois Alzheimer in 1911: historical, histological and molecular genetic analysis. Neurogenetics. 1997;1:73–80.
8. Stefanacci RG. The costs of Alzheimer's disease and the value of effective therapies. Am J Manag Care. 2011;17:S356–62.
9. Helzner EP, Scarmeas N, Cosentino S, et al. Survival in Alzheimer disease: a multiethnic, population-based study of incident cases. Neurology. 2008;71:1489–95.
10. Nalivaeva NN, Turner AJ. The amyloid precursor protein: a biochemical enigma in brain development, function and disease. FEBS Lett. 2013;587(13):2046–54.
11. Satpute-Krishnan P, Degiorgis JA, Conley MP, et al. A peptide zipcode sufficient for anterograde transport within amyloid precursor protein. Proc Natl Acad Sci U S A. 2006;103(44):16532.
12. Zhou J, Yu Q, Zou T. Alternative splicing of exon 10 in the tau gene as a target for treatment of tauopathies. BMC Neurosci. 2008;9 Suppl 2:S10.
13. Noda K, Sasaki K, Fujimi K, et al. Quantitative analysis of neurofibrillary pathology in a general population to reappraise neuropathological criteria for senile dementia of the neurofibrillary tangle type (tangle-only dementia): the Hisayama Study. Neuropathology. 2006;26:508–18.
14. McKee AC, Cantu RC, Nowinski CJ, et al. Chronic traumatic encephalopathy in athletes: progressive tauopathy following repetitive head injury. J Neuropathol Exp Neurol. 2009;68:709–35.
15. Mosconi L, Mistur R, Switalski R, et al. FDG-PET changes in brain glucose metabolism from normal cognition to pathologically verified Alzheimer's disease. Eur J Nucl Med Mol Imaging. 2009;36:811–22.
16. Meyer M, Koeppe RA, Frey KA, Foster NL, Kuhl DE. Positron emission tomography measures of benzodiazepine binding in Alzheimer's disease. Arch Neurol. 1995;52:314–7.
17. Ma Y, Zhang S, Li J, et al. Predictive accuracy of amyloid imaging for progression from mild cognitive impairment to Alzheimer disease with different lengths of follow-up: a meta-analysis. [Corrected]. Medicine (Baltimore). 2014;93(27), e150.
18. Leinonen V, Rinne JO, Virtanen KA, et al. Positron emission tomography with [18F]flutemetamol and

[11C]PiB for in vivo detection of cerebral cortical amyloid in normal pressure hydrocephalus patients. Eur J Neurol. 2013;20:1043–52.

19. Kondo M, Tokuda T, Itsukage M, et al. Distribution of amyloid burden differs between idiopathic normal pressure hydrocephalus and Alzheimer's disease. Neuroradiol J. 2013;26(1):41–6.
20. Hamilton R, Patel S, Lee EB, et al. Lack of shunt response in suspected idiopathic normal pressure hydrocephalus with Alzheimer disease pathology. Ann Neurol. 2010;68(4):535–40.
21. Graff-Radford NR. Alzheimer CSF, biomarkers may be misleading in normal-pressure hydrocephalus. Neurology. 2014;83(17):1573–5.

8 Neurodegenerative Diseases

Progressive degenerative illnesses that affect the central nervous system represent a frustrating and tragic area of neurology that leads to major disability for the patient and is often untreatable. Although our knowledge about the molecular pathophysiology is growing at exponential rates, modern medicine still is unable to effectively halt or reverse neuronal damage incurred by mutations within specific genes. For example, although medications such as carbidopa-levodopa may provide temporary symptomatic relief from tremor and rigidity due to the central dopamine deficiency incurred by Parkinson's disease, there still is no safe and effective treatment for the underlying degenerative process that leads to premature dopaminergic cell death. To complement the detailed pathophysiologic discussion in Chap. 7 on Alzheimer's as the most common type of neurodegenerative disease, this chapter focuses on disease pathophysiology of Parkinson's disease (PD) as the second most common degenerative brain disease and contrasts this to the less common problem of Huntington's (HD) and even rarer diseases such as DRPLA (dentatorubral-pallidoluysian atrophy). Neurodegenerative illness is such a broad topic that only major examples are highlighted here across the spectrum of common (PD) to infrequent (HD) to rare (DRPLA) with common pathophysiologic themes tied to gene mutations illustrated by reviewing other related diseases such as fronto-temporal dementia and the ALS-Parkinson dementia complex of Guam; the most common autosomal recessive neurodegenerative disease of childhood is also reviewed (neuronal ceroid lipofuscinosis, or NCLF).

Although written descriptions of PD date back to Chinese texts from 1000 BC, the first formal medical report was published in 1817 by Dr. James Parkinson. The characteristic bradykinesia and tremor in combination with altered gait became widely recognized as hallmarks of the disease (see 1886 illustration in Fig. 8.1). Almost one century later, Tretiakov confirmed the earlier microscopic changes described by Fredrich Lewy, including neuronal loss of pas compacta neurons of the substantia nigra within the midbrain and named the intraneuronal protein aggregate type inclusions after their discoverer and named them Lewy bodies. As shown in Fig. 8.2, the typical Lewy body inclusion represents an aggregate of a protein known as alpha-synuclein [1, 2]. Other major components are ubiquitin and neurofilament protein. Minor components include LRRK2 which is found normally within the endoplasmic reticulum of dopaminergic neurons, HDAC6, which is a key protein linked to autophagy, and CHMP2B, which is part of the endosomal sorting complex for protein degradation [3].

The key component, alpha-synuclein, is a protein normally concentrated within presynaptic nerve terminals. Mutations within the SNCA gene encoding the protein have been linked to PD

M.A. Meyer, *Neurologic Disease*, DOI 10.1007/978-3-319-39581-4_8

and appear to induce the altered synuclein protein to self-aggregate into beta pleated sheets which then form lengthy fibrils and eventually a spherical aggregate in the form of a Lewy body. A prion-like transmission of alpha-synuclein aggregates has been hypothesized; after being liberated to the extracellular space after a diseased neuron dies, the misfolded α-synuclein could then enter other neurons and act as a template, seeding the aggregation of other synuclein molecules and initiating the formation of other Lewy bodies [4].

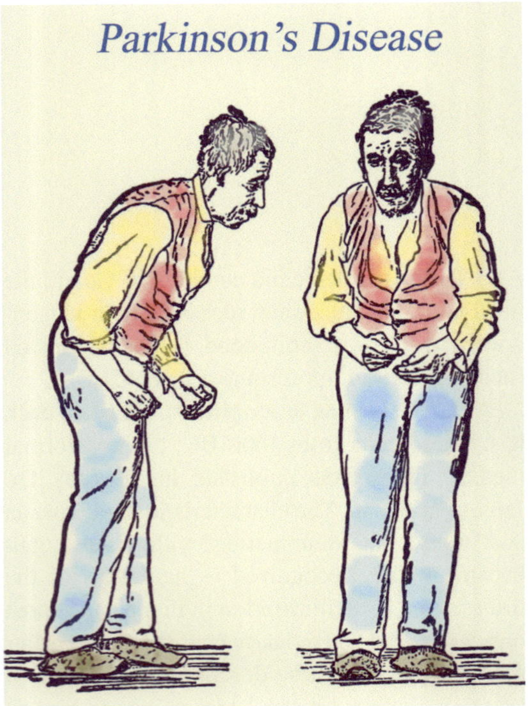

Fig. 8.1 Illustration of Parkinsonian gait and posture from the classic 1886 text of Gowers

Mutations within the LRRK2 gene are found in 10 % of autosomal dominant familial PD cases, versus 3.6 % of sporadic PD cases; it is important to note however that mutations also occur in 1.8 % of healthy controls [5]. Normally found in the endoplasmic reticulum, the large LRRK2 protein may serve as a scaffold for the assembly of other proteins; PD-related mutations seem to alter the enzymatic activity of the kinase portion of the protein or may alter the GTPase functional aspect.

In general, genetic factors are important considerations as 10–30 % of PD patients have a first-degree relative also affected by the disease. Genetic factors are especially important for familial juvenile and early-onset PD, where mutations in the Parkin gene are found 80 % in patients with onset before the age of 20 but very rarely found in those with PD onset after age 50 [6]. The Parkin protein transfers ubiquitin to specific protein substrates for proteasomal and autophagic degradation; mutations may thereby reduce the clearance of toxic proteins [3]. However, substantia nigra cell loss is noted with

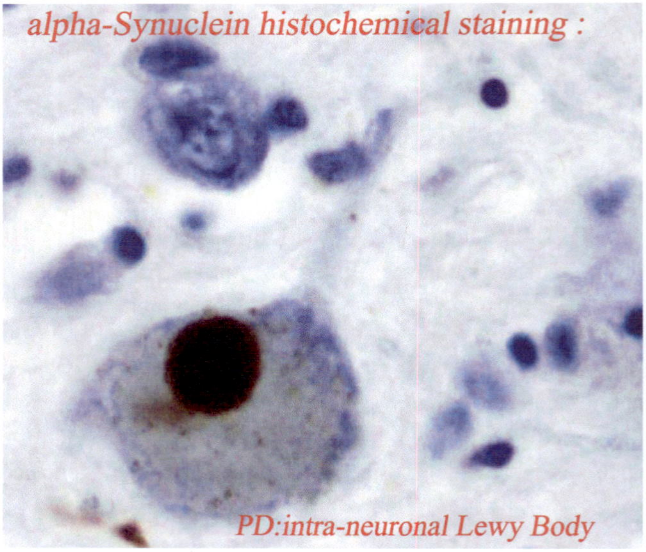

Fig. 8.2 Histochemical staining for alpha synuclein showing Lewy Body as a PD-related intraneuronal inclusion (adapted from Wikipedia)

symptomatic Parkin mutations yet without Lewy body formation.

Other genetic defects linked to early-onset PD include glucocerebrosidase (GBA) mutations in Gaucher's disease [7]. Known to be a recessive lysosomal storage disease, Gaucher's disease display features of Parkinsonism, and show numerous Lewy bodies within the cerebral cortex. Glucocerebrosidase mutations in PD patients are linked to earlier disease onset as well as a tendency for other family members to be affected [8].

As dopamine cannot be readily absorbed, the cornerstone of treatment for PD relies on the use of L-dopa in combination with carbi-dopa to enhance absorption. Orally administered L-dopa can then readily be absorbed from the gut and then be extracted from the circulation as a precursor for affected nigro-striatal neurons to then synthesize dopamine and overcome deficient stores of this necessary transmitter (Fig. 8.3); chirality of the dopa molecule is important as the dextrorotary form will not be absorbed. The necessary enzyme to convert L-dopa into dopamine is dopa decarboxylase, which relies on pyridoxine (vitamin B6) as a necessary cofactor.

Much advancement in understanding Parkinson's disease has taken place since its original 1817 description, including the ability to evaluate disease biology with SPECT (Fig. 8.4) and PET (Fig. 8.5) imaging. Using 18F-Fluorodopa, dopaminergic presynaptic terminals can be visualized with PET, whereas radio-iodinated ligands that bind to the presynaptic dopamine reuptake transporter can be visualized with SPECT (Fig. 8.4) [9]. Imaging the density of postsynaptic terminals using various 18F-labeled ligands that bind to D2 dopaminergic receptors can be accomplished using PET (see Fig. 8.5 for example of 18F-spiroperodol brain PET imaging of an individual with a writing dystonia—note diminished binding for the posterior left putamen).

Dopaminergic deficiencies in Parkinson's disease can affect activation of neurons outside the basal ganglia where D2 receptors predominate;

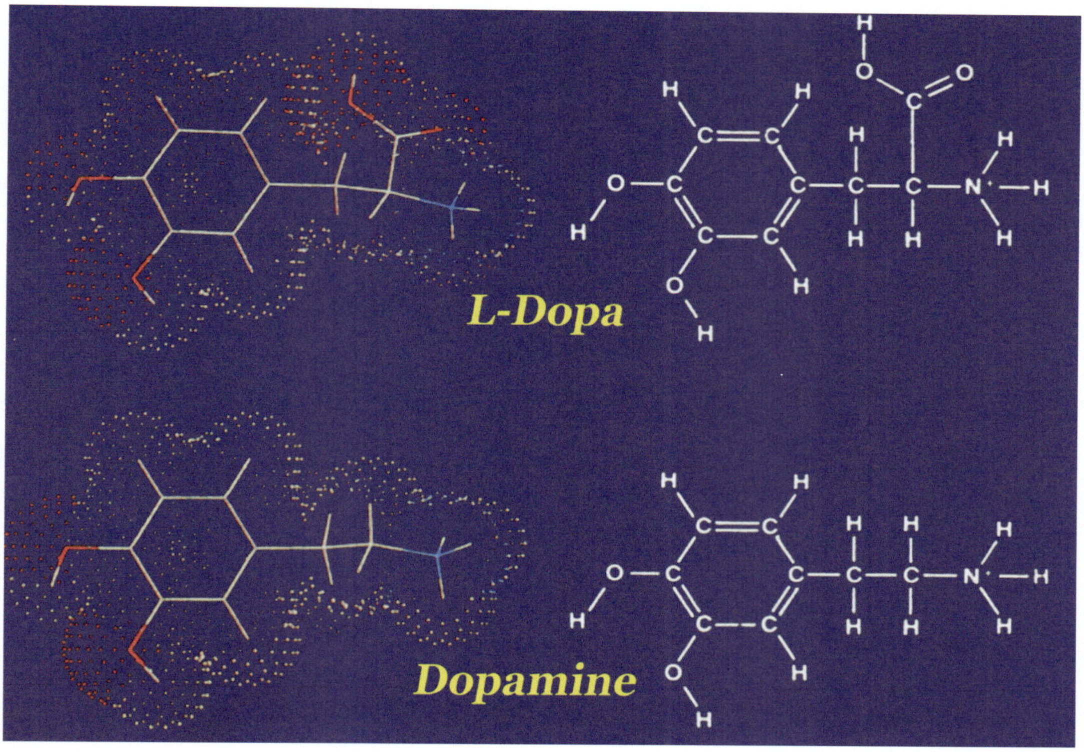

Fig. 8.3 L-dopa is converted to dopamine by dopa decarboxylase

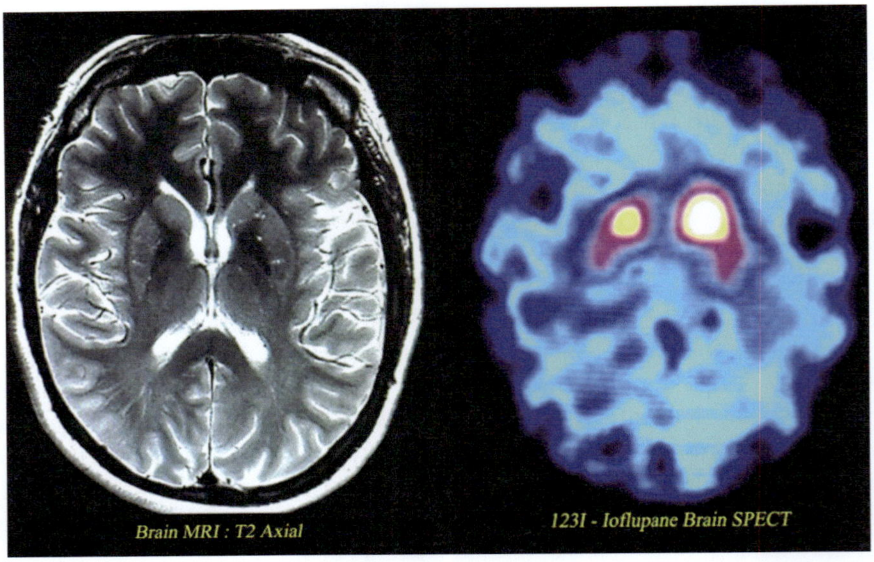

Fig. 8.4 Case example: New onset of left-hand tremor with minor involvement in left leg over time in a 59-year-old female with a family history of Alzheimer's disease. Using the presynaptic ligand Ioflupane that binds to the dopamine reuptake site, the scan reveals normal dopaminergic synaptic terminal density with the left basal ganglia yet markedly reduced on the *right*, corresponding to the tremor of new onset on the contralateral side. No obvious structural defects are evident on brain MRI shown at *right*

Fig. 8.5 18F-spiroperodol brain PET imaging of an individual with a writing dystonia—note diminished binding for the posterior left putamen

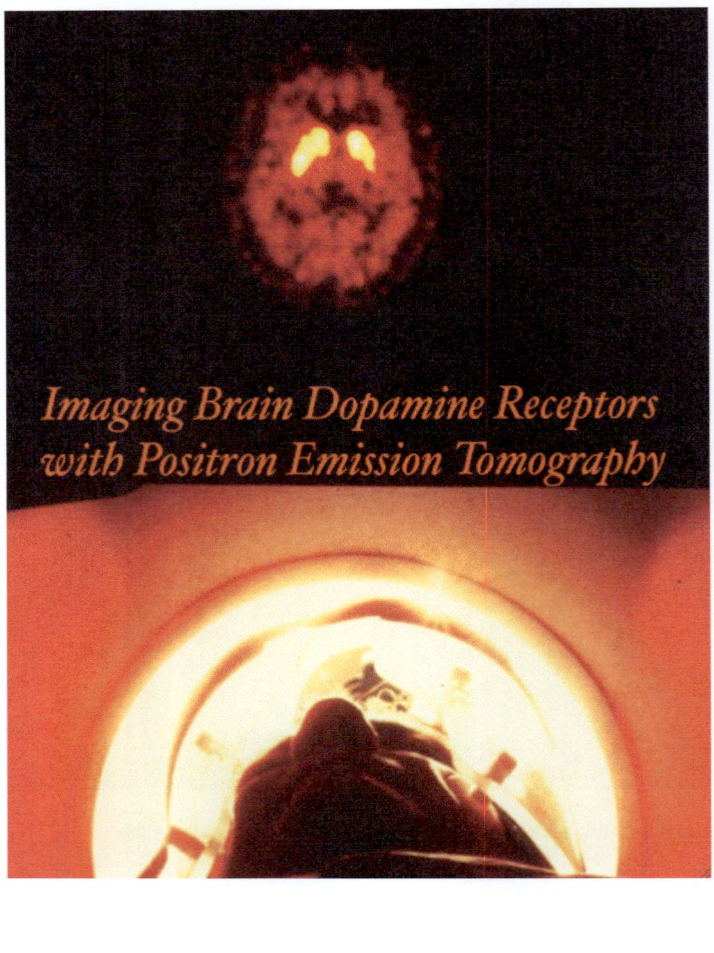

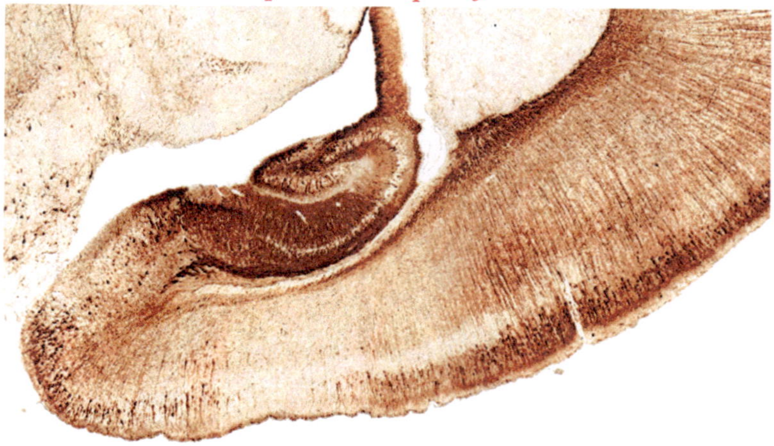

Fig. 8.6 It is important to note that dopamine deficiency in Parkinson's disease affects not only activation of D1 and D2 type receptors within the basal ganglia, but may also affect dopaminergic activation of cerebral cortex neurons that use D3 and D4 receptors, or other structures, such as the hippocampus, which has a dense population of neurons that use the D3 receptor subtype as shown here for the mouse hippocampus

as shown in Fig. 8.6, D3 receptors are found in the hippocampus and other cortical areas of the temporal lobes. As cognitive impairment can also occur in PD, altered activation of hippocampal D3 receptors may explain some of the behavioral and cognitive changes seen in advanced PD. D3 receptor imaging may be of importance not only in Parkinson's disease, but also in studying schizophrenia, anxiety, depression; D3 receptor imaging may be of help as well in assessing substance use disorders as there appears to be a role for the D3 receptor in drug-seeking behaviors [10].

Parkinson's disease with dementia has been found to coexist in unfortunate natives of Guam afflicted by ALS, leading to the description of a fatal progressive combined illness known as the amyotrophic lateral sclerosis—parkinsonism-dementia complex (ALS-PDC). Although surprisingly frequent amongst Chamorro families on the Pacific island of Guam, where the illness is termed Lytico-Bodig, a number of Japanese families located on the Kii peninsula of Japan and the Auyu and Jakai people of New Guinea have a similar illness [11]. The neuropathological changes consists of predominantly neurofibrillary tangles (NFTs) in both the brain and spinal cord; in this regard, it has been noted that mutations in the microtubule-associated protein Tau may be responsible for the illness [12]. The clinical features for the Guamanian form of the disease may show prominent ALS-like features with extensive arm and leg muscle atrophy (Fig. 8.7) coupled with fasciculation and progressive weakness. In contrast to the low incidence rate of 2.2 cases of ALS per 100,000 in the US population [13], ALS may occur more than 100 times more frequently in certain Guamanian villages, such as Umatac as noted by the pioneering field work of Mayo Clinic Neuro-Epidemiologist Dr. Leonard Kurland. In addition to adding support for linking ALS-PDC to tau mutations, a recent study also found linkage to a chromosome number 12 marker that is very close to the LRRK2 gene (leucine-rich repeat kinase 2) which is implicated to cause autosomal dominant parkinsonism and sporadic Parkinson disease.

Another neurodegenerative illness that has a well-defined pathophysiology is Huntington's disease, which runs within families as autosomal dominant problem that also shows anticipation, where age of onset seems to be at progressively earlier ages. Originally described within a Long Island, NY family by Dr. George Huntington in 1872, much has been discovered about this disease after localizing the mutated gene from an intensive 1983 study of affected families within two isolated Venezualan villages in the Lake Maracaibo region where HD incidence is 100 times higher than anywhere else, with overall study population comprised 18,000 people [14]. HD was later found to be attributable to an unstable trinucleotide mutation within the Huntingtin protein gene at chromosomal site 4p16.q3, with extra copies of CAG sequences encoding the

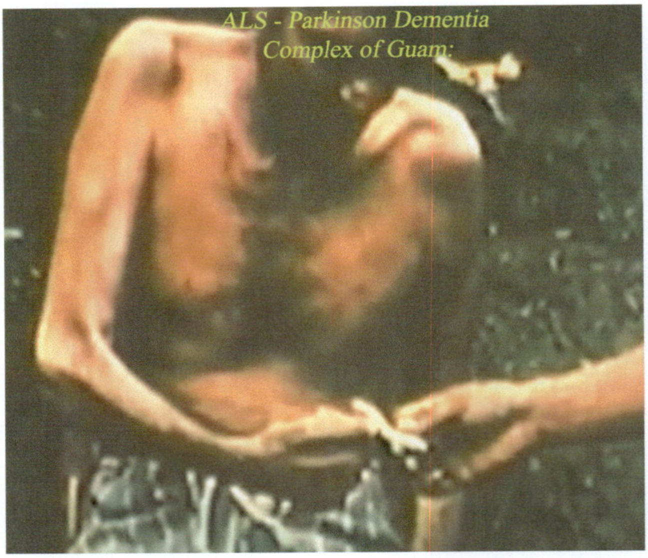

Fig. 8.7 Marked muscle atrophy with weakness in an individual affected by ALS-PDC

amino acid glutamine; it is hypothesized the expanded polyglutamine tracts within the protein causes it to misfold and assume a toxic conformation. Normal individuals have fewer than 26 repeats versus affected individuals having 40 copies or more of the CAG repeat sequence, with age of onset and disease severity inversely correlating to the number of repeats.

The toxic form of the misfolded huntingtin protein induces degeneration and loss of neurons within the caudate nuclei, thereby producing jerky, random, and uncontrollable movements known as choreiform movements; as the disease progresses, prominent cognitive changes take place along with neuropsychiatric changes of depression and anxiety. Degeneration of the caudate is very evident not only on MRI examinations, but also by PET imaging studies of glucose metabolic activity where the caudate head nuclei are barely visible (Fig. 8.8). Although no approved medication is available to halt the progression of this tragic disease, promising animal research has shown that antisense oligonucleotide infusion into the cerebrospinal fluid of symptomatic HD mouse models can be effective [15].

Members from a kindred from Northeastern Tennessee that traditionally had been thought to carry the clinical diagnosis of familial Huntington's disease presented to the University of Tennessee Medical Center in Knoxville in the year 1992 for further evaluation (Fig. 8.9). Although choreiform movements were present along with progressive cognitive and neuropsychiatric symptoms were present, many family members reported having seizures, which is unusual for HD; furthermore, close inspection of MR imaging studies disclosed extensive deep subcortical white matter changes (Figs. 8.10 and 8.11). As all these findings were not typical for HD, subsequent direct molecular testing failed to identify the HD expansion mutation in affected individuals. Although dentatorubral-pallidoluysian atrophy (DRPLA) was thought at that time to be a strictly oriental disease from Japan, molecular testing did demonstrate the presence of the characteristic CAG trinucleotide DRPLA expansion mutation in all affected individuals; furthermore, the size of the expansion correlated with the age of onset of clinical symptoms [16]. Since the original 1993 study of this Tennessee kindred, DRPLA has been recognized as a progressive neurodegenerative disorder with a worldwide distribution.

This rare degenerative illness has a disease pathophysiology that is similar to HD, and is caused by a toxic gain of function to the Atrophin-1 (ATN1) protein, presumably due to abnormal misfolding due to the presence of

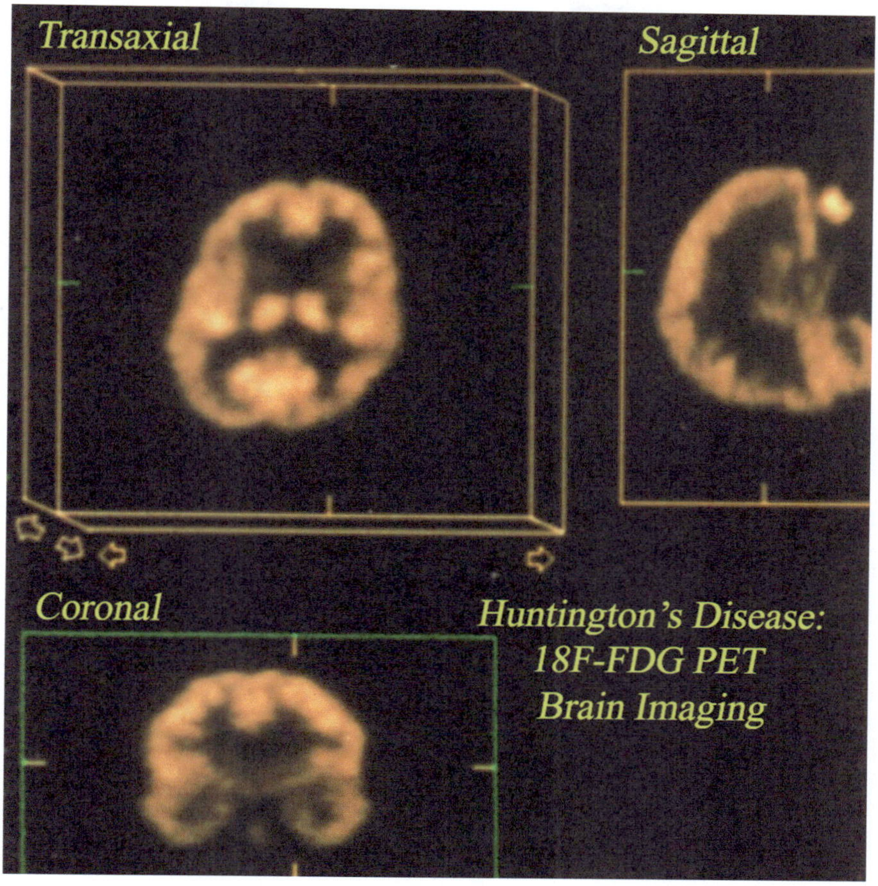

Fig. 8.8 Brain PET scan of patient affected by HD: marked hypometabolism of degenerated atrophic caudate head nuclei

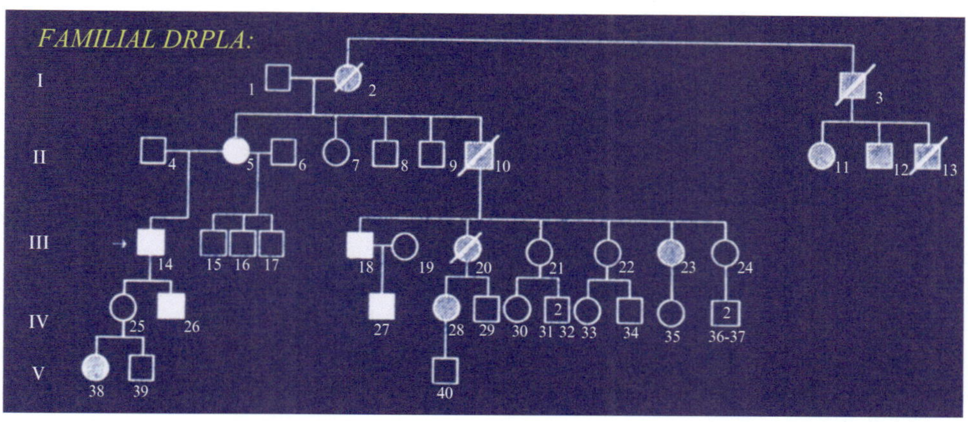

Fig. 8.9 DRPLA family pedigree showing autosomal dominant inheritance as well as genetic anticipation and phenotypic heterogeneity

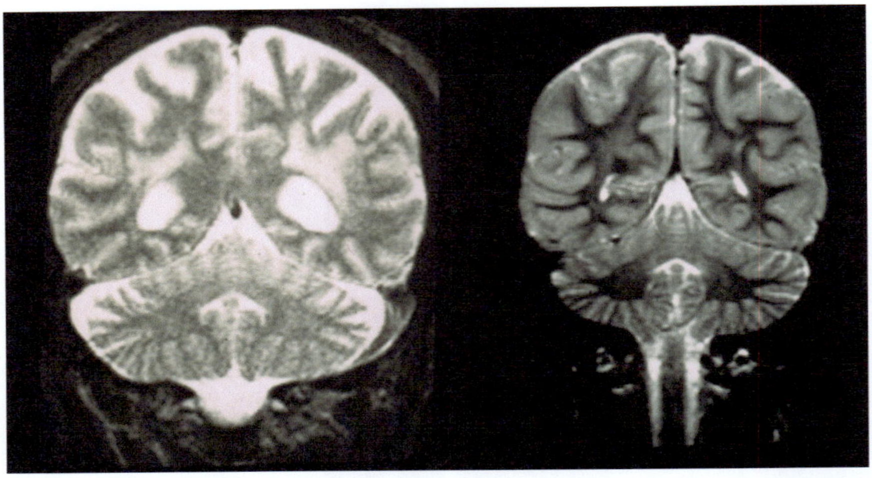

Fig. 8.10 DRPLA: confluent white matter MR signal abnormalities evident for both father (*left*) and son (*right*)

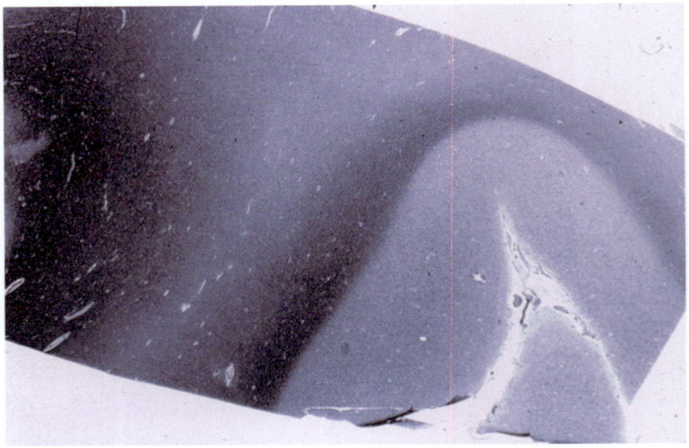

Fig. 8.11 Corresponding pathologic change of demyelination due to DRPLA for an affected relative who came to autopsy

extensive expanded polyglutamine tracts; normal individuals have fewer than 34 CAG repeats, whereas affected individuals display 49 or more repeats [17]. Normally found as a hydrophilic 1184 amino acid protein with several repetitive motifs including a variable length polyglutamine tract, ATN1 contains nuclear import and export sequences and normally acts as a transcriptional co-repressor and is expressed in all tissues including the brain. In DRPLA, abnormal accumulations of ATN1 can be found within the nucleus of neurons which appear deformed with nuclear membrane indentations [18].

Clinical evaluation of affected individuals show extensive white matter changes on MRI (Fig. 8.10), whereas PET imaging of those with advanced disease reveals extensive cortical hypometabolism with relative preservation of the occipital cortex (Fig. 8.12).

Whereas HD and DRPLA involve a toxic gain of function within an altered misfolded protein, alternate forms of dementia known as frontotemporal dementia (FTD) have their molecular basis in mutations that induce an incapacitating loss of function and are collectively known as tauopathies. Mutations within the gene on chromosome 17 encoding the key protein Tau induce a destabilization of microtubules within neurons that are vital to the process of axonal transport; without the normal stabilizing effect of Tau, microtubules that form the neuronal cytoskeleton disassemble and fall apart, inducing major neuronal

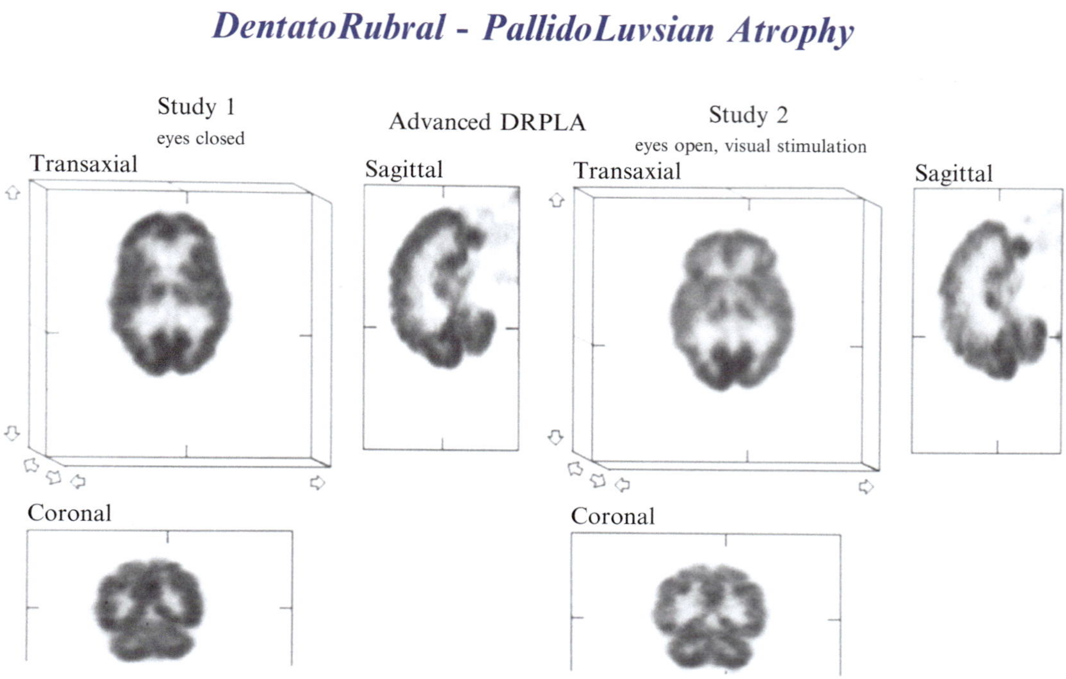

Fig. 8.12 DRPLA case example: cortical hypometabolism sparing the visual cortex is evident from this PET study, with caudate head hypometabolism noted as well

dysfunction and subsequent degeneration. In FTD, degeneration is remarkably severe in the frontal lobes, and is evident both on CT and PET imaging (Figs. 8.13 and 8.14); frontal lobe atrophy is very evident at autopsy (Fig. 8.13). The disease is found in less than 5 % of all autopsy cases of dementia yet accounts for 20 % of young onset dementia cases; survival after diagnosis averages only about 8 years [19].

First described in 1892 by neurologist Dr Arnold Pick, the disease was generally referred as Pick's disease until only recently when the preferred term of fronto-temporal dementia (FTD) was adopted to more accurately describe a broader spectrum of cases. As Pick body inclusions are seen only in the less common type of 3R repeat tau variant, it is important to note that exon 10 of the tau (MAPT) gene is alternatively spliced to generate either three (3R) or four (4R) conserved amino acid repeats in the microtubule binding domain of the tau protein; typical neurofibrillary tangles in FTD is comprised of both 3R and 4R variants [20]. When the mutation within the tau gene occurs within the splice junction of exon 10, tau depositions clump together not only within neurons but also in glial cells. Other classifications of the disease include FTDP-17T, which is frontotemporal dementia and Parkinsonism linked to chromosome 17 MAPT mutations versus FTDP-17U due to progranulin gene mutations with ubiquitin-positive, TDP-43 immunoreactive inclusions.

Although there are many molecular variants, there are shared clinical signs and symptoms that are fairly common amongst FTD patients, and collectively reflect frontal lobe dysfunction. Behavioral changes are evident with defects in cognitive skills for planning and organizing are noted along with poor impulse control. In contrast, perceptual and visual-spatial skills are relatively intact reflecting preservation of the occipital cortex; however, some patients will display progressive speech impairment. In this regard, some patients show language deficits as the initial presenting symptom in the form of slowly progressive aphasia (SPA, otherwise known as primary

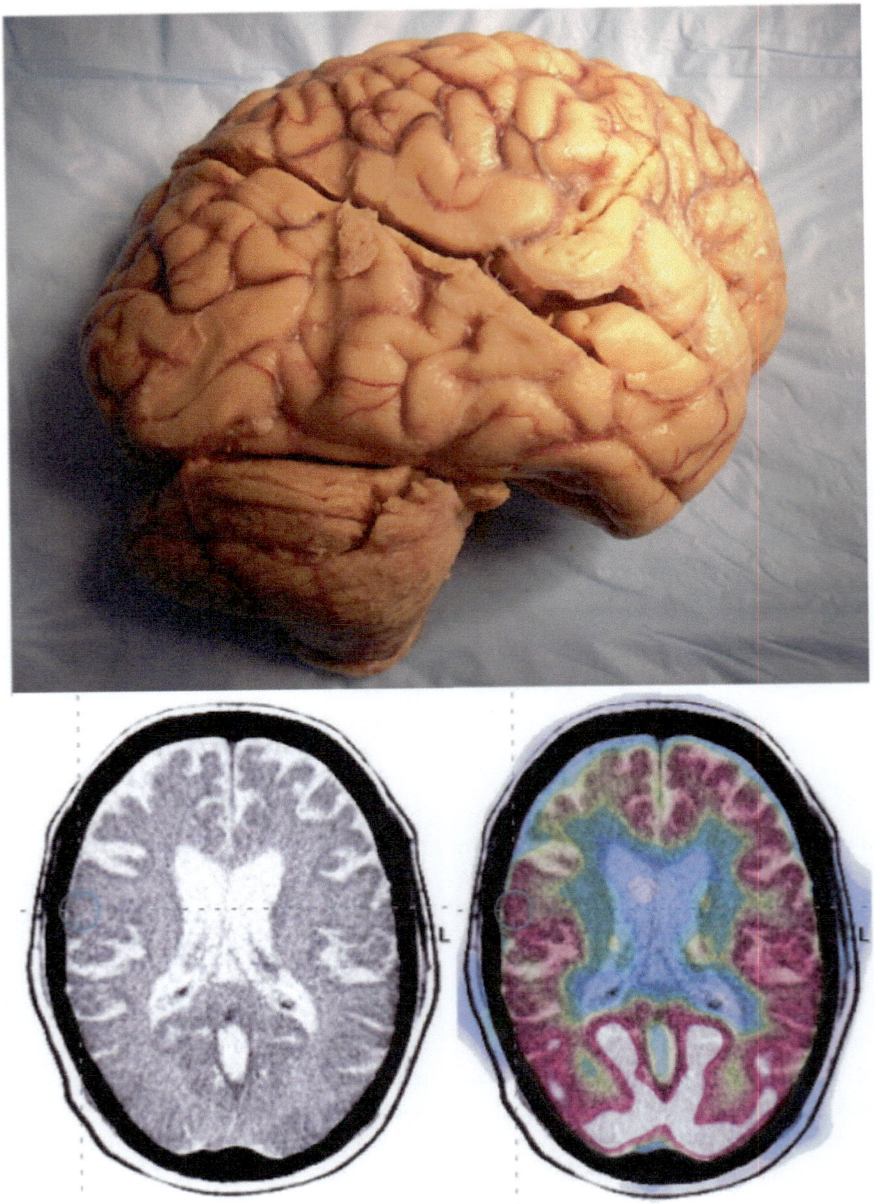

Fig. 8.13 Fronto-temporal dementia: PET detection of right frontal hypometabolism with corresponding right frontal atrophy seen on CT and later at autopsy

progressive aphasia; Fig. 8.15). Although some SPA patients progress to develop Alzheimer's disease, a disproportionate number seem to develop FTD with three subtypes noted: (1) progressive non-fluent aphasia, (2) semantic dementia, and (3) logopenic progressive aphasia [21].

Whereas FTD seems to develop at an age that is younger than that for Alzheimer's, with one study citing a mean onset of age 53 [21], there are a variety of rare neurodegenerative illnesses that produce dementia in young adults. Aside from early-onset cases of HD or DRPLA with large trinucleotide repeat expansions, there is a spectrum of neurodegenerative illnesses that can affect children and young adults known as neuronal ceroid lipofuscinoses (NCLF) that involve the

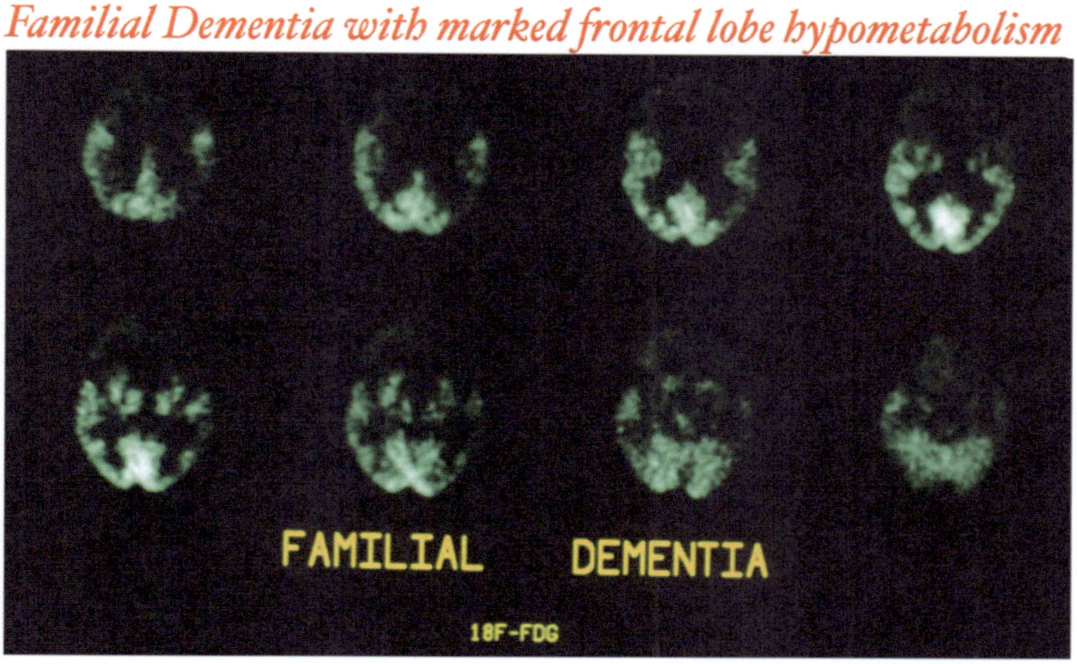

Fig. 8.14 Familial fronto-temporal dementia (FTD): Presumed FTD in a 82-year-old patient with progressively severe dementia presenting in an identical form experienced by an older brother who also had a FDG PET examination revealing an identical pattern of frontal hypometabolism; both had prominent frontal lobe atrophy on CT examination

pathologic intracellular accumulation of autofluorescent lipofucsin material due to defective lysosomal enzymes (Fig. 8.16). Although at least 10 different types have been identified, the most aggressive type has an infantile onset with myoclonic jerks, delayed psychomotor development with progressive deterioration and seizures. Collectively, NCLF is the most common autosomal recessive neurodegenerative disease of childhood [22]. The infantile form has the most rapid progression and is due to a gene defect within DNA encoding the enzyme PPT-1 (palmitoyl-protein hydrolase 1) that mediates lysosomal catabolism of lipid-modified proteins. Early visual loss leading to blindness occurs by age 2 years that progresses to a vegetative state by age 3. A later onset lysosomal defect occurs in Batten's disease, which is a fatal NCLF illness that first begins to affect young children between ages 2 and 5, and causes progressive mental impairment and seizures, with eventual loss of sight, speech, and motor skills. Animal models of NCLF have demonstrated early and prominent synaptic pathology which is particularly evident in the thalamus in advance of any major changes within the cortex [23]. An adult form of NCLF exists and is known as Kuf's disease with average onset age being age 30.

Another lysozomal disorder that strike infants and young children that produces severe neurologic degeneration with death by age 4 is the feared Tay-Sachs disease (TSD). First described in the 1880s by British ophthalmologist Dr. Waren Tay and New York Neurologist Dr. Bernard Sachs, the disease is now known to be caused by an ultimately fatal mutation in the gene HEXA that encodes thee alpha subunit of the beta-hexosaminidase enzyme which normally degrades GM2 gangliosides in central nervous system cell lysosomes [24]. In TSD, toxic accumulation of these autofluorescent gangliosides results in progressive neuronal dysfunction with eventual cell death (Fig. 8.17). Although TSD infants appear healthy at birth, neurological decline becomes evident by age 6 months. Like many other lysosomal storage diseases, early

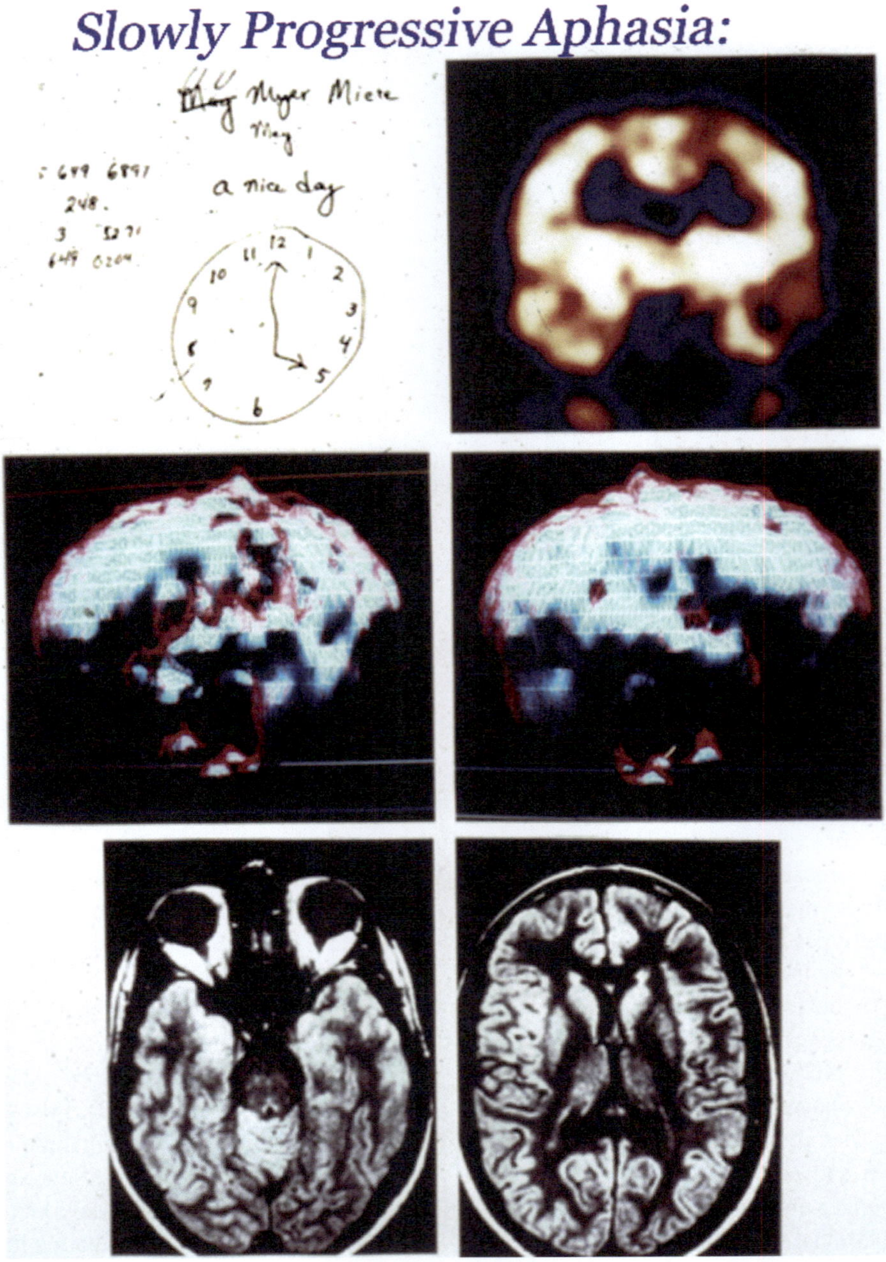

Fig. 8.15 Case example: slowly progressive aphasia in a 60–year-old female who had worked as a telephone receptionist, but then had progressive difficulty with expressing herself with difficulty writing as well, referable to SPECT defined left temporal dysfunction (MR negative for focal atrophy or other lesions). SPA is known to lead into FTD or AD, with a predilection for the former

pathologic MRI signal changes are prominently evident in the thalamus. At the same time that neuronal lipid accumulation occurs within the brain, a chalky white central halo within the macula becomes evident on examination of the retina, reflecting sphingolipid accumulation within the normally dense concentration of retinal ganglion cells; it is the central foveal pit that

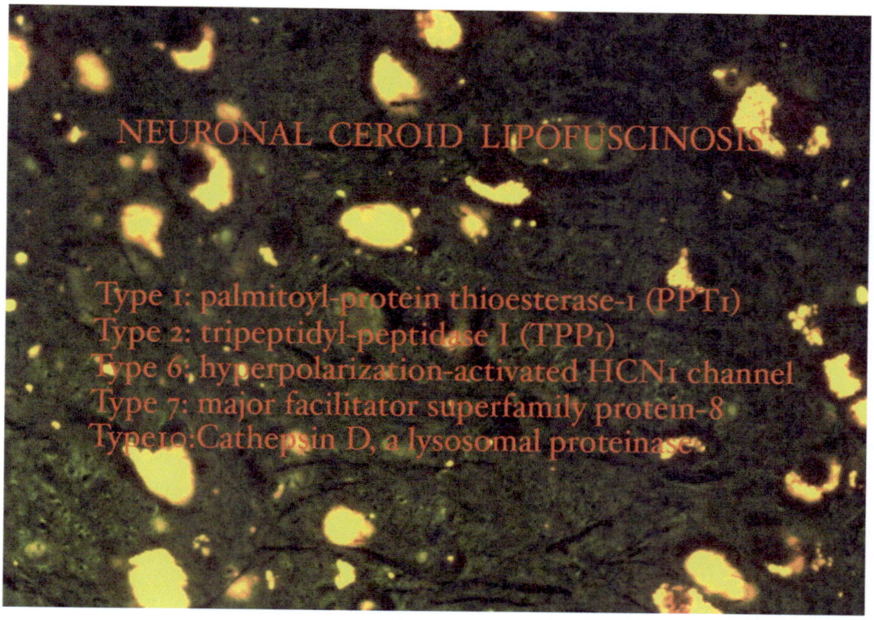

Fig. 8.16 NCLF: intensely autofluorescent intra-neuronal granules of lipofuscin-type material

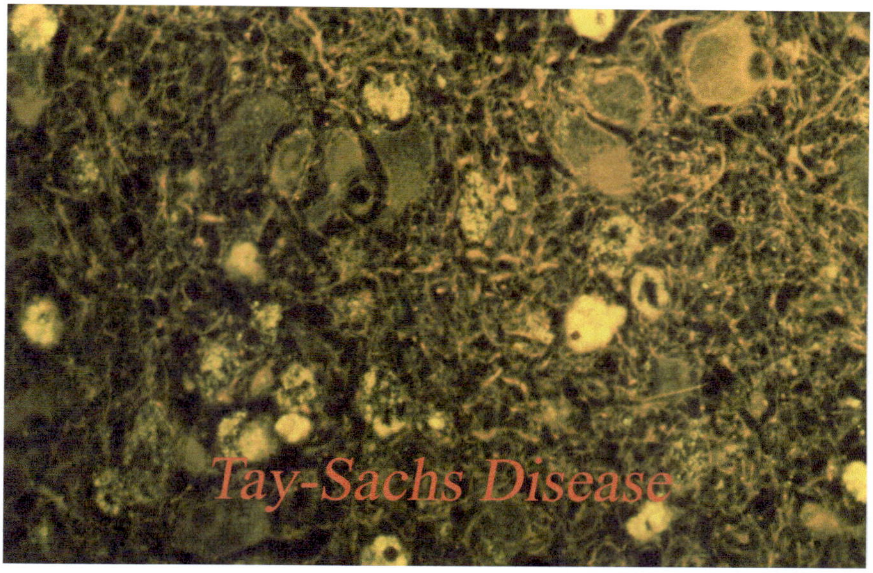

Fig. 8.17 Tay-Sachs disease: postmortem analysis revealing autofluorescent intra-neuronal aggregates of ganglioside material

lacks ganglion cells which retains its red hue that gives rise to the characteristic "cherry red spot" seen in the disease. Found more commonly amongst Ashkenazi Jews, Louisiana Cajuns, and French Canadians, the disease still has no treatment that is available.

In contrast to these degenerative diseases that affect the central nervous system, there are a variety of progressive hereditary illnesses that selectively affect the peripheral nervous system. As illustrated in Fig. 8.18, a good example of this would be the Dejerine-Sottas neuropathy.

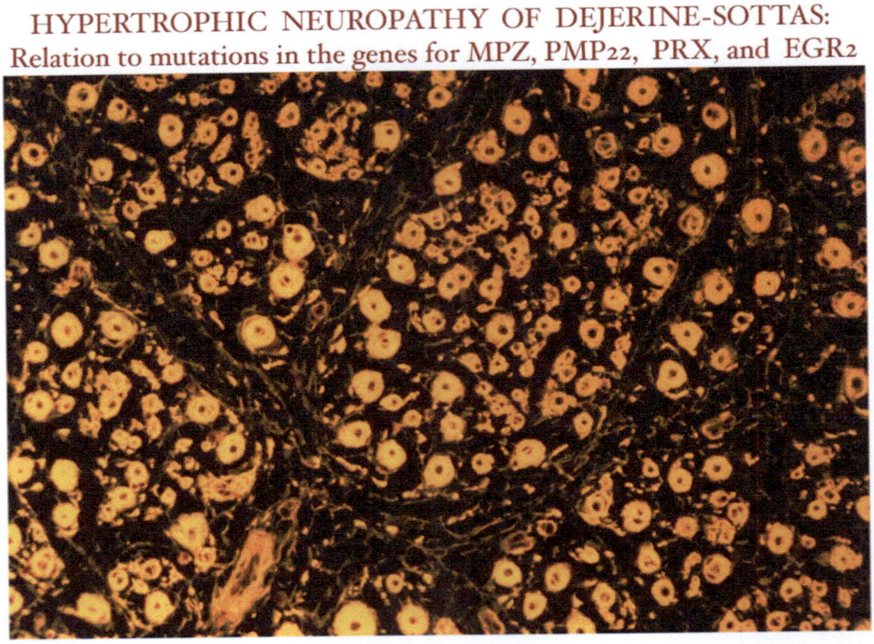

Fig. 8.18 Cross-sectional view of hypertrophied axons from a case of Dejerine-Sottas neuropathy

Originally described in an 1893 autopsy study of an affected sibling pair by Joseph Jules Dejerine and Jules Sottas, the essential features can be summarized by the long title of their initial publication, "On the interstitial hypertrophic and progressive neuritis of childhood; often a familial affection beginning in infancy, characterized by a muscular atrophy of the extremities with marked disturbances of sensation and ataxia of movement and caused by an interstitial hypertrophic neuritis that ascends with consecutive medullary [cord] lesions" [25, 26]. Both brother and sister index cases had clubfeet, kyphoscoliosis, weakness and muscular atrophy with fasciculations, areflexia, marked distal sensory loss and incoordination with Romberg's sign, miosis, and decreased pupillary reaction to light. Modern-day classification schemes place it as autosomal recessive hereditary motor sensory neuropathy (HMSN) type III. Known today as a severe, demyelinating neuropathy, lab testing reveals very slow nerve conduction velocities (<10 m/s) and high CSF protein. Onset is early in infancy with hypomyelination and classic onion bulbs found on pathological examination; the classic onion bulb appearance relates to repeated cycles of demyelination and remyelination of surviving axons with extensive Schwann cell proliferation. Although hereditary motor and sensory neuropathies with onset in infancy such as Dejerine-Sottas are rare disorders, much has come to be known about their molecular pathogenesis [27]. The underlying defect can often be traced to mutations within the myelin protein zero gene (MPZ), the peripheral myelin protein gene (PMP22), the periaxin gene (PRX), and the early growth response gene (EGR2).

References

1. Parent M, Parent A. Substantia nigra and Parkinson's disease: a brief history of their long and intimate relationship. Can J Neurol Sci. 2010;37(3):313–9.
2. Spillantini MG, Schmidt ML, Lee VM, et al. Alpha-synuclein in Lewy bodies. Nature. 1997;388(6645):839–40.
3. Giráldez-Pérez R, Antolín-Vallespín M, Muñoz M, et al. Models of α-synuclein aggregation in Parkinson's disease. Acta Neuropathol Commun. 2014;2:176.
4. George S, Rey NL, Reichenbach N, et al. α-Synuclein: the long distance runner. Brain Pathol. 2013;23(3):350–7.
5. Paisán-Ruíz C, Nath P, Washecka N, et al. Comprehensive analysis of LRRK2 in publicly available

Parkinson's disease cases and neurologically normal controls. Hum Mutat. 2008;29(4):485–90.
6. Corti O, Lesage S, Brice A. What genetics tells us about the causes and mechanisms of Parkinson's disease. Physiol Rev. 2011;91(4):1161–218.
7. Neumann J, Bras J, Deas E, et al. Glucocerebrosidase mutations in clinical and pathologically proven Parkinson's disease. Brain. 2009;132(Pt 7):1783–94.
8. Sidransky E, Nalls MA, Aasly JO, et al. Multicenter analysis of glucocerebrosidase mutations in Parkinson's disease. N Engl J Med. 2009; 361(17):1651–61.
9. Tatsch K, Poepperl G. Nigrostriatal dopamine terminal imaging with dopamine transporter SPECT: an update. J Nucl Med. 2013;54(8):1331–8.
10. Le Foll B, Wilson AA, Graff A, et al. Recent methods for measuring dopamine D3 receptor occupancy in vivo: importance for drug development. Front Pharmacol. 2014;5:161.
11. Sieh W, Choi Y, Chapman NH, et al. Identification of novel susceptibility loci for Guam neurodegenerative disease: challenges of genome scans in genetic isolates. Hum Mol Genet. 2009;18(19):3725–38.
12. Sundar PD, Yu CE, Sieh W, et al. Two sites in the MAPT region confer genetic risk for Guam ALS/PDC and dementia. Hum Mol Genet. 2007;16(3):295–306.
13. Kiernan MC, Vucic S, Cheah BC, et al. Amyotrophic lateral sclerosis. Lancet. 2011;377(9769):942–5.
14. Gusella JF, Wexler NS, Conneally PM, et al. A polymorphic DNA marker genetically linked to Huntington's disease. Nature. 1983;306(5940): 234–8.
15. Kordasiewicz HB, Stanek LM, Wancewicz EV, et al. Sustained therapeutic reversal of Huntington's disease by transient repression of huntingtin synthesis. Neuron. 2012;74(6):1031–44.
16. Potter NT, Meyer MA, Zimmerman AW, et al. Molecular and clinical findings in a family with dentatorubral-pallidoluysian atrophy. Ann Neurol. 1995;37(2):273–7.
17. Yazawa I, Nukina N, Hashida H, et al. Abnormal gene product identified in hereditary DRPLA brain. Nat Genet. 1995;10(1):99–103.
18. Takahashi J, et al. Neuronal nuclear alterations in dentatorubral-pallidoluysian atrophy: ultrastructural and morphometric studies of the cerebellar granule cells. Brain Res. 2001;919(1):12–9.
19. Neary D, Snowden J, Mann D. Frontotemporal dementia. Lancet Neurol. 2005;4(11):771–80.
20. Hardy J, Momeni P, Traynor BJ. Frontal temporal dementia: dissecting the aetiology and pathogenesis. Brain. 2006;129(Pt 4):830–1.
21. Kirshner HS. Frontotemporal dementia and primary progressive aphasia, a review. Neuropsychiatr Dis Treat. 2014;10:1045–55.
22. Cooper JD. Progress towards understanding the neurobiology of Batten disease or neuronal ceroid lipofuscinosis. Curr Opin Neurol. 2003;16(2):121–8.
23. Kielar C, Wishart TM, Palmer A, et al. Molecular correlates of axonal and synaptic pathology in mouse models of Batten disease. Hum Mol Genet. 2009; 18:4066–80.
24. Lew RM, Burnett L, Proos AL, Delatycki MB. Tay-Sachs disease: current perspectives from Australia. Appl Clin Genet. 2015;8:19–25.
25. Krishnamoorthy KS, Eichler F, Rapalino O, Frosch MP. Case records of the Massachusetts General Hospital. Case 14-2014. An 11-month-old girl with developmental delay. N Engl J Med. 2014;370(19): 1830–41.
26. Pearce JMS. Dejerine-Sottas disease (progressive hypertrophic polyneuropathy). Eur Neurol. 2006; 55:115–7.
27. Baets J, Deconinck T, De Vriendt E, et al. Genetic spectrum of hereditary neuropathies with onset in the first year of life. Brain. 2011;134:2664–76.

9 Diseases of Skeletal Muscle

9.1 Introduction

The History of Neuroscience begins with the study of muscle, both from the anatomic perspective as shown from the 1543 dissection studies of Vesalius (Fig. 9.1) to the 1658 functional studies by the Dutch physiologist Swammerdam on the neural activation of skeletal muscle, later published in 1670, as shown in Fig. 9.2. This important study was able to discount the ancient theory of Galen that muscle contraction was based on inflow of a vital fluid pumped through nerves that were regarded only as conduit pipes for the fluid. By enclosing the nerve-muscle preparation in a sealed tube, no change in volume was deduced from the failure of a bubble to move at the top of the chamber when the nerve was irritated, causing the muscle to contract [1]. Great advances have since been made to not only understand the electrophysiologic aspects and ultrastructural details of the neuromuscular junction and muscle, but also to understand the molecular pathogenesis of disease, which is now apparent for major muscle illnesses, such as myasthenia gravis.

Before discussion of myasthenia gravis as a key muscle disease, it is important to fully understand the structure of the neuromuscular junction (Fig. 9.3), and to fully understand and appreciate pre- versus postsynaptic relationships, with acetylcholine receptor molecules embedded within the postsynaptic membrane (Fig. 9.4). To make muscles contract, the nerves form specialized contacts with individual muscle fibers called neuromuscular junctions. In the process of development, multiple nerve fibers reach out to individual muscle fiber but eventually all but one is eliminated. The final successful nerve fiber embeds into the muscle membrane to strongly innervate and activate the muscle fiber through the synaptic release of the neurotransmitter acetylcholine, which transmit the activation signal to the muscle by the postsynaptic pentameric nicotinic acetylcholine receptor (Fig. 9.4). Autoimmune T-cell-dependent attack by antibodies can bind to the acetylcholine receptor and block the normal biding of the released acetylcholine neurotransmitter, thereby producing the profound weakness associated with myasthenia gravis (MG).

The first described case of MG is from 1664 regarding the Native American Chief Opechancanough, who was observed by a Virginia settler, "….the excessive fatigue he encountered wrecked his constitution; his flesh became macerated; his sinews lost their tone and elasticity; and his eyelids were so heavy that he could not see unless they were lifted up by his attendants … he was unable to walk; but his spirit rising above the ruins of his body directed from the litter on which he was carried by his Indians" [2]. In the late 1800s, the first modern publications on the disease emerged that used the name myasthenia gravis; the term had been invented by

M.A. Meyer, *Neurologic Disease*, DOI 10.1007/978-3-319-39581-4_9

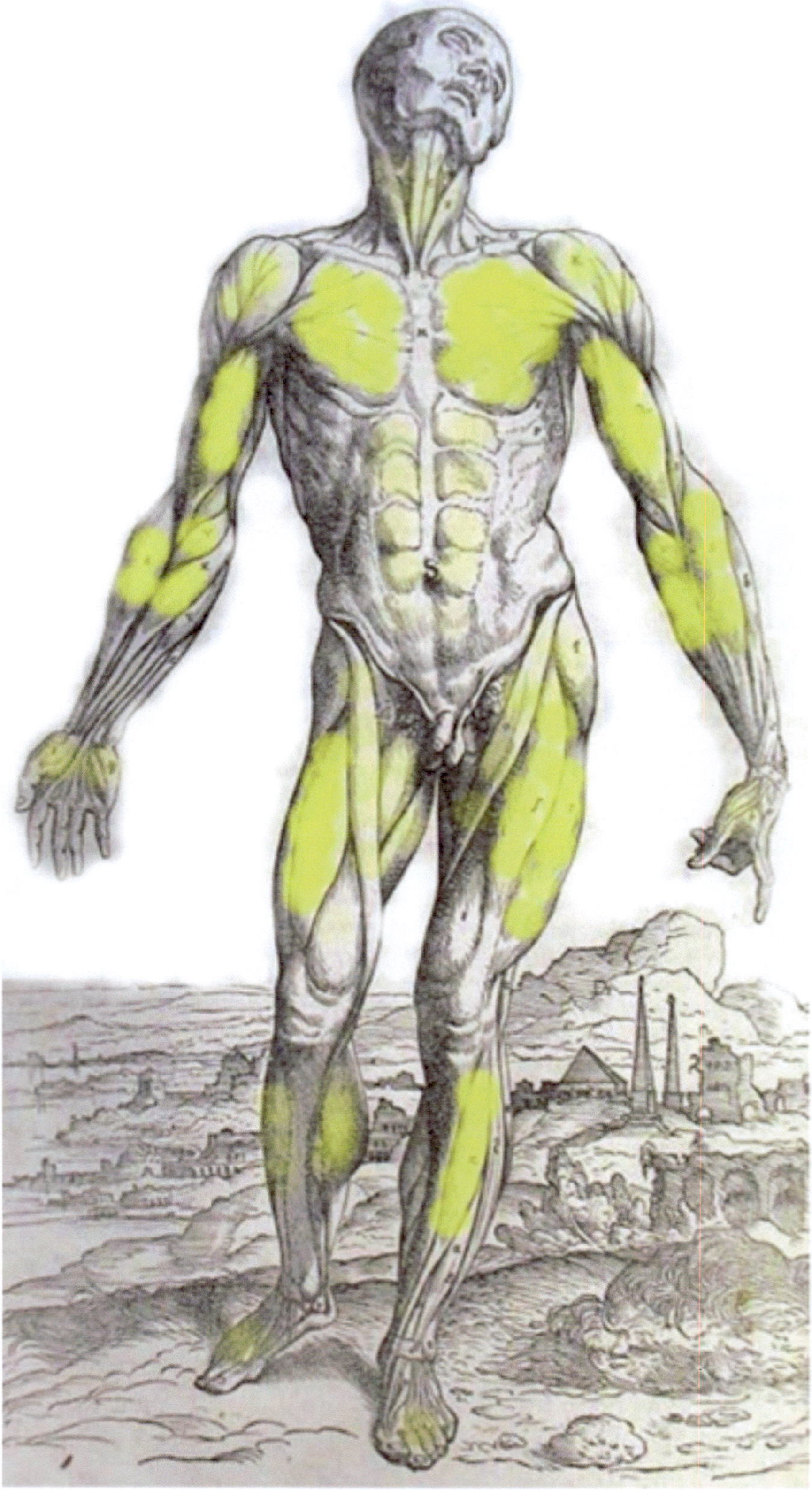

Fig. 9.1 1543 study of muscle anatomy by Vesalius

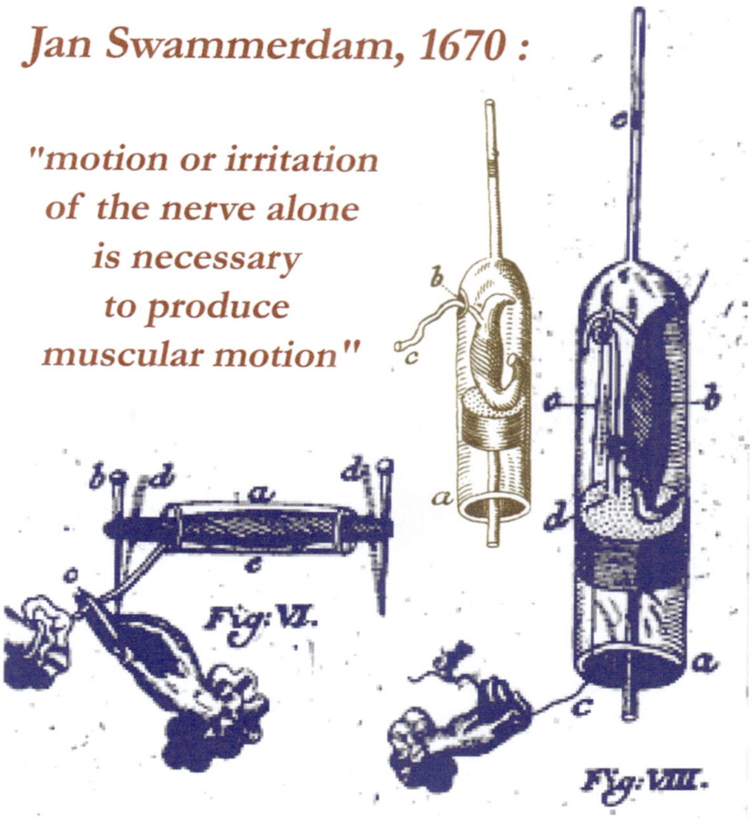

Fig. 9.2 1670 study of muscle contraction by Swammerdam

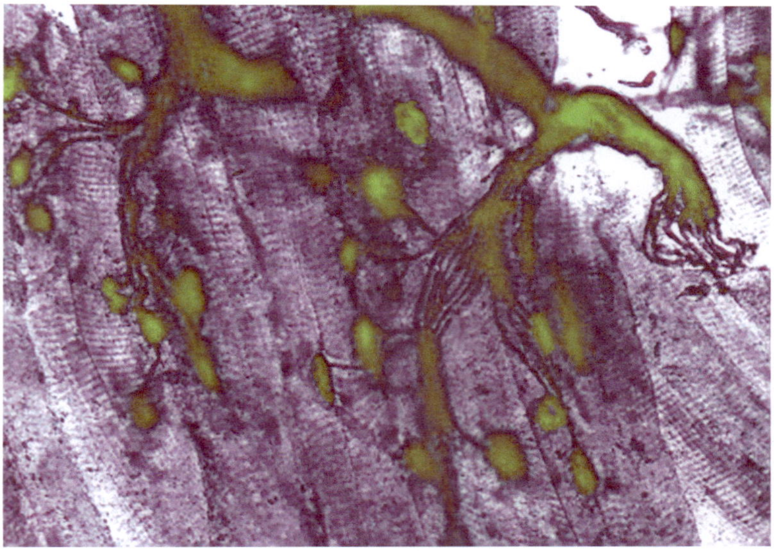

Fig. 9.3 Motor endplates in muscle, with gross view of neuromuscular junctions (adapted from Wikipedia)

fusing the Greek expressions for muscle and weakness with the Latin term for severe. Overall, the disease is fortunately uncommon, with a 1 in 5000 prevalence rate. The incidence can vary between 2 per million per year in Virginia versus ten times higher in Barcelona, Spain; with regards to age, a 7 to 3 predominance of women over men is noted for those under 40 versus a 3 to 2

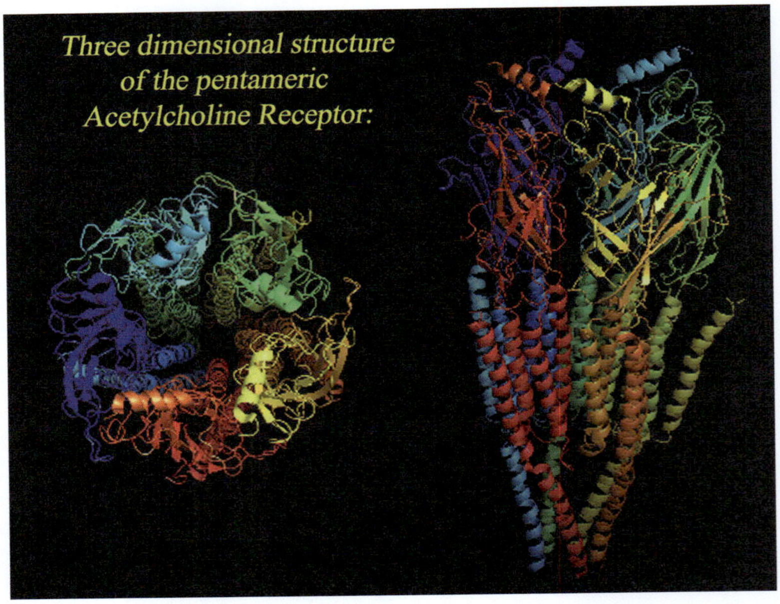

Fig. 9.4 The acetylcholine receptor molecule (adapted from Wikipedia)

predominance for men over women for those over 50 years of age [3].

MG presents fluctuating levels of weakness that seems to worsen as the day progresses and can be activity-related; ocular weakness with asymmetric drooping of one of both eyelids with episodic double vision are common initial symptoms that progress to involve weakness in arms and/or legs. The course is variable, and most developing bulbar or limb weakness within 3 years after the onset of initial ocular symptoms. Inspection of whole-body 18F-FDG PET scans of metabolic activity for individuals at rest yield insight as to why ocular muscles are so commonly involved, as the orbital eye muscles light up brightly on PET scans indicating their constant motion, even with seemingly stationary gaze where microsaccades are constantly active to prevent saturation and extinction of visual purple retinal photoreceptor pigments.

In patients suspected of having MG with fatigable muscle weakness, the diagnosis can be supported by a clear and definite response to oral doses of the cholinesterase inhibitor pyridostigmine. Other forms of testing include the use of edrophonium test infusions to check for improvement in strength or repetitive nerve stimulation studies and/or single-fiber electromyography; acetylcholine receptor (AChR) or muscle-specific tyrosine kinase (MuSK) antibody lab testing is critically important as well.

Depending on the individual patient and their profile of risk factors, differential diagnostic possibilities might include malignancy-associated Lambert Eaton syndrome, brainstem ischemia, motor neuron disease, botulism, organophosphate intoxication, mitochondrial disorders, and acute inflammatory demyelinating polyradiculoneuropathy.

Treatment must be individualized according to diseases severity that most often relies upon the use of the cholinesterase inhibitor pyridostigmine, but may require additional use of corticosteroids, azathioprine, cyclosporine, and mycophenolate mofetil. Unfortunately, dose-dependent self-limited side effects with cholinestersase inhibitors occur by activation of cholinergic muscarinic receptors, giving rise to nausea, vomiting, abdominal cramping, diarrhea, diaphoresis, increased lacrimation, salivation, and bronchial secretions. For emergent problems with myasthenic crisis events, rapid improvement can be gained via plasma exchange or intravenous immunoglobulin (IVIG). With the advent of these immunomodulatory techniques in intensive care units within hospitals, mortality from this serious disease can be minimized to less than 5 %, with most patients now able to enjoy a near normal life expectancy.

With regards to diagnosis, it is important to note that lack of acetylcholine receptor antibodies does not rule out MG as antibodies to muscle-specific tyrosine kinase (MuSK) have been found in over 40 % of patients in this group. MG patients with MuSK antibodies show patterns of weakness and electrophysiologic findings that are quite similar to those with definite AChR antibodies. Although pathophysiologic details are still unclear, it is known that MuSK initiates aggregation of AChRs within the formation of the neuromuscular junction during development.

An additional therapeutic consideration is the unusual association of thymoma with the disease. MG patients with thymoma have a more severe disease course with more severe weakness and higher AChR antibody titers; fortunately, most thymic tumors are benign and well differentiated (reference 3). Regardless, patients with MG should still undergo CT and/or PET/CT to evaluate for the possible presence of thymoma; if present, thymectomy is recognized as one way to achieve a medication-free remission in selected MG cases, with the best chances for improvement if thymectomy is performed early in the course of MG. Thymic hyperplasia is found in about 65 % of MG patients, and thymomas are noted in 10 % of cases [4]. However, there is no convincing evidence for the role of thymectomy in MuSK-associated myasthenia, which is a relatively small group of cases, as only 5–8 % of myasthenia gravis patients test positive for antibodies against muscle-specific tyrosine kinase (MuSK) receptors [5].

In an effort to illustrate normal muscle structure and function, it is worthwhile to consider disease pathophysiology in the uncommon yet highly serious problem of malignant hyperthermia that arises acutely with general anesthesia in certain predisposed individuals with ryanodine gene mutations. Normally, ryanodine receptors found in skeletal muscle function as a calcium release channel in the sarcoplasmic reticulum but also serves to connect the sarcoplasmic reticulum and transverse tubule. Normally, after acetylcholine binds to its receptor and depolarizes the muscle membrane, a muscle action potential is propagated into the transverse tubule (Fig. 9.5, T

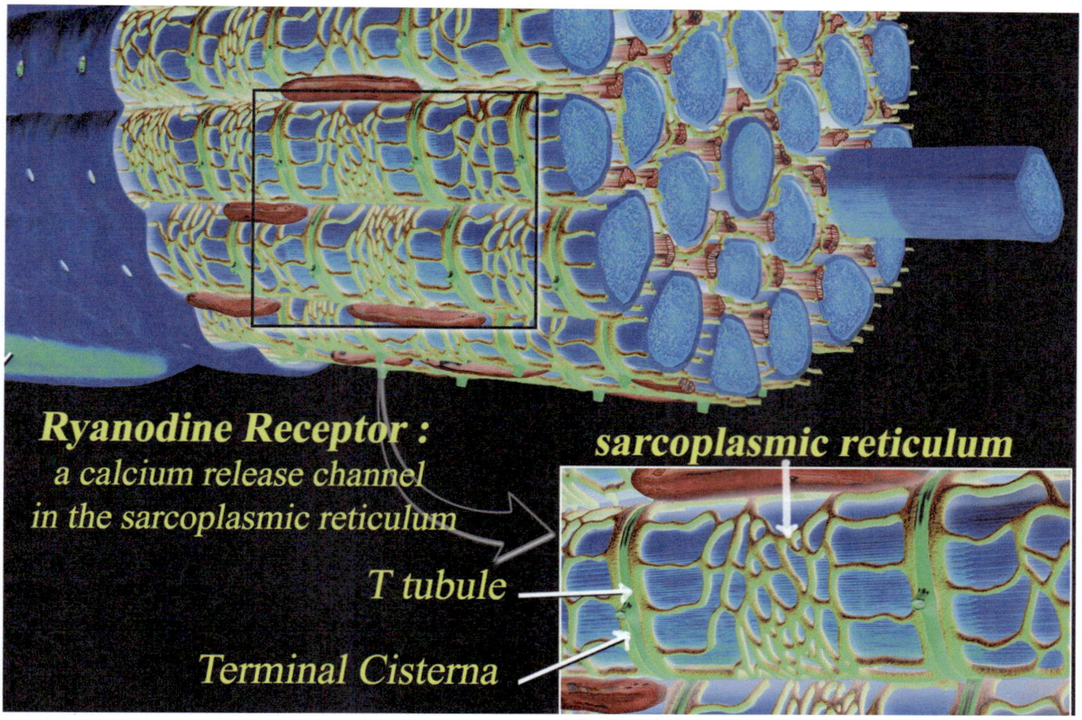

Fig. 9.5 The sarcoplasmic reticulum and ryanodine receptors within the T tubules (adapted from Wikipedia)

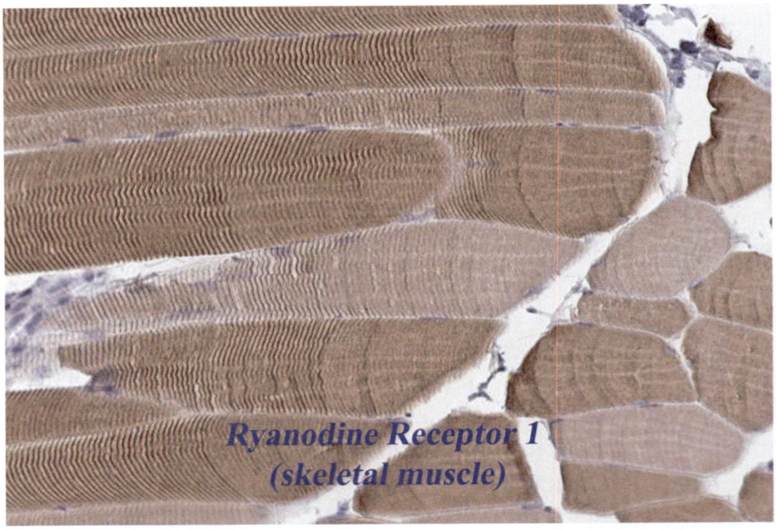

Fig. 9.6 Ryanodine receptor 1 localization within normal human muscle fibers

tubule) where dihydropyridine receptors open up to then activate the ryanodine receptors located on the terminal cisternae of the sarcoplasmic reticulum (Figs. 9.5 and 9.6), which release calcium from the sarcoplasmic reticulum. Mutations in the ryanodine receptor gene are associated with malignant hyperthermia susceptibility during general anesthesia, where an uncontrolled and overwhelming calcium release from the sarcoplasmic reticulum causes sustained muscle contractile activity with a dangerous depletion of ATP occurring with excess heat production, inducing muscle breakdown and rhabdomyolysis as the muscle rigidity continues [6]. Emergent use of dantrolene is indicated in these situations as it is a muscle relaxant that depresses excitation–contraction coupling by binding to the ryanodine receptor and stopping the pathologic leak of calcium into the intracellular compartment. Although dantrolene is a hydantoin derivative like phenytoin, it does not have anti-epileptogenic activity; however, dantrolene is also useful in treating neuroleptic malignant syndrome, and ecstasy intoxication.

Although malignant hyperthermia (MH) is usually triggered by volatile anesthetics including all halogenated inhalative agents and depolarizing muscle relaxants like succinylcholine, heat or vigorous exercise can bring on the problem in predisposed individuals; MH episodes are also known for those with other myopathies such as central core disease [6]. Overall, MH is very uncommon, with the prevalence in Japan was calculated to be 1:73,000 [7]. Ryanodine mutations do not account for all cases, as molecular genetic investigations have confirmed this only in about 70 %. Other gene mutations have been described in the gene encoding the main subunit of dihydropyridine-sensitive voltage-gated calcium channel, known as the CACNA1S gene [8].

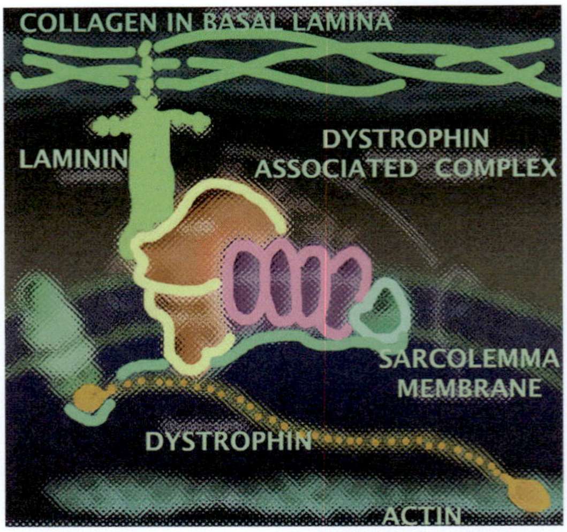

Fig. 9.7 Dystrophin links intra-membranous proteins with actin filaments

As shown in Fig. 9.7, a cross-sectional view of the sarcolemmal membrane reveals a complex

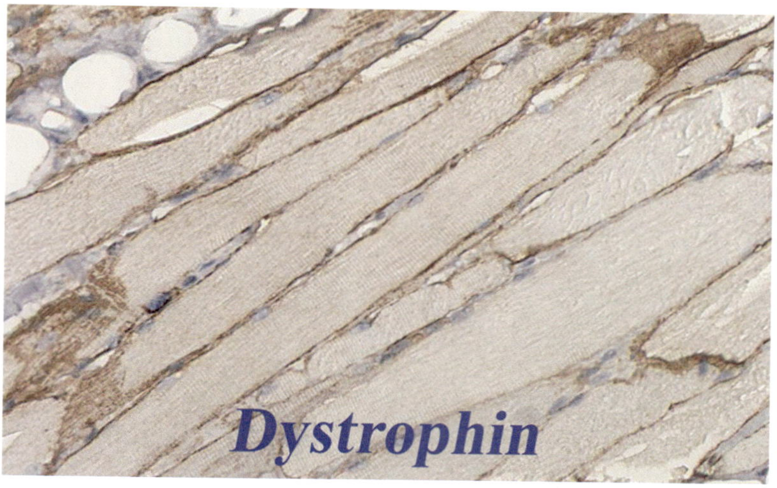

Fig. 9.8 Localization of dystrophin within normal human skeletal muscle fibers

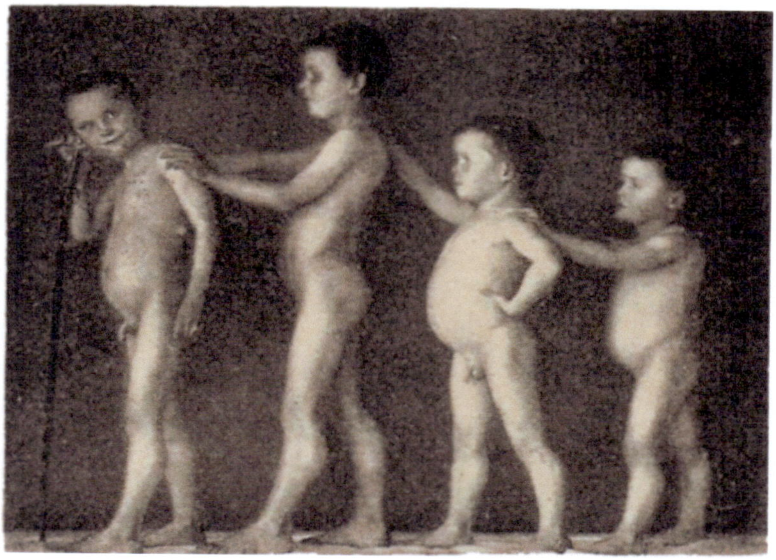

Fig. 9.9 Duchene muscular dystrophy is an X-linked defect within the dystrophin gene that affects young boys. Pseudohypertrophic muscular dystrophy. Four brothers aged 12, 11, 8, and 7 years. The calves and anterior surface of the thighs are hypertrophied. The muscles of the back are atrophied. The eldest has so much weakness of the muscles of the neck that he cannot hold up his head

variety of structural support proteins that helps insure mechanical stability of the muscle under states of strain and stress with mechanical contraction. In essence, this complex interconnects the inner cytoskeleton with the extracellular matrix through the cell membrane, and comprises of alpha-dystrobrevin, syncoilin, synemin, sarcoglycan, dystroglycan, and sarcospan to collectively form the dystrophin-associated complex, as it is linked to the underlying mobile actin filaments through the key linking protein known as dystophin (Fig. 9.8). This fundamentally important protein supports muscle fiber strength—its absence causes increased muscle injury and sarcolemmal deformability, and compromises the mechanical stability of connections within the extracellular matrix to adjacent muscle fibers.

Loss of successful dystrophin production from mutations within the very large gene for dystrophin results in the debilitating and ultimately fatal disease Duchenne muscular dystrophy (DMD). The dystrophin gene is one of the longest, comprising 0.08 % of the human genome; located at chromosome Xp21, it takes 16 h to transcribe the 79 exons to finally assemble a huge protein with over 3500 amino acids [9]. Although comprising only 0.002 % of total muscle protein, its absence causes a progressively severe and diffuse muscle degeneration and weakness in affected young boys (Fig. 9.9), causing muscle to

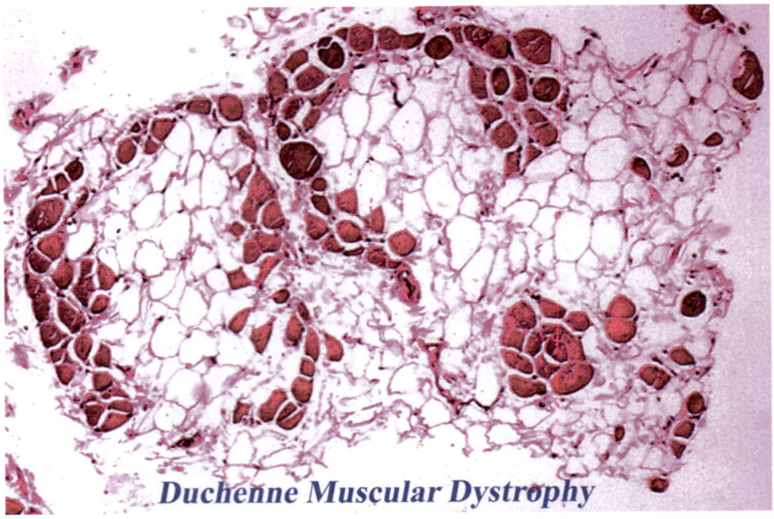

Fig. 9.10 Degenerated muscle fibers replaced by fat cells in DMD (from Wikipedia)

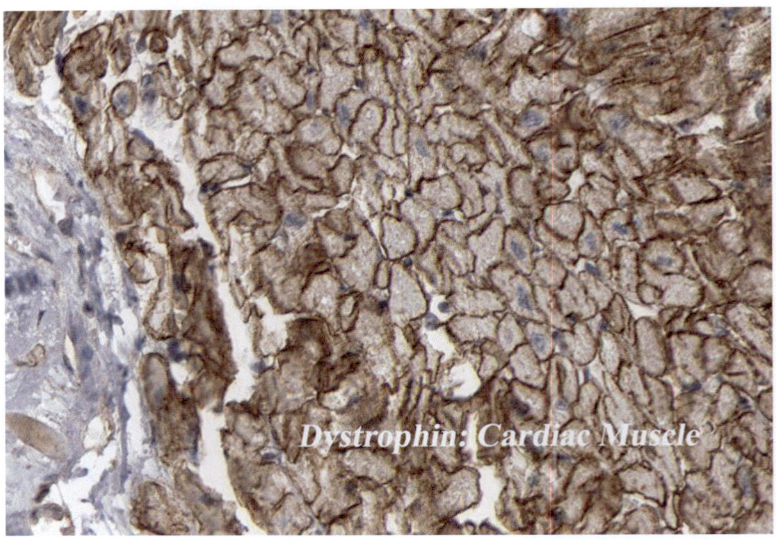

Fig. 9.11 Dystrophin localization to normal human cardiac muscle

be replaced by fat cells (Fig. 9.10) giving rise to the false appearance of hypertrophy to affected muscles. Affecting 1 in 3500 newborn boys, DMD causes not only progressive weakness of the skeletal muscles, it also produces a significant cardiomyopathy (see Fig. 9.11 for normal intense pattern of dystrophin expression for cardiac muscle); almost all are wheelchair-dependent by 12 years of age, and most die in early adulthood from respiratory failure.

Duchenne's muscular dystrophy is caused by deletions in 72 % of cases and duplications in 7 % of one or more exons, versus point mutations being the cause in about 20 %; these mutations can prematurely stop dystrophin synthesis by disrupting the open reading frame. A milder form of the disease is known as Becker's muscular dystrophy which arises from the assembly of a shorter yet still functional dystrophin, possibly due to a spontaneous ability to skip over a defective exon yet still maintain the reading frame. It is this phenomenon along with rare finding in DMD of dystrophin-positive "revertant" fibers that has lead to the brilliant therapeutic idea of using antisense oligonucleotides for frame-restoring skipping of defective exons to induce the formation of abbreviated yet still functional dystrophin molecules [10–12]. Subcutaneous injection of an antisense oligonucleotide designed to skip exon 51 was recently studied in young DMD patients with a mean age of 9 years: new dystrophin expression was found in a dose-dependent manner for 60–100 % of muscle fibers in 10 of the 12 patients; furthermore, a significant increase of 35 m from the baseline of 384 m was observed for the 6-min walk test [12].

In addition to these examples of autoimmune (MG) and genetic causes (DMD) of primary muscle disease, inflammatory diseases of muscle deserve attention and discussion (Fig. 9.12). The three major immune-mediated inflammatory myopathies that may be encountered in clinical practice include dermatomyositis (DM), polymyositis (PM), and inclusion body myositis (IBM); both DM and PM can occur as isolated primary muscle syndrome or may be part of a larger systemic connective tissue disease. DM and IBM are more common than PM to present as isolated syndromes, with sporadic IBM being the most common progressive myopathy for patients over 40 years old. In general, patients are likely to present with proximal muscle pain and weakness, and in particular may show difficulty in ascending stairs or rising from a chair. When these proximal signs present along with an elevated muscle CK value, an inflammatory myopathy may be in the differential diagnosis; when these changes are seen in conjunction with dermatologic changes, DM may be a consideration.

DM pathogenesis focuses on endothelial cell antibodies that produce a microangiopathic ischemic changes within muscles, giving rise to proximal muscle weakness and pain, along with characteristic cutaneous changes on the face (heliotrope rash), hands and elbows (Gottron's patches), and trunk (shawl sign). Of concern is the associated higher risk of underlying malignant neoplasm with DM, and therefore careful screening for this is needed for any patient newly diagnosed with DM. Diagnostic biopsies in DM show interstitial and perivascular inflammatory changes consisting of B cells, CD4+ T cells as well as plasmacytoid dendritic cells. In contrast, muscle biopsy in polymyositis shows endomysial inflammatory infiltration and consists of CD8+ and CD4+ cells as well as dendritic cells, macrophages, and plasma cells. Special stains for amyloid and phosphorylated tau are helpful for the histologic diagnosis of IBM [13].

In general, a pathologic T-cell response with invasion of muscle fibers by CD8+ lymphocytes is more characteristic for PM and IBM along with perforin-mediated cytotoxic necrosis. Special stains for amyloid and phosphorylated tau are helpful for the histologic diagnosis of IBM, where degenerative changes are noted

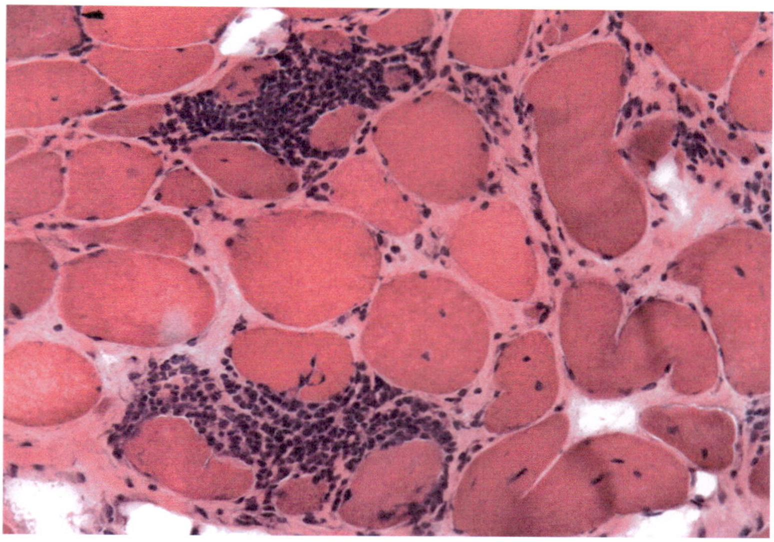

Fig. 9.12 Muscle biopsy findings revealing an inflammatory myopathy (from Wikipedia)

along with beta-amyloid inclusions reflecting proteasomal dysfunction. Whereas resistance to conventional forms of immunotherapy is often encountered in IBM, those with DM or PM usually respond to treatment with steroids and immunosuppressive agents [13].

References

1. Meyer MA. Swammerdam's experiments on neuromuscular physiology. Neurology. 1985;35:1431.
2. Conti-Fine BM, Milani M, Kaminski HJ. Myasthenia gravis: past, present, and future. J Clin Invest. 2006;116(11):2843–54.
3. Juel VC, Massey JM. Myasthenia gravis. Orphanet J Rare Dis. 2007;2:44.
4. Namba T, Brunner NG, Grob D. Myasthenia gravis in patients with thymoma, with particular reference to onset after thymectomy. Medicine (Baltimore). 1978; 57(5):411–33.
5. El-Salem K, Yassin A, Al-Hayk K, et al. Treatment of MuSK-associated myasthenia gravis. Curr Treat Options Neurol. 2014;16(4):283.
6. Bandschapp O, Girard T. Malignant hyperthermia. Swiss Med Wkly. 2012;142:w13652.
7. Sumitani M, Uchida K, Yasunaga H, et al. Prevalence of malignant hyperthermia and relationship with anesthetics in Japan: data from the diagnosis procedure combination database. Anesthesiology. 2011;114:84–90.
8. Monnier N, Procaccio V, Stieglitz P, Lunardi J. Malignant-hyperthermia susceptibility is associated with a mutation of the alpha 1-subunit of the human dihydropyridine-sensitive l-type voltage-dependent calcium-channel receptor in skeletal muscle. Am J Hum Genet. 1997;60:1316–25.
9. Tennyson CN, Klamut HJ, Worton RG. The human dystrophin gene requires 16 hours to be transcribed and is cotranscriptionally spliced. Nat Genet. 1995; 9(2):184–90.
10. van Deutekom JC, Janson AA, Ginjaar LB, et al. Local dystrophin restoration with antisense oligonucleotide PRO051. N Engl J Med. 2007;357:2677–86.
11. Falzarano MS, Scotton C, Passarelli C, Ferlini A. Duchenne muscular dystrophy: from diagnosis to therapy. Molecules. 2015;20(10):18168–84.
12. Goemans NM, Tulinius M, van den Akker JT, et al. Systemic administration of PRO051 in Duchenne's muscular dystrophy. N Engl J Med. 2011;364:1513–22.
13. Mastaglia FL. Inflammatory muscle diseases. Neurol India. 2008;56(3):263–70.

10 Diseases of the Spinal Cord

The spinal cord is a relatively thin and small yet highly compact and complex collection of ascending and descending fibers that serve as a vital link between the brain and the outer world. Although we can easily survive without a few cubic centimeters of non-dominant right frontal cortex for example, a similar sized lesion within the spinal cord could be devastating and perhaps fatal. It is therefore critically important to be able to recognize the signs and symptoms of spinal cord compression, especially for those patients who present acutely (for example, with lower extremity weakness with abrupt sensory changes below a segmental dermatomal level). Immediate intervention is required in these acute cases to relive mechanical pressure upon the corticospinal tract and its delicate blood supply, whether that pressure effect is from trauma, neoplasm, or abscess. At the other end of the time spectrum is slowly progressive spinal motor neuron degeneration that can arise from neurodegenerative processes, such as from amyotrophic lateral sclerosis (ALS). In order to arrive at the correct diagnosis, a fundamental knowledge of spinal cord anatomy is needed, which will be reviewed here (Figs. 10.1, 10.2, and 10.3).

The most fundamentally important fiber tract within the entire nervous system is shown in Fig. 10.1. Known as the corticospinal tract, it arises from pyramidal motor neurons within the motor cortex, and descends down into the brainstem where it decussates at the level of the lower pons and upper medulla, where the crossed tract descends further in the contralateral dorsolateral aspects of the spinal cord, giving off branches at each level to innervate alpha motor neurons in the ventral horn of the spinal cord (Figs. 10.1, 10.2, and 10.3); uncrossed fibers descend in the anterior ventral corticospinal tract (Fig. 10.3). The actual course of the corticospinal tract can be traced in occasional cases by MRI where Wallerian degeneration of a selectively injured fiber tract can be seen as a circumscribed continuous areas of T2 signal abnormality, as shown in Fig. 10.2, which illustrates chronic MRI changes in a patient with a remote, chronic right pyramidal tract lesion arising within the right semicentrum ovale. As shown in Fig. 10.3, there is a somatotopic laminar organization to the descending motor tracts with the sacral fibers being outermost versus the cervical fibers running in the most medial inner parts of the corticospinal tract. A similar somatotopic organization is seen for the ascending sensory fibers arising from the dorsal roots carrying sensory impulses into the medial placed dorsal columns (lower extremity sensory fibers placed medially within the gracilus tract versus upper extremity fibers within the more lateral yet adjacent cuneatus tract); motor action potentials travel through exiting ventral root axons to innervate and activate muscle. Rare cases have been described where hemispheric subcortical stroke can result in ipsilateral paralysis [1]; pathophysiologic explanations relate to the fact that up to 30 % of descending motor fibers may remain ipsilaterally within the anterior ventral corticospinal tract (Fig. 10.3) [2].

M.A. Meyer, *Neurologic Disease*, DOI 10.1007/978-3-319-39581-4_10

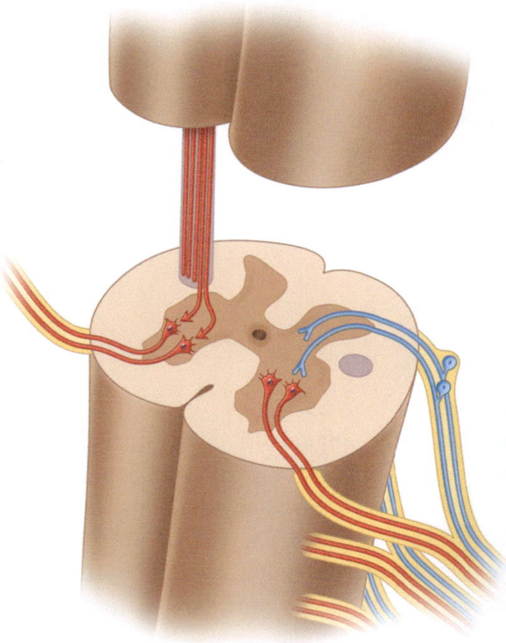

Fig. 10.1 The descending corticospinal tract

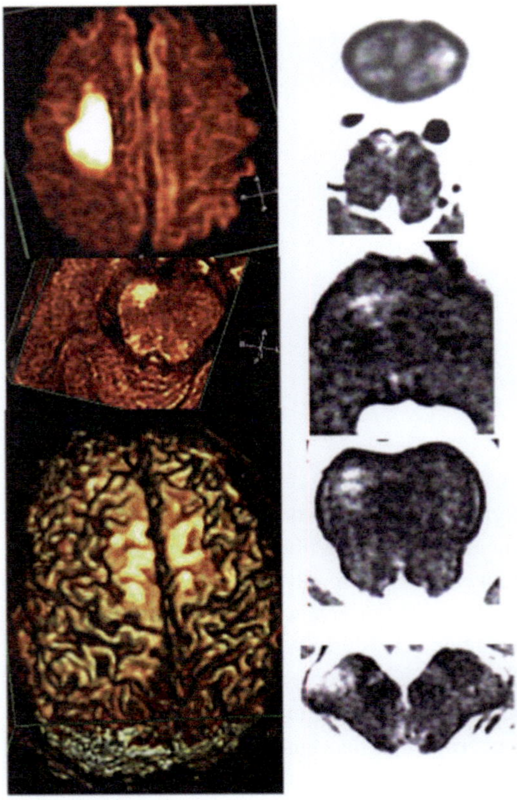

Fig. 10.2 Tracing the extent of Wallerian degeneration of the corticospinal tract with MRI in a patient with a chronic right parietal subcortical infarct

With regards to spinal cord pathophysiology, it is important to note that a critical factor in proper neuronal functioning is a balance of inhibitory versus excitatory input upon the motor neuron; should inhibitory transmission become impaired, over-excitation with rigidity results as shown Fig. 10.4 for retrogradely absorbed intra-neuronal Tetanus toxin, which produces life-threatening rigidity and spasm as inhibitory neurons cannot release glycine or GABA to inhibit the alpha motor neurons. Tetanus toxin is a zinc-dependent metalloproteinase that targets VAMP (synaptobrevin/vesicle-associated membrane protein) that allows fusion of synaptic vesicles with the neuronal plasma membrane [3]. Tetanus toxin ultimately reaches its spinal cord target via extensive retrograde axonal transport from the infected peripheral wound; once it is within the spinal cord, it is transported across synapses and then taken up by inhibitory GABAergic and/or glycinergic neurons that normally inhibit alpha motor neurons; intraneuronal tetanus toxin then cleaves VAMP, thereby inhibiting the release of GABA and glycine. As illustrated in the 1809 painting shown in Fig. 10.4 by Sir Charles Bell, life threatening and often fatal lack of inhibition upon motor neurons results in opisthotonus, which was not uncommon in the pre-tetanus vaccination era. However, despite modern health care delivery advances, tetanus cases persist worldwide as shown in the global map within Fig. 10.4 for the 1990–2004 time frame.

A major spinal cord disease is amyotrophic lateral sclerosis (ALS), which is a fatal degeneration of motor neurons disorder that can also involve motor neurons at bulbar and cortical levels. First reported in 1869 by Charcot, the disease became more well known after baseball player Lou Gehrig was diagnosed with this by the Mayo Clinic in 1939. The most common form is sporadic in nature yet remaining 5–10 % of the cases are identified as having an obvious familial pattern.

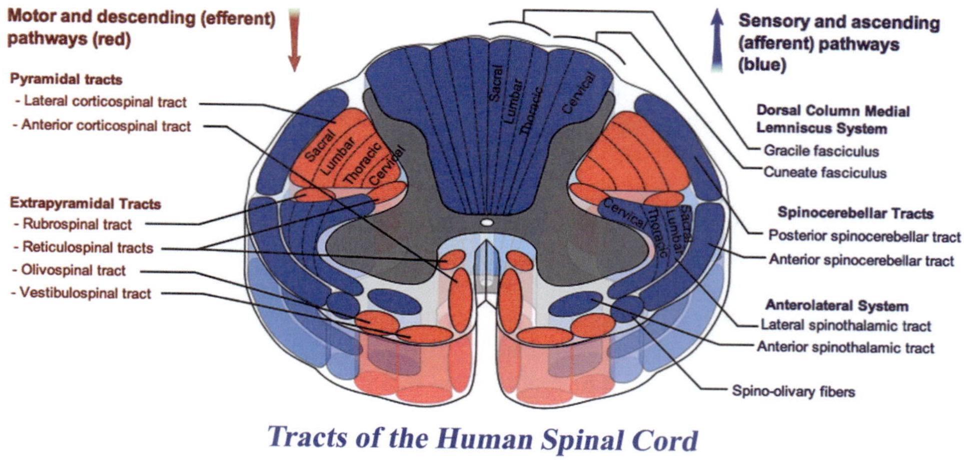

Fig. 10.3 Ascending versus descending tracts within the spinal cord (from Wikipedia)

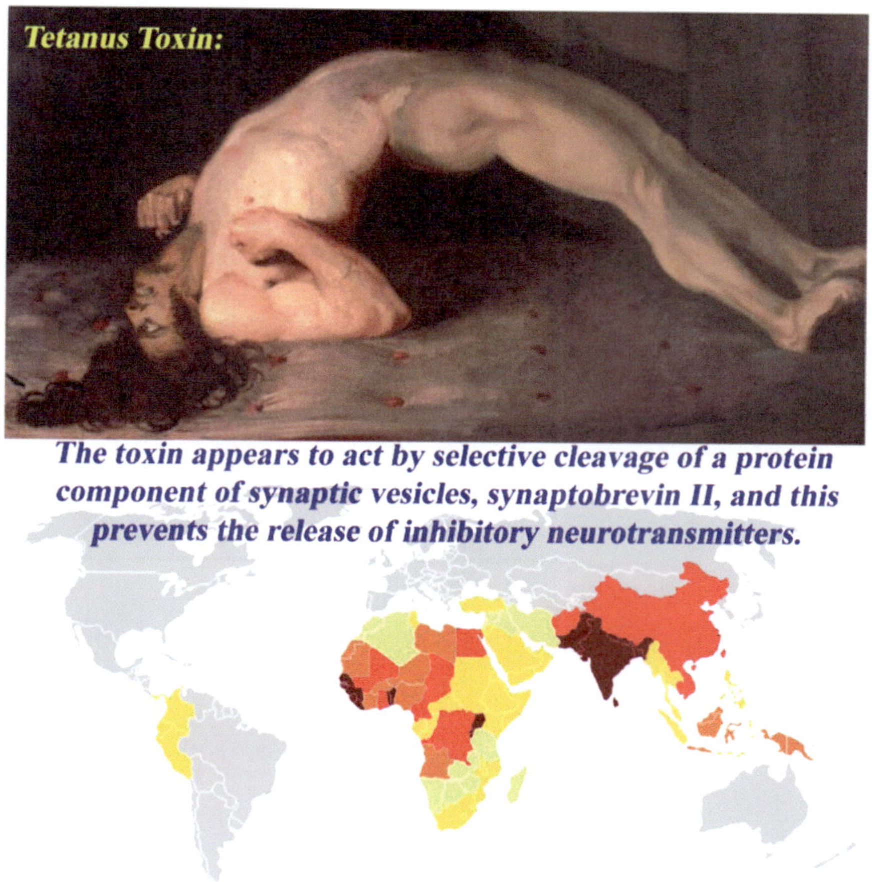

Fig. 10.4 Tetanus toxin-related opisthotonus (1809 painting by Sir Charles Bell); *lower panel* shows global map of persistent occurrence of tetanus cases (adapted from Wikipedia)

Onset is typically between the ages of 50 and 65 with the median age at diagnosis being 64; initial symptoms include muscle weakness and twitching known as fasciculations; progressive disease has fatal compromise of respiratory muscle function.

With regard to well defined gene defects in ALS, the most common cause is a mutation of the gene encoding the antioxidant enzyme superoxide dismutase 1 (SOD1) which causes the protein to misfold and produce toxic aggregation in the motor neurons, resulting in impaired axonal transport and other associated defects. SOD1 mutations can account for 20 % of familial cases [4].

In 1995, the heavy neurofilament (NF-H) gene was proposed as a probable site of pathogenic mutation in ALS [5]; subsequent studies confirmed this to be true in rare occasional cases [6]. Deletions in the KSP repeat region of the NF-H gene were found in addition to a novel insertion in the NF-H gene that produces extra KSP repeat elements in a highly conserved repetitive region of the gene. Furthermore, a NF-H based animal model of ALS had been developed [7].

As for prognosis of ALS patients as a collective group, more than half of patients diagnosed do not survive the first 30 months after symptom onset; only one out of five survive between 5 and 10 years after symptoms onset. Advanced age of symptom onset, early respiratory muscle dysfunction, and bulbar onset are adverse factors whereas limb-onset at younger ages predictor longer survival [5].

As shown in Fig. 10.5, histologic examination of postmortem specimens of the spinal cord from patients with both upper and lower motor neuron involvement by ALS will often reveal sclerotic degenerative changes within the remnants of the bilateral corticospinal tracts (hence the name for the disease: lateral sclerosis). As illustrated in Fig. 10.6, FDG PET scans of affected ALS patients can help confirm whether there is a substantial upper motor neuron component to the disease within the parietal primary motor cortex; in the illustrated example, focal defects in metabolism are noted bilaterally within the motor cortex, as seen in the coronal plane.

To further investigate other candidate genes that have the potential to generate an ALS phenotype should a mutation or deletion develop, a comprehensive review was made of the ventral horn patterns of expression for 3430 genes [8]. From this large group, 17 genes were found to be highly expressed within the anterior horn suggesting localization to its primary cellular constituent, the alpha spinal motor neuron. For some genes, an inter-relationship to ALS was already known, such

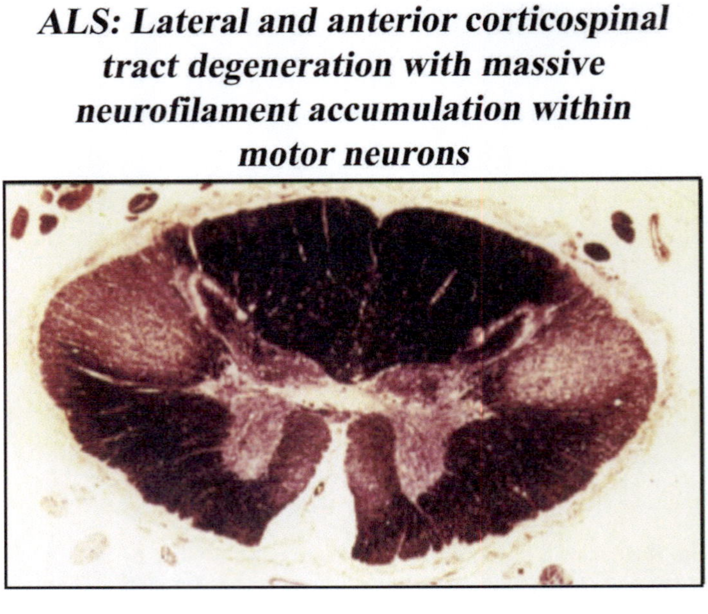

Fig. 10.5 ALS histology showing sclerosis of the bilateral corticospinal tracts

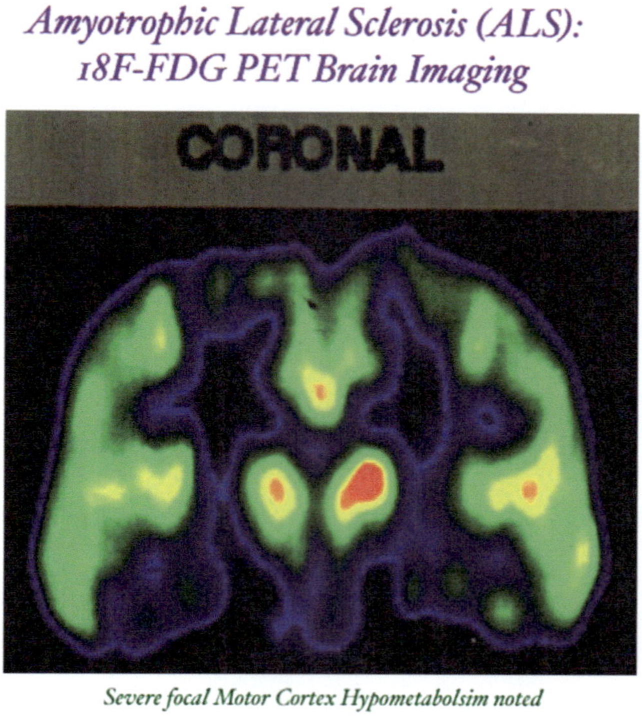

Fig. 10.6 18F-FDG PET findings in a ALS patient with upper motor neuron involvement as well as lower motor neuron clinical findings: coronal view

as for heavy, medium, and light neurofilaments, and peripherin. Other genes identified include: Gamma Synuclein, GDNF, SEMA3A, Extended Synaptotagmin-like protein 1, LYNX1, HSPA12a, Cadherin 22, PRKACA, TPPP3 as well as Choline Acetyltransferase, Janus Kinase 1, and the Motor Neuron and Pancreas Homeobox 1 (Fig. 10.7).

With regards to peripherin, a neuronal intermediate filament associated with inclusion bodies in motor neurons of patients with amyotrophic lateral sclerosis (ALS), a possible peripherin gene alteration in ALS was hypothesized [9]. As reported by Gros-Louis et al., two unique peripherin gene variants were discovered in ALS cases but not in 380 control individuals; one variant was an intron 8 insertion and the other was exon 1 deletion [10]. As expression of the mutation in culture disrupted neurofilament network assembly, it was concluded that peripherin gene mutations account for a small percentage of ALS cases, and that neurofilament disorganization continues to be a common pathogenic theme. One overall impression of the clinical syndrome of ALS is that it may be a common phenotype for uncommon mutations and/or deletions within a variety of genes responsible for encoding proteins involved in the neuronal cytoskeleton and/or axonal transport system.

Although motor neuron diseases like ALS are a group of neurological diseases that are typically thought to involve older adults, they also can occur in childhood in the form of spinal muscular atrophy (SMA) or early adult years for spinal and bulbar muscular atrophy (SBMA). Presenting as a severe, autosomal recessive disease with onset in infancy or early childhood involving lower motor neuron loss and skeletal muscle weakness, SMA is now known to be caused by lack of the survival of motor neuron (SMN) protein, with alterations in spliceosome assembly. In contrast, SBMA is caused by a highly toxic polyglutamine expansion in the androgen receptor (similar toxic trinucleotide expansion disease mechanism also noted for Huntington's and DRPLA—see Chap. 8). SBMA is milder than SMA, and has an X-linked pattern of inheritance [10].

Aside from slowly evolving neurodegenerative hereditary causes for spinal cord dysfunction, an

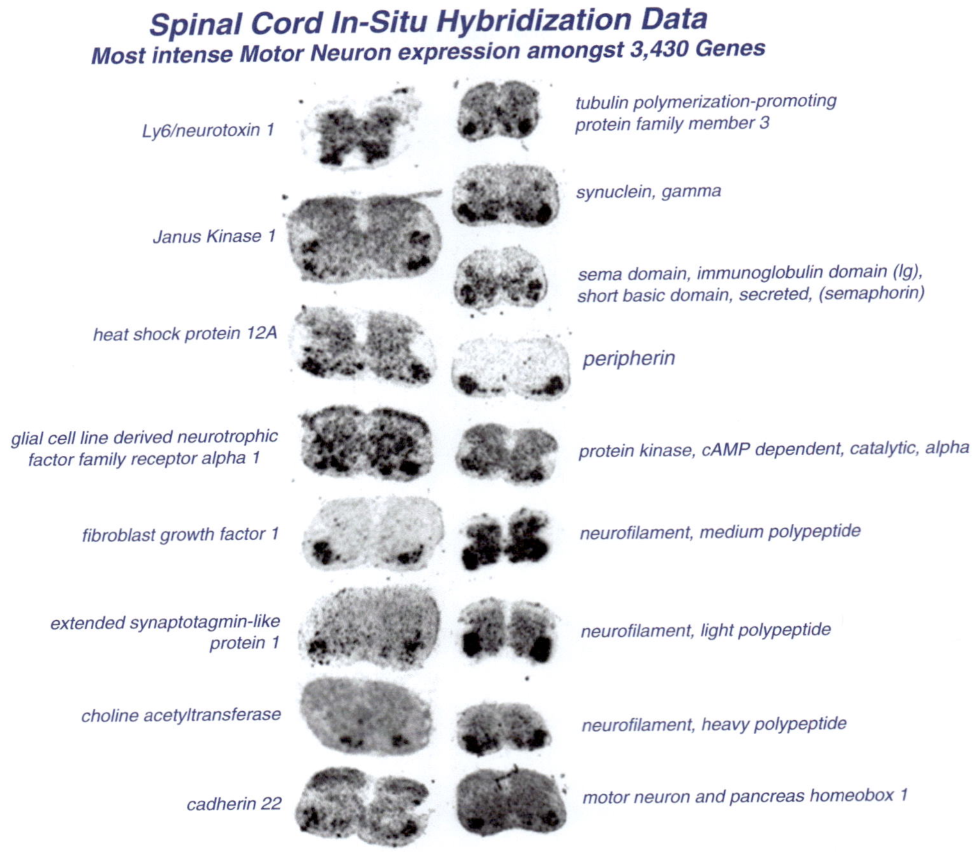

Fig. 10.7 17 candidate genes that may be involved in ALS

important differential diagnostic consideration for weakness in an elderly patient involves compressive effects from arthritic and degenerative changes within the surrounding spinal elements. In this regard, important considerations arise in evaluating elderly patients with symptoms potentially referable to the spinal cord itself, with the important need to determine whether life-threatening compression of the cord is present. Rapid decline in gait can signal a thoracic compression if bowel and bladder dysfunction are present, especially when a sensory level is found on examination along with bilateral plantar extensor reflexes being noted. The concerns become even greater with four limb involvement, suggesting a high cervical compression, as shown in Fig. 10.8. Whereas the recommendation for urgent surgical decompression are clear for extreme cases such as the type shown in Fig. 10.8, many cases of degenerative cervical spondylolisthesis are not as clear cut. In this regard, a systematic review has been carried out on the topic of degenerative cervical spondylolisthesis; from a study group of over 100 cases, nearly two-thirds presented with myelopathy or myeloradiculopathy. Degenerative cervical spondylolisthesis was most common in C3/4 and C4/5, with 46 % found to have segmental instability on flexion-extension views [11]. The decision to intervene surgically must be individualized; the patient illustrated in Fig. 10.8 had slowly progressive symptoms over many months and ultimately declined surgery due to the perceived risks at the advanced age of 87 years.

With regards to acute spinal cord trauma, high-dose steroid treatment may be helpful (Table 10.1), but its uniform use is controversial. Methylprednisolone can attenuate peroxidation of membrane lipids and post-traumatic inflam-

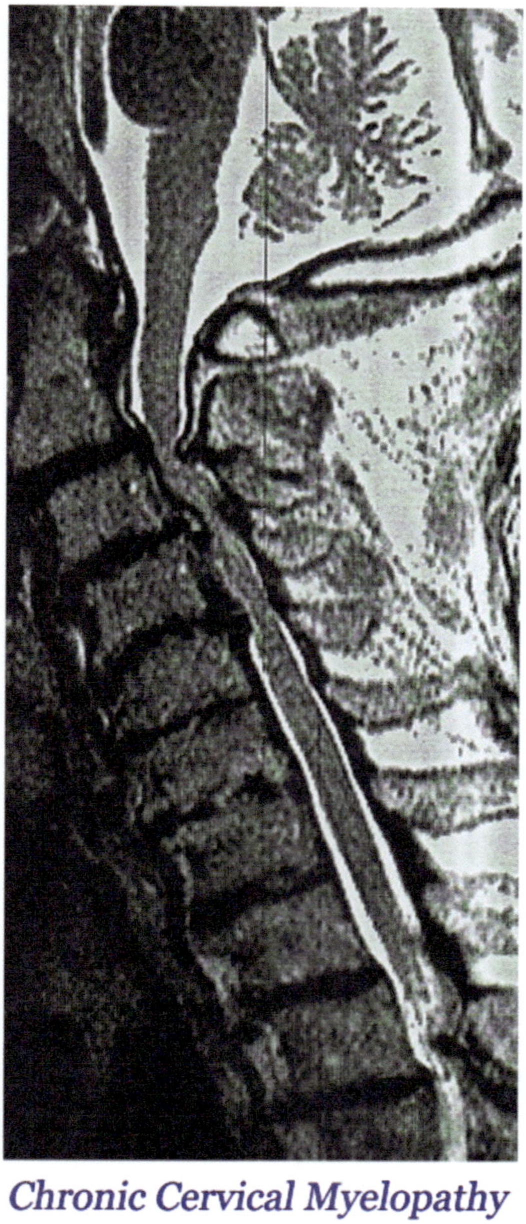

Fig. 10.8 High cervical cord compression in a 87-year-old male

Table 10.1 Spinal cord trauma

• Methylprednisolone IV at 30 mg/kg within first 6 h of trauma may improve long-term outcome
• MR imaging is essential
• Neurologic intensive care unit required
• Neurosurgical consultation in the ER

mation [12]. Although a Cochrane meta-analysis review of three studies found no effect for a high-dose 24-h infusion of methylprednisolone in terms of motor recovery at 6 months, methylprednisolone was associated with an additional 4-point improvement in NASCIS motor score when steroids were started within 8 h after injury; as noted by Wilson et.al., "….consensus guidelines recommend that 24-h infusion of methylprednisolone, started within 8 h after injury, is a treatment option that should only be undertaken with knowledge of the potential complications….. Intravenous methylprednisolone has been used as a neuroprotective strategy based on limited evidence, but this is not a standard of care and may be associated with an increased risk of complications." Therapeutic hypothermia has not yet been proven to be of help.

As noted by Ki et al. spinal cord infarction is a relatively rare problem [13], but can occur in cocaine users, cardiac and aortic surgery, aortic angiography, arteriovenous malformation, polyarteritis nodosa, and systemic hypotension. However, as also noted by Ki et al. and shown in Fig. 10.9, spinal cord infarction can spontaneously occur due to asymptomatic aortic aneurysm with intraluminal thrombus. As shown in Fig. 10.9, MR is helpful in visualizing the extent and site of cord ischemia, with CT angiography employing 3D reconstruction techniques helpful in revealing the patency of segmental radicular arterial branches from the abdominal aorta.

Intraspinal fluid cavities known as syringomyelia are readily detected by MRI (Fig. 10.10) and may enlarge over time and cause progressive neurologic dysfunction; many but not all are associated with cerebellar tonsilar herniation (Chiari malformation). Recent studies suggest a pathophysiologic mechanism based on the idea that in primary spinal syringomyelia, exaggerated spinal subarachnoid pressure waves "…act on the spinal cord above the block to drive CSF into the spinal cord and create a syrinx. After a syrinx is formed, enlarged subarachnoid pressure waves compress the external surface of the spinal cord, propel the syrinx fluid, and promote syrinx progression." [14].

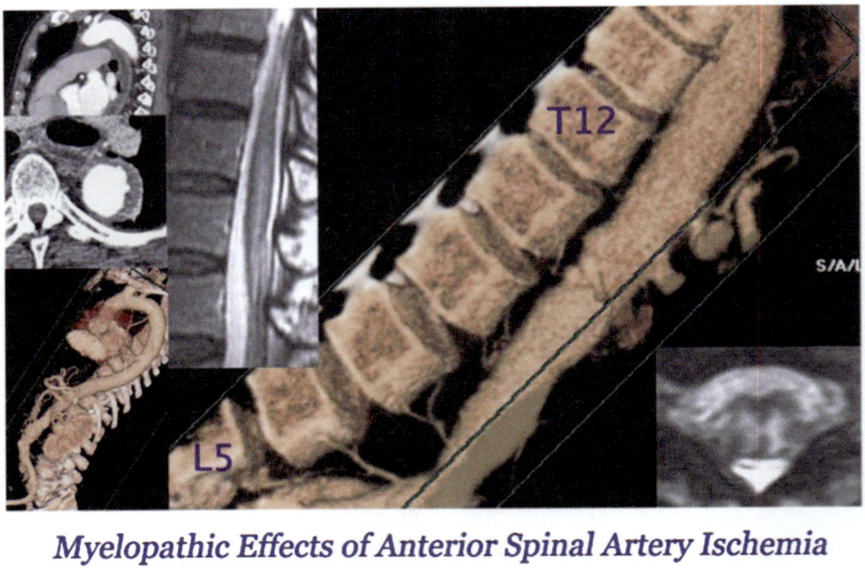

Fig. 10.9 Embolic spinal cord infarct with non-visualization of T12-L1 radicular artery

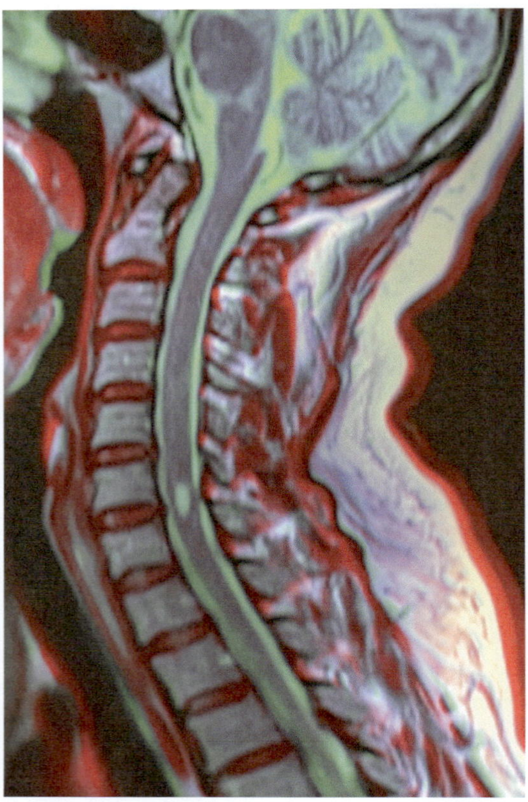

Fig. 10.10 Syringomyelia at C6–C7 (adapted from Wikipedia)

Syringomyelia associated with spinal pathology is known as primary spinal syringomyelia and accounts for about 17 % of all cases and may be due to trauma, inflammation, or compressive lesions that compromise the subarachnoid space. Posttraumatic syringomyelia usually presents with symptoms above the level of injury that starts months to years after initial trauma; paraplegia rates are at least 4 %. Compression of the CSF pathways by tumors, osteophytes, or herniated disks have been linked to syrinx formation, as well as herniated cerebellar tonsils that can act as pistons to produce cervical subarachnoid pressure waves that leads to progressive syrinx expansion.

References

1. Saada F, Antonios N. Existence of ipsilateral hemiparesis in ischemic and hemorrhagic stroke: two case reports and review of the literature. Eur Neurol. 2014;71:25–31.
2. Weiller C, Chollet F, Frinston KJ, et al. Functional reorganization of the brain in recovery from striatocapsular infarction in man. Ann Neurol. 1992;31:463–72.

3. Hassel B. Tetanus: pathophysiology, treatment, and the possibility of using botulinum toxin against tetanus-induced rigidity and spasms. Toxins (Basel). 2013;5(1):73–83.
4. Zarei S, Carr K, Reiley L, et al. A comprehensive review of amyotrophic lateral sclerosis. Surg Neurol Int. 2015;6:171.
5. Meyer MA, Potter NT. Sporadic ALS and chromosome 22: evidence for a possible neurofilament gene defect. Muscle Nerve. 1995;18(5):536–9.
6. Tomkins J, Usher P, Slade JY, et al. Novel insertion in the KSP region of the neurofilament heavy gene in amyotrophic lateral sclerosis (ALS). Neuroreport. 1998;9(17):3967–70.
7. Kriz J, Meier J, Julien JP, Padjen AL. Altered ionic conductances in axons of transgenic mouse expressing the human neurofilament heavy gene: a mouse model of amyotrophic lateral sclerosis. Exp Neurol. 2000;163(2):414–21.
8. Meyer MA. Identification of 17 highly expressed genes within mouse lumbar spinal cord anterior horn region from an in-situ hybridization atlas of 3430 genes: implications for motor neuron disease. Neurol Int. 2014;6(2):5367.
9. Gros-Louis F, Larivière R, Gowing G, et al. A frameshift deletion in peripherin gene associated with amyotrophic lateral sclerosis. J Biol Chem. 2004; 279(44):45951–6.
10. Bricceno KV, Fischbeck KH, Burnett BG. Neurogenic and myogenic contributions to hereditary motor neuron disease. Neurodegener Dis. 2012;9(4):199–209.
11. Jiang SD, Jiang LS, Dai LY. Degenerative cervical spondylolisthesis: a systematic review. Int Orthop. 2011;35(6):869–75.
12. Wilson JR, Forgione N, Fehlings MG. Emerging therapies for acute traumatic spinal cord injury. CMAJ. 2013;185(6):485–92.
13. Ki YJ, Jeon BH, Bang HJ. Spinal cord infarction caused by non-dissected and unruptured thoracoabdominal aortic aneurysm with intraluminal thrombus. Ann Rehabil Med. 2012;36(2):297–302.
14. Heiss JD, Snyder K, Peterson MM, et al. Pathophysiology of primary spinal syringomyeli. J Neurosurg Spine. 2012;17(5):367–80.

The Cerebellum

11

11.1 Introduction

The cerebellum is an amazing structure that mediates motor coordination on an automatic unconscious basis. Analogous to a computer dedicated to sensing all aspects of movement, the neurons within the cerebellum receive and processes a variety of somatotopically organized sensory inputs with a well defined modular circuitry endlessly repeated within its cortical folds. To extend the analogy a little more, the basic computational element within the cerebellar cortex is the complex dendritic tree of the large Purkinje neuron which contain about 200,000 dendritic spines; input comes from a multitude of relatively weak inputs from parallel fibers versus singular strong glutaminergic inputs from climbing fibers that arise from the inferior olive, where a single climbing fiber can excite a single Purkinje neuron at 500 synaptic points of contact throughout the dendritic tree. The final output is from Purkinje cell axons that converges upon the deep cerebellar nuclei in the form of inhibitory GABAergic synapses.

A remarkable feature to the cerebellum is the highly cellular nature, where 50 billion small granule cells form a compact inner layer to the three-layer cortex. Although literally translated from the Latin terminology as "The Little Brain", it is anything but small as the highly compact and infolded cerebellum holds 80 % of the total number of nerve cells in the entire brain! The middle layer is Purkinje cell layer, whereas the outer layer is known as the molecular layer, which contains the highly branched dendritic trees of the Purkinje neurons along with. Whereas the cerebral cortex comprises 84 % of total human brain mass, cerebellar neurons outnumber cortical neurons by 3.6 to 1 despite the fact that the cerebellum comprises about 10 % of the total brain weight [1].

It was not until the early 1800s that it became apparent that the cerebellum was critical for motor coordination and balance. As revealed by the studies of Flourens, surgical removal of the cerebellum resulted in severe ataxia and imbalance (see Fig. 11.1 for the 1842 illustration on the effects of cerebellum removal in the pigeon; [2]). At about the same time, the gifted Czech anatomist Johann Evangelist Purkinje performed the first microscopic histologic examinations of the cerebellum, leading to his discovery of the dominantly large neurons that now bear his name.

The gross anatomy for the cerebellum is shown in Figs. 11.2 and 11.3, which illustrate the large fiber peduncular tracts that interconnects the cerebellum with the brain stem; rich interconnections exist between the highly infolded inferior olive within the anterior aspects of the medulla. Although midline cerebellar cortex projects to the cluster of small deep nuclei known as the emboliform, globose, and fastigial nuclei, the remainder of the cerebellar cortex projects to the highly infolded all important dentate nucleus (Fig. 11.4). As the main output center of the cer-

M.A. Meyer, *Neurologic Disease*, DOI 10.1007/978-3-319-39581-4_11

Fig. 11.1 Jean Pierre Flourens (1794–1867) Cerebellar Ataxia: adaptation of a 1842 publication by Flourens on the role of the cerebellum in maintaining balance and coordination. Pigeon from which the cerebellum has been removed is markedly ataxic and incoordinated

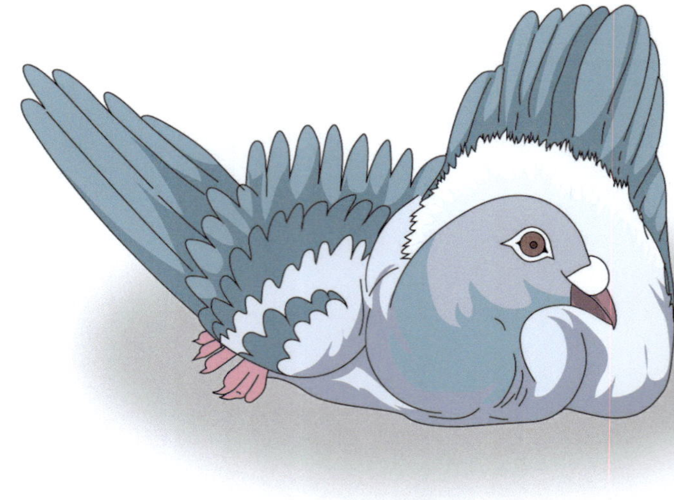

Fig. 11.2 Gross anatomy of the cerebellum; note the cerebellar peduncles attaching the cerebellum to the brain stem

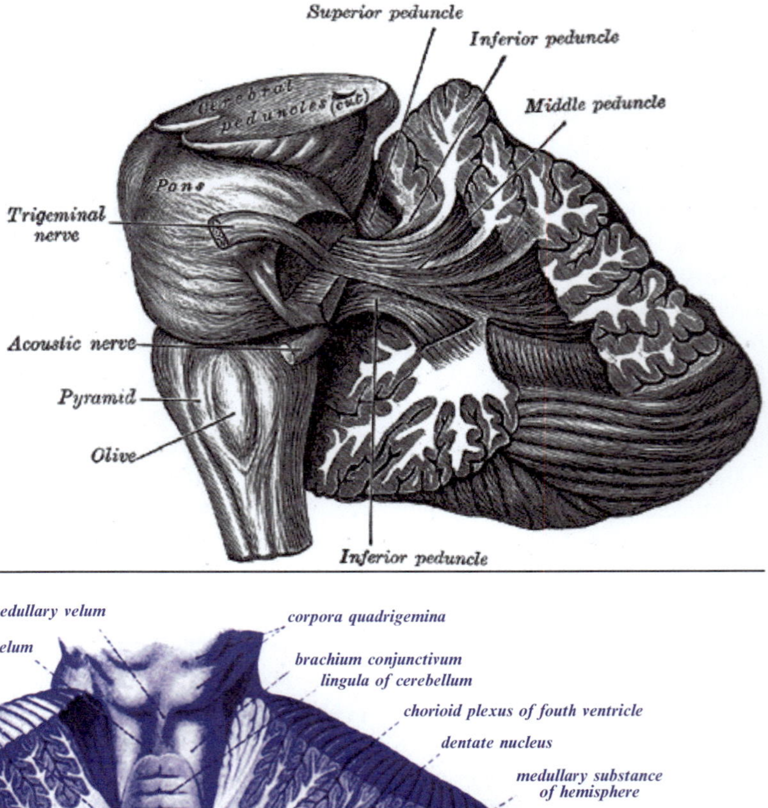

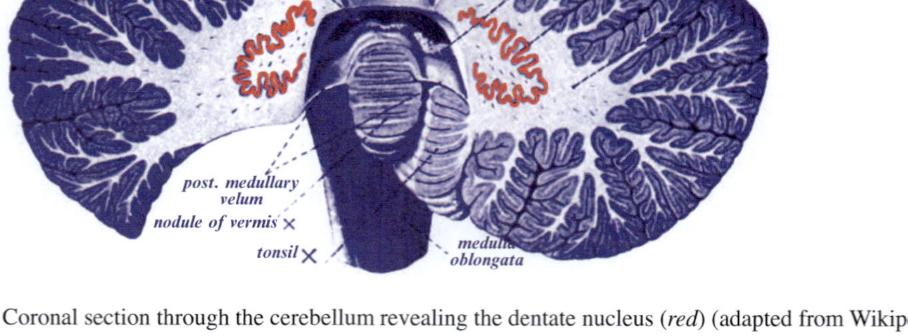

Fig. 11.3 Coronal section through the cerebellum revealing the dentate nucleus (*red*) (adapted from Wikipedia)

ebellum, the dentate neurons project not only to the ventrolateral thalamus, and red nucleus, but also to the cerebral cortex; the dorsal aspects of the dentate project to the primary motor and premotor cortices whereas ventral aspects project to the posterior parietal and prefrontal cortices [3]. With regards to the cortical projections, it has been proposed that the cerebellum is also involved in maintaining a sense of direction and navigating motor activities within a mental representation of space [4]. Other functions include a proposed role in associative learning and memory, as well as modulation of cognitive and emotional processes [5, 6].

The functional organization of the cerebellum is illustrated in Fig. 11.4, where the inferior olive projects excitatory input to the dendritic tree of the large Purkinje neuron, which is activated as well by a network of parallel fibers that derive from the multitude of small granule cells that form axons that split in two to resemble a "T"; the small granule cells receive their activating input from mossy fibers. GABAergic inhibitory cells within the cerebellum include basket cells

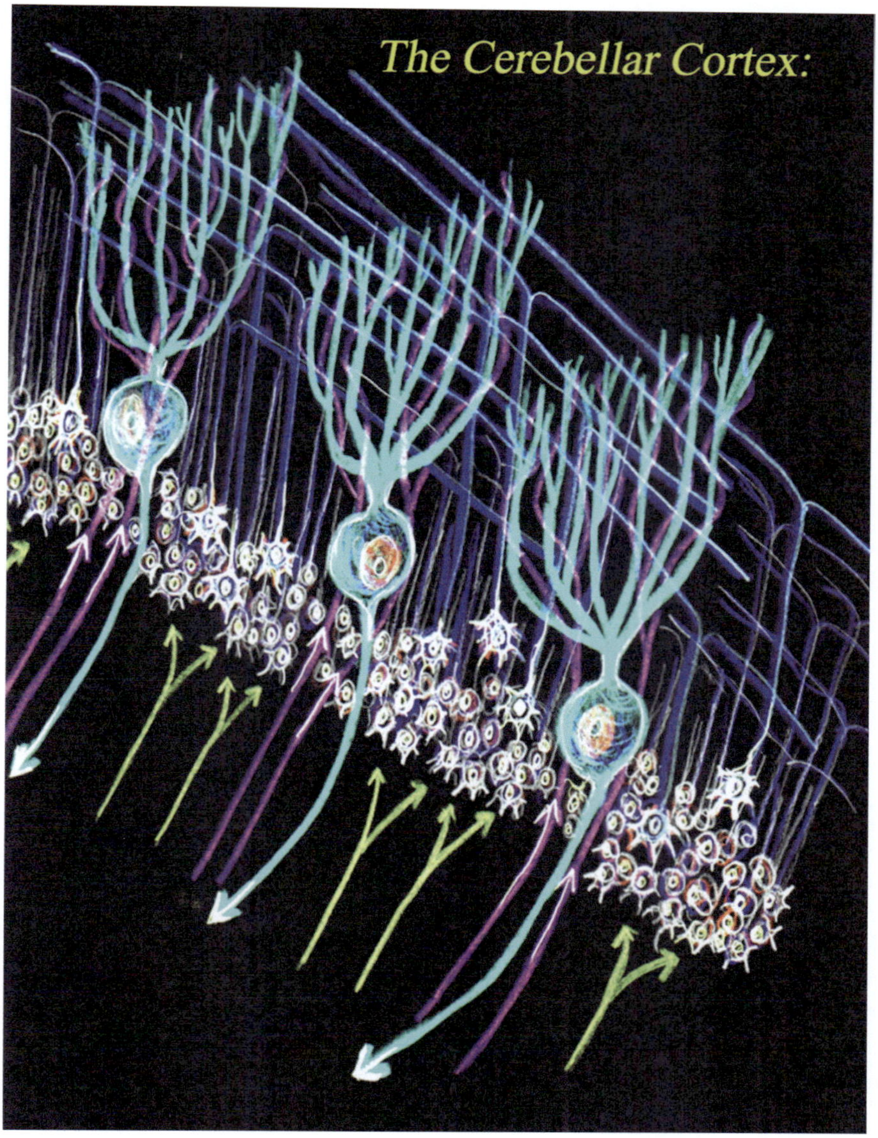

Fig. 11.4 Cerebellar neuronal circuitry, showing mossy fiber input in *yellow* versus climbing fiber input in *purple*

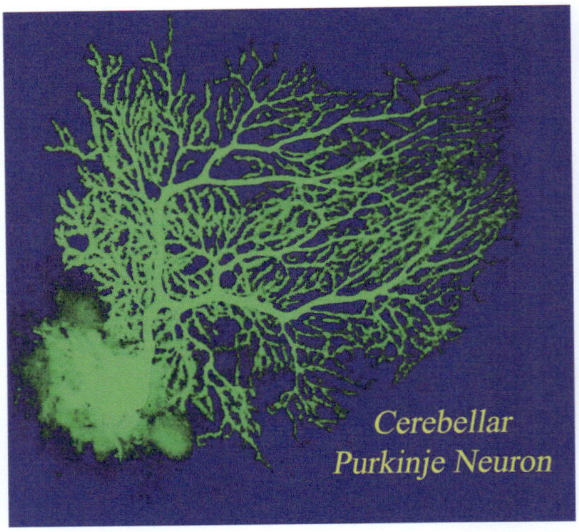

Fig. 11.5 Intracellular injection of a fluorescent tracer to reveal Purkinje cell dendritic arborization details (adapted from Wikipedia)

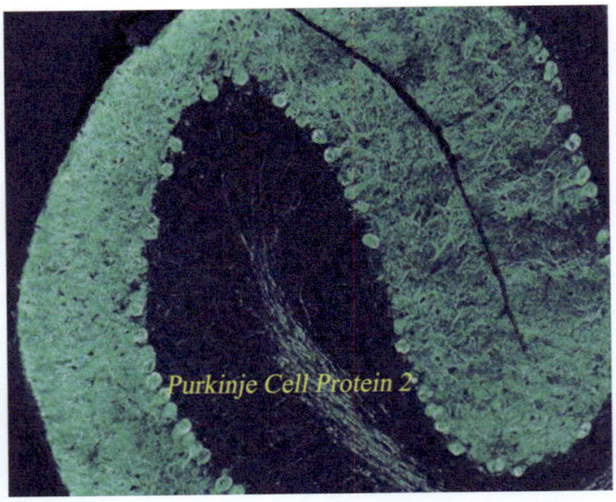

Fig. 11.6 Cerebellar expression of Purkinje cell protein 2

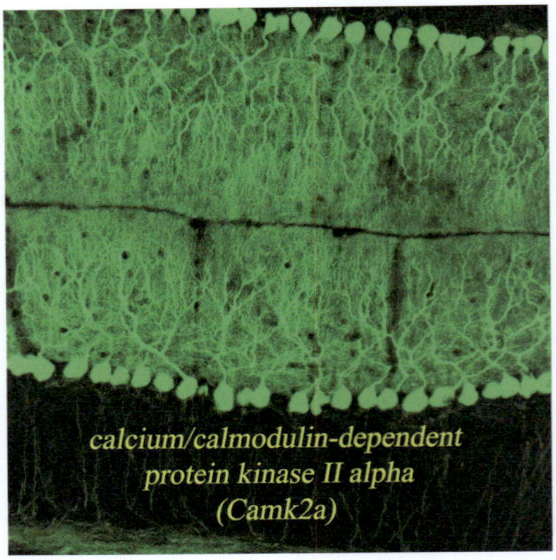

Fig. 11.7 Cerebellar expression of CamK2a

that have axonal branches that surround the Purkinje cell body in the shape of a basket and mediate inhibition along with the stellate cell interneurons.

The intricate morphology of the Purkinje neuron dendritic tree is shown in Fig. 11.5 after direct intracellular injection of a fluorescent dye. Although very elaborate, the dendritic tree is compacted into one flat plane that is perpendicular to the cortical folds and oriented at right angles to the network of parallel fibers that pass through the tree, forming about 20,000 synaptic contacts with each Purkinje neuron. Histochemical techniques can reveal biochemical details of gene expression within the Purkinje neuron, as shown in Fig. 11.6 for one of many proteins that are selectively expressed within Purkinje neurons. In contrast, other proteins expressed throughout the brain and other organs may also be strongly expressed within Purkinje neurons, as shown in Fig. 11.7 for the case of CAMK2A, otherwise known as calcium/calmodulin-dependent protein kinase II, which is a ubiquitous serine/threonine protein kinase found throughout the brain as a major component of the postsynaptic density; of additional note, inhibitory phosphorylation of this protein seems to play a critical role in neural plasticity and learning [7].

Normal expression of the cerebellar protein Ataxin-2 is illustrated in Fig. 11.8. Normally, this protein is involved in regulation of the epidermal growth factor receptor and the inositol 1,4,5-triphosphate receptor as well as linked with functioning of the endoplasmic reticulum and the Golgi complex [8]. However, when mutations arise that expand the CAG trinucleotide repeat in exon 1 of the Ataxin-2 gene causing extra glutamine residues within the assembled protein, the protein misfolds and undergoes a toxic gain of function. Accumulation of these toxic misfolded Ataxin-2 proteins induce a progressive degeneration of cere-

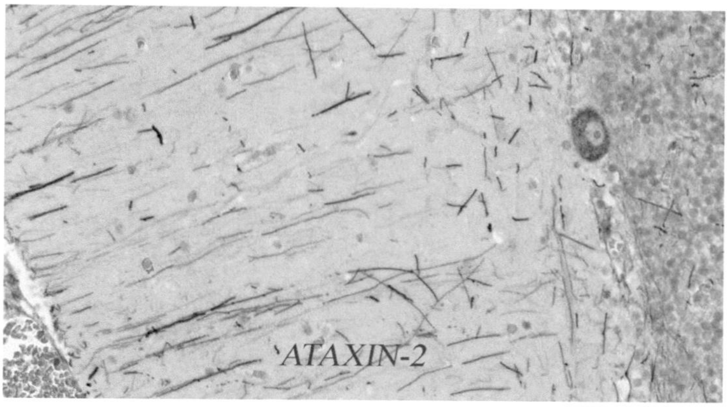

Fig. 11.8 Cerebellar expression of the Ataxin-2 protein; trinucleotide gene expansions linked to OPCA (SCA2)

bellar Purkinje cells, and selective loss of neurons within the brainstem and spinal cord, along with developing progressive incoordination, gait ataxia, slurred speech, with cognitive impairment. Known as a form of olivo-pontocerebellar atrophy (OPCA) and classified as spino-cerebellar atrophy type 2 (SCA2), the age of onset is known to be inversely correlated to the length of the trinucleotide repeat, as with other similar trinucleotide repeat disorders such as Huntington's and DRPLA.

Symptomatic cerebellar degeneration can also arise as a paraneoplastic effect, especially with ovarian cancer or small cell lung carcinoma. Known as one of the most frequent paraneoplastic syndromes affecting the CNS, paraneoplastic cerebellar degeneration (PCD) presents with cerebellar symptoms of gait ataxia, incoordination, or dysarthria with nystagmus, and may actually be the presenting problem in a previously healthy individual in advance of any known symptoms referable to an occult malignancy. PCD is associated with antibodies targeting intracellular neuronal antigens not thought to be directly pathogenic (e.g., Hu, Yo, Ri), versus known association with antibodies to surface antigens that could be potentially pathogenic such as Delta/Notch-like epidermal growth factor-related receptor (DNER). Recently, the case of a poorly differentiated squamous cell lung carcinoma patient was reported with symptoms of progressive dizziness, vomiting, oscillopsia, dysarthria, with nystagmus, plus severe cerebellar dysarthria, limb incoordination and gait ataxia that was so severe, he was unable to walk. Eventually diagnosed with PCD, he was found to have autoantibodies to a novel neuronal antigen termed plasticity-related gene 5 (PRG5), which is a transmembrane protein expressed in the hippocampus and cerebellum and involved in dendritic spine formation [9].

This unusual phenomenon of paraneoplastic cerebellar degeneration raises questions about how Purkinje neurons become the target for autoimmune attack. In this regard, it is important to note that fluorescent antibodies specific for the pan T lymphocyte marker CD3 will also selectively stain Purkinje neurons (Figs. 11.9 and 11.10) [10, 11]. Considering this surprising expression of a key immune system protein in the cerebellum, it is tempting to speculate that this leaves the Purkinje predisposed to attack by altered antigen presentation. As the CD3 subunits on T lymphocytes normally bind with the T-cell receptor to form an immunologic synapse that recognizes specific antigens bound to major histocompatibility complex present on antigen-presenting cells, it is possible that a similar immunological synapse forms on Purkinje neural membranes, predisposing the cerebellum to autoimmune attack.

With regards to other disease states that link Purkinje cells with immune deficits is the rare pediatric cerebellar degeneration known as ataxia telangiectasia. Caused by a defect within the ATM gene (Fig. 11.11), the autosomal recessive disorder is characterized by progressive cerebellar dysfunction, oculocutaneous telangiectasia, and immune deficiency. Other features are chromosomal instability, high sensitivity to ionizing radiation plus susceptibility to malignancies, especially leukemia and lymphoma. The normal human cerebellar expression of the ATM gene is

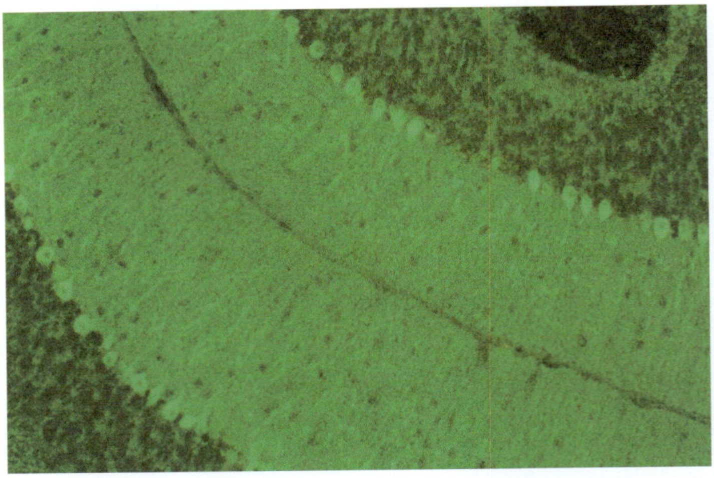

Fig. 11.9 Purkinje cell localization using fluorescent tagged monoclonal antibody to CD3

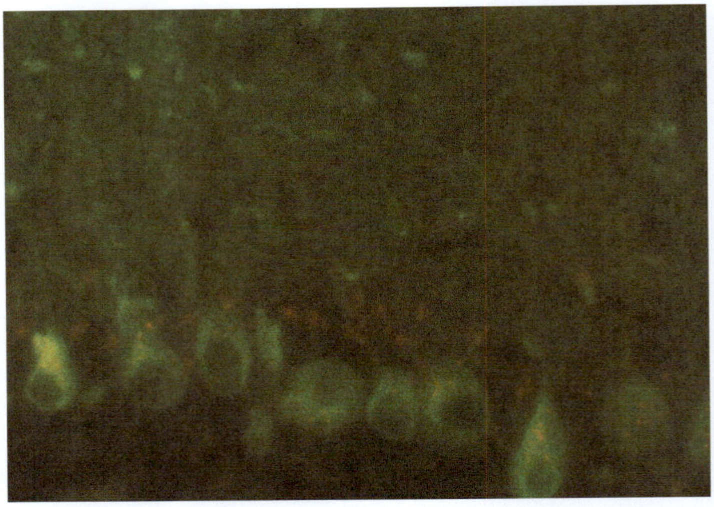

Fig. 11.10 Close-up view of CD3 localization to Purkinje neurons

shown in Fig. 11.11; the protein is involved in numerous pathways including cell cycle checkpoint control and DNA repair [12]. More specifically, ATM protein is an important cell cycle checkpoint kinase that phosphorylates and thereby regulates many downstream proteins such as tumor suppressor proteins p53 and BRCA1, and DNA repair protein NBS1; in essence, ATM is essential for cell response to DNA damage and for genome stability. As ATM is found in other areas of the brain, it still remains unclear why the cerebellum is preferentially affected.

A fairly common problem in clinical practice is the question of cerebellar Chiari malformation as it relates to the evaluation of patients with headaches who show prominence to the cerebellar tonsils on MRI. When clinically significant, the cerebellar tissue may actually herniate through the cisterna magna, creating what is commonly termed the Chiari malformation (Fig. 11.12), which is graded one through four for severity, with type one being the most common and least severe. Although the condition can arise in certain cases due to trauma, most are thought to be congential, and may be asymptomatic during childhood, but often manifest in early adulthood with headaches secondary to alterations in the flow of cerebrospinal fluid as the cerebellar tonsil can crowd the limited space within the foramen magnum and partially obstruct normal flow of spinal

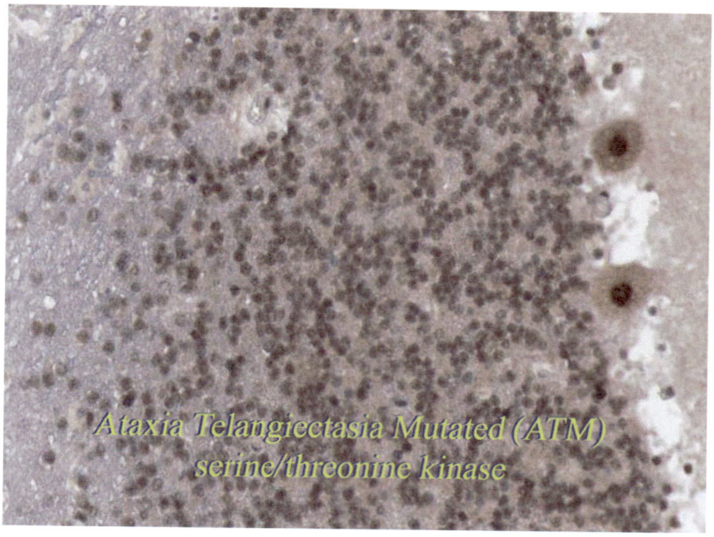

Fig. 11.11 Human cerebellum localization of ATM protein to granule cell nucleus and Purkinje cell nucleus

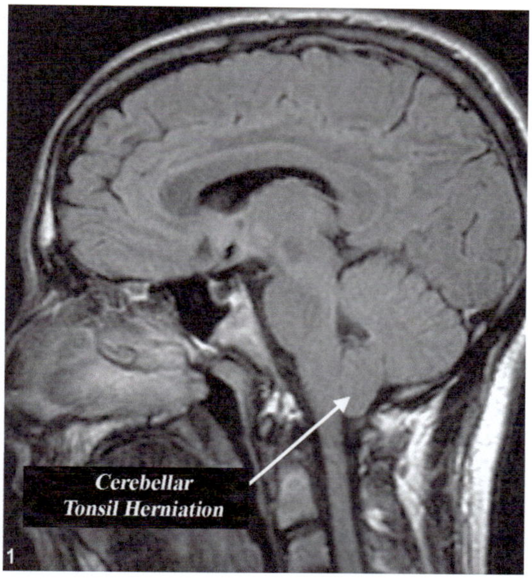

Fig. 11.12 MRI revealing Chiari type 1 malformation (from Wikipedia)

fluid. First described in the late nineteenth century by the Austrian pathologist, the symptoms of the Chiari malformation predominantly involve headache, but can also include fatigue with poor sleep and generalized weakness, and in severe cases may have associated nausea with vomiting, dizziness, tinnitus, impaired coordination, neck pain, and unsteady gait. Severe cases can rarely present as a neurosurgical emergency with signs of increased intracranial pressure with obstruction, requiring a decompressive craniectomy with the placement of a shunt, as shown in Fig. 11.13. In about one-fourth of all Chiari cases is the coexistence of a spinal cord syrinx; syringomyelia in these cases is often seen between the C-4 and C-6 levels and likely arises from pressure waves transmitted through the central canal from intermittent partial obstruction of normal spinal flow at skull base.

Finally, this overview on cerebellar disease pathophysiology would be incomplete without discussing the paroxysmal familial disorder known as episodic ataxia (EA) which is generally autosomal dominant and characterized by sporadic bouts of severe incoordination; seven types are known but two forms predominate. It is important to note that some patients with episodic ataxia also have migraine (particularly the uncommon familial hemiplegic form) or progressive cerebellar degenerative disorders; some patients also respond to the use of acetazolamide. As the disorder can be based upon defects within potassium channels expressed within inhibitory basket cells that wrap around Purkinje neurons, as in type 1 EA, alteration of cerebellar electrical activity with alteration of Purkinje cell mediated inhibition upon the deep cerebellar nuclei explain the symptoms of episodic generalized ataxia; however, myokymia is also present, leading to alternate names for the disorder as episodic ataxia with myokymia (EAM), or hereditary paroxysmal ataxia with neuromyotonia (Isaacs-Mertens syndrome). EA1 attacks last from seconds to minutes, and are caused by potassium channel gene mutations (KCNA1) encoding the $K_V1.1$ protein.

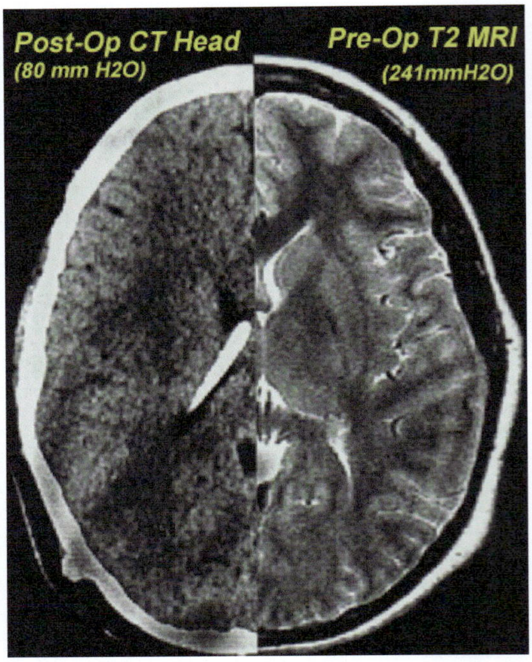

Fig. 11.13 Pre-op versus post-op imaging of Chiari patient requiring emergent neurosurgical decompression

Episodic ataxia can also be caused by hereditary defects within calcium channels, as in EA2, which is characterized by acetazolamide-responsive attacks of cerebellar ataxia with or without migraine. As with EA1, attacks can be brought on by stress, but also by alcohol or caffeine. The disorder is brought on by mutations within the gene CACNA1A (Fig. 11.14) which codes for the pore-forming alpha1A subunit of voltage-gated P/Q calcium channel; the gene is also linked to familial hemiplegic migraine and spinocerebellar ataxia type 6. The gene is expressed throughout the brain and particularly in the cerebellar Purkinje and granule cells. EA2 is also known as acetazolamide-responsive hereditary paroxysmal cerebellar ataxia (AHPCA). Electrophysiologic recordings of cultured cells that coexpressed the mutagenized human alpha1A-2 subunit showed complete loss of calcium channel activity [13].

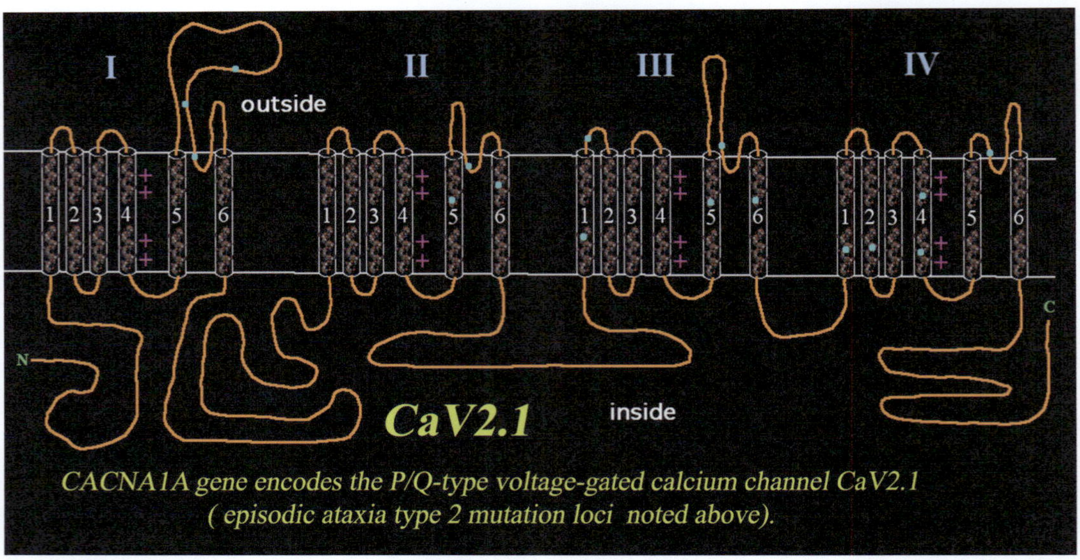

Fig. 11.14 CACNA1A gene mutation loci (*light blue*) responsible for episodic ataxia (adapted from Wikipedia)

References

1. Herculano-Houzel S. Coordinated scaling of cortical and cerebellar numbers of neurons. Front Neuroanat. 2010;4:12.
2. Flourens MJP. Recherches expérimentales sur les propriétés et les functions du système nerveux dans les animaux vertébrés. Paris: JB Ballière; 1842.
3. Dum RP, Strick PL. An unfolded map of the cerebellar dentate nucleus and its projections to the cerebral cortex. J Neurophysiol. 2003;89(1):634–9.
4. Rondi-Reig L, Paradis AL, Lefort JM, et al. How the cerebellum may monitor sensory information for spatial representation. Front Syst Neurosci. 2014;8:205.
5. Popa LS, Hewitt AL, Ebner TJ. The cerebellum for jocks and nerds alike. Front Syst Neurosci. 2014; 8:113.
6. Bernard JA, Seidler RD. Moving forward: age effects on the cerebellum underlie cognitive and motor declines. Neurosci Biobehav Rev. 2014;42:193–207.
7. Elgersma Y, Fedorov NB, Ikonen S, et al. Inhibitory autophosphorylation of CaMKII controls PSD association, plasticity, and learning. Neuron. 2002;36: 493–505.
8. Dansithong W, Paul S, Figueroa KP, et al. Ataxin-2 regulates RGS8 translation in a new BAC-SCA2 transgenic mouse model. PLoS Genet. 2015;11(4), e1005182.
9. van Coevorden-Hameete MH, de Graaff E, Titulaer MJ, et al. Plasticity-related gene 5: a novel surface autoantigen in paraneoplastic cerebellar degeneration. Neurol Neuroimmunol Neuroinflamm. 2015;2(5), e156.
10. Gerloff C, Knoth R, Volk B. Cytoplasmic expression of the leu-4 (CD3) antigen in developing Purkinje cells in the rat cerebellum. Neuropathol Appl Neurobiol. 1993;19(4):313–23.
11. Nakamura K, Hirai H, Torashima T, et al. CD3 and immunoglobulin G Fc receptor regulate cerebellar functions. Mol Cell Biol. 2007;27(14):5128–34.
12. Chopra C, Davies G, Taylor M, et al. Immune deficiency in Ataxia-Telangiectasia: a longitudinal study of 44 patients. Clin Exp Immunol. 2014;176(2): 275–82.
13. Guida S, Trettel F, Pagnutti S, et al. Complete loss of P/Q calcium channel activity caused by a CACNA1A missense mutation carried by patients with episodic ataxia type 2. Am J Hum Genet. 2001;68(3):759–64.

12 The Visual Cortex

The visual system of human beings form a crowning achievement to the process of evolution. The visual system is perhaps the most important aspect of neurologic functioning and forms the basis of what we do as humans—life without the ability to see is hard to imagine, as we are so dependent on this amazing gift many of us take for granted. The process of how light striking the retina becomes transformed into a three-dimensional perception within the visual cortex is truly amazing; most of what will be discussed in this chapter focuses on the primary and secondary occipital cortices, with an emphasis on the columnar organization, basic review of the retina in health and disease will be presented along with a discussion of the lateral geniculate nucleus as the key intermediary way station between the retina and the cortex.

The primary topic of the visual cortex serves as a gateway to a major section that reviews one of the most fundamental neurologic problems: migraine. When developing as a classic migraine, with premonitory and/or associated visual symptoms, modern neuroimaging techniques such as PET and MRI confirm that spreading depression with a wave of reduced cerebral blood flow propagates outward and forward from the occipital poles. Complex migrainous aura symptoms with glowing lines, columns, and bars reflect the underlying columnar organization of the visual cortex.

Starting out in the periphery, the visual system has its basis within the retina, where the entire human retina contains about seven million cones to encode color vision versus 150 million rods that transduce even very faint and weak light stimuli; it is quite remarkable that a single rod photoreceptor cell can respond to a single photon, and the brain requires fewer than 10 such responses to register the sensation of a flash of light. The molecular basis for this is outlined in Fig. 12.1; light stimulation actually hyperpolarizes the photoreceptor membrane in graded shifts. Intracellular cyclic GMP keeps sodium channels open until the light photon hits the 11-cis retinal molecule and induces molecular motion within the photoreceptor membrane from the isomerization into all-trans retinal thereby activating multiple G proteins and a phosphodiesterase that then degrades cyclic GMP, prompting closure of sodium channels that cause hyperpolarization; photoreceptor neurotransmitter release is thereby reduced. Through the network of inter-connected horizontal, amacrine, and bipolar cells, these receptors influence retinal ganglion cells (Fig. 12.2); these retinal ganglion cells can be of the ON or OFF type and have special central receptive fields with annular surround effects, where light has the opposite effect on the firing of the cell. In ON cells, central light stimulation activates the firing rate whereas light stimulation to the center of the receptive field diminishes firing of OFF cells. Likewise, linear spatial summation effects are encoded in X versus Y cells. Collectively, these ganglion cells funnel their output toward the optic disk (the "blind spot")

M.A. Meyer, *Neurologic Disease*, DOI 10.1007/978-3-319-39581-4_12

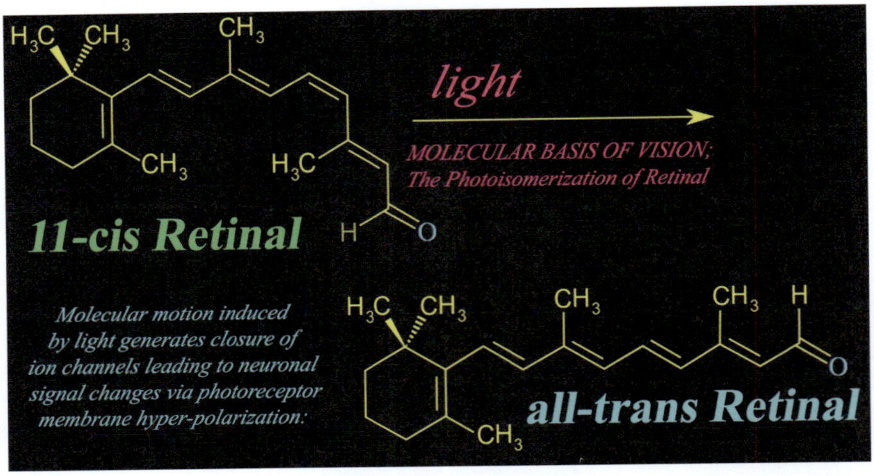

Fig. 12.1 Molecular motion induced by light generates closure of ion channels leading to neuronal signal changes via membrane hyperpolarization

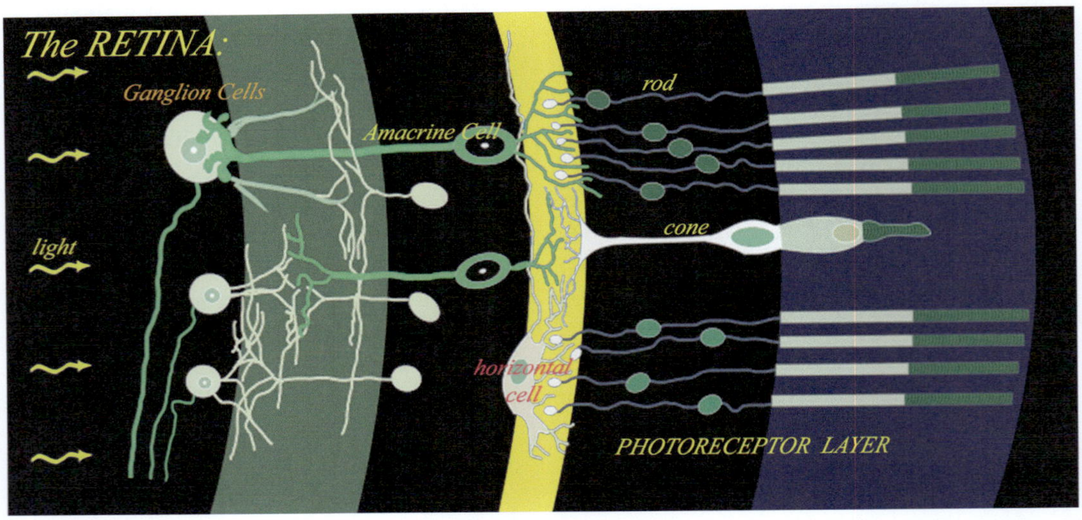

Fig. 12.2 Neuronal circuitry of the retina (adapted from Wikipedia)

as a nasally located zone where the optic nerve fibers exit to form the optic nerves. As significant pre-processing takes place within the retinal layers, the numerous 130 million retinal receptors funnel their activity into a more compact output bundle of only 1.2 million axonal nerve fibers that form the optic nerve.

In about 1 in 1000 individuals, the optic nerves degenerate on a hereditary basis, forming a collective group termed optic neuropathies. The dominant forms for this disease involve the loss of retinal ganglion cells, as seen in Leber hereditary optic neuropathy (LHON) caused by maternally inherited mitochondrial DNA (mtDNA) mutations; another retinal ganglion degenerative disease includes autosomal-dominant optic atrophy (DOA) caused by mutations within the OPA1 gene, which codes for a mitochondrial inner-membrane protein [1]. LHON is rare but is important to recognize as it can present as acute, painless loss of central vision, with the other eye invariably affected within a year; patients often become symptomatic in the second and third decades of life, and over 90 %

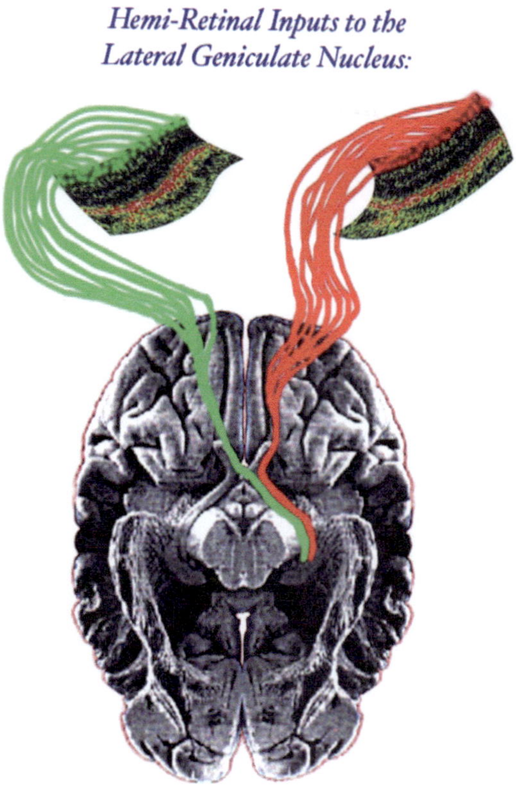

Fig. 12.3 Unification of fibers from each hemi-retinas at the optic chiasm radiate back to innervate the lateral geniculate of the thalamus

of those with the gene mutation have visual failure by age 50.

As shown in Fig. 12.3, the ganglion cells of the temporal retina (red) project ipsilaterally to the lateral geniculate nucleus (LGN) of the thalamus along with fibers from the nasal hemi-retina of the opposite eye (green), providing a unified sense of depth perception of the same aspects of the visual field projected by the lens upon each hemi-retina in an inverted fashion from slightly different angles. Their projections upon the LGN is segregated into layers, where the ipsilateral eye transmits input to LGN layers 2, 3, and 5 (Fig. 12.4, red), whereas the eye on the opposite side sends information to layers 1, 4, and 6 (Fig. 12.4, green). The inner two layers are termed magnocellular as they are comprised of large neurons that get their retinal input from ganglion cells interconnected to rods and help mediate perception of depth and movement along with small differences in brightness, while the outer four layers (layers 3, 4, 5, and 6) are parvocellular layers made up of small neurons that mediate the perception of color via their connections from ganglion cells supplied by cones. A third set of neurons, known as the koniocellular type, are more obscure and comprise very small neurons that are intralaminar in location between large cell and small cell layers; these very small neurons mediate not only some aspects of color vision but integrate somatosensory and proprioceptive information with visual input from the retina [2]. Much of the input in the LGN comes from sources other than the retina and include the visual cortex, superior colliculus, pretectum, thalamic reticular nuclei, and local LGN interneurons; brainstem input arises from the mesencephalic reticular formation, dorsal raphe nucleus, periaqueductal grey matter, and the locus coeruleus [3]. Feedback input from higher cortical regions of the visual cortex play important roles in modulating LGN activity, with some corticogeniculate axons conducting signals back to the LGN in less than 10 ms [4].

As shown in Fig. 12.4, the output of the LGN segregates into ocular dominance columns within the primary visual cortex, otherwise known as V1 or the primary striate cortex, which lies medial to progressively higher levels of cortical integration and processing termed V2 through V5, which comprise lateral segments of the extra-striate cortex. Ocular dominance columns represent a fundamental organization to the visual cortex, and were discovered by Nobel laureates David Hubel and Torsten Wiesel. By correlating their electrophysiologic recordings with functional autoradiographic studies using 14C-labeled deoxyglucose administered during unilateral visual stimulation, they were able to demonstrate in their animal studies that cortical neurons are arranged into alternating columns that not only demonstrate ocular selectivity but also show a columnar organization in terms of their selectivity in being tuned to specific angles of orientation for visual stimuli. Ocular dominance columns within the monkey occipital cortex were also demonstrated by unilateral intra-ocular injection of radioactively tagged

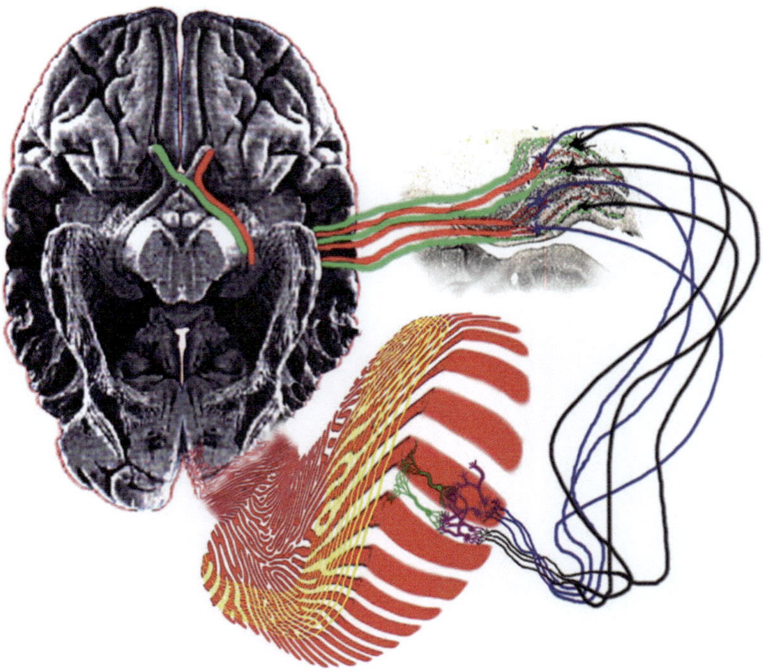

Fig. 12.4 Occular dominance columns within the occipital cortex—ocular dominance columns form a basic organizational theme to the occipital cortex (*red* versus *white stripes*), where serpiginous strips of input from one eye alternate with same for the other eye. Superimposed on this anatomic parcelization are functional columns tuned for orientation of the visual stimulus (*yellow lines*)

amino acids and then later autoradiographing retained cortical activity after trans-synaptic transfer had taken place within the LGN with subsequent anterograde axonal transport depositing tagged proteins within synaptic terminals arranged in columnar fashion [5].

Since Hubel and Weisel's original formulation of ocular dominance and orientation columns, it has been recognized that higher levels of other columnar organization are superimposed upon this basic map that include aspects of color and other spatial frequencies of visual stimuli. Electrophysiologic recordings show that visual cortex neurons selectively fire according to specific properties of the visual stimuli, with the most basic being tuned to the angle of movement yet other showing more complex properties of selectively firing according to sharp changes in contrast (edge detection). Current research efforts now focus on higher levels of visual processing in extrastriate cortical regions V2 through V6. Although specific regions of the extra-striate visual processing centers have been identified that mediate complex tasks such as facial recognition, the neurophysiologic basis at the cellular level for accomplishing this task remains a mystery. In this regard, the acquired inability to recognize previously familiar faces (prosopagnosia) can be traced to lesions within the inferior occipital cortex (occipital face area), fusiform gyrus (fusiform face area within the inferior occipital-temporal cortex), and the anterior temporal cortex [6]. However, the actual molecular mechanism by which interconnected neurons in these regions accomplish this amazing task of facial recognition remains obscure, and raises questions about the molecular basis of perception, and even ultimately the human imagination. Contemplating Fig. 12.5, our brains are so complex that unique patterns can be perceived with minimal information, as neurons within the human occipital cortex are so richly interconnected.

The columnar organization to the human visual cortex can be revealed by postmortem histochemical staining of the mitochondrial enzyme cytochrome oxidase within the striate cortex of individuals who suffered unilateral loss of one eye; this unilateral loss of afferents to the lateral geniculate (LGN) results in functional inactivation of the LGN efferent pathways to the visual cortex corresponding to absent cytochrome oxidase staining, as shown in Fig. 12.6.

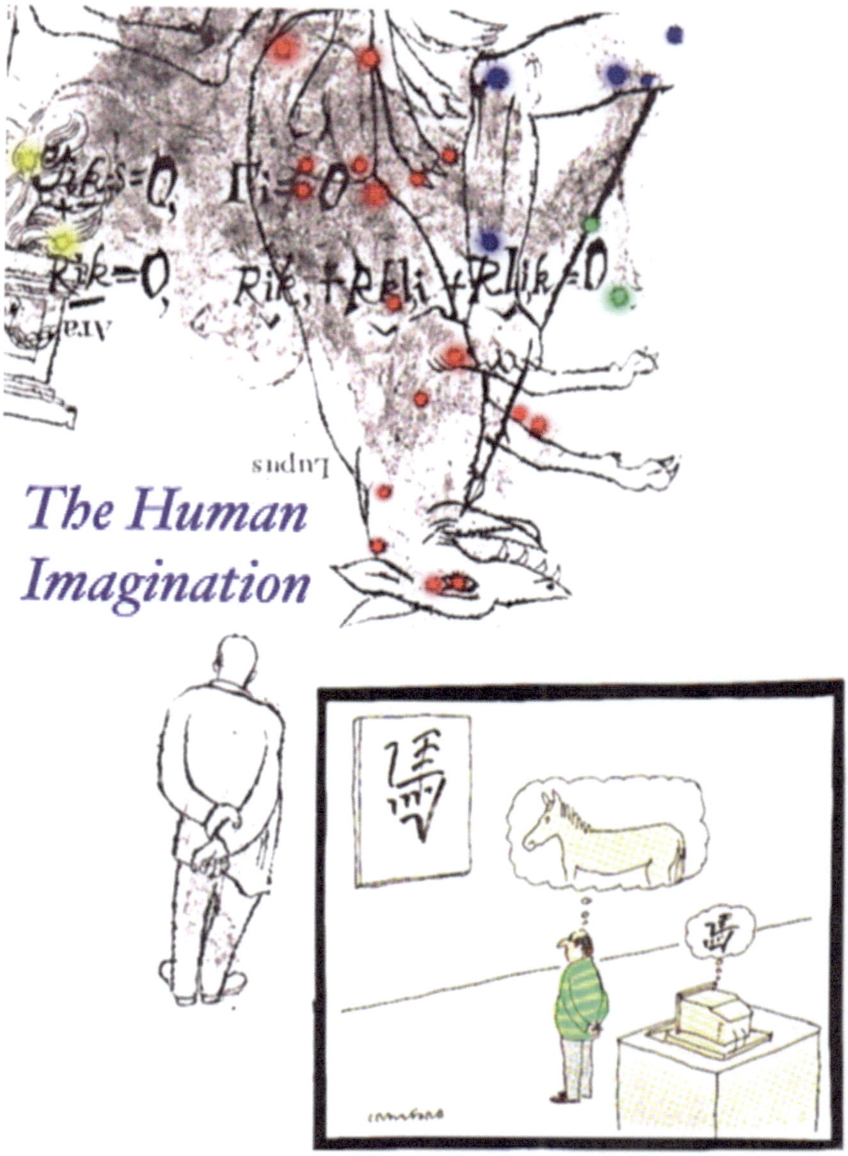

Fig. 12.5 The occipital cortex is not a simple computer that displays visual information as it is richly interconnected to other higher levels of cortical processing and posterior parietal association cortex, generating complex abstract thought and imagination

The primary visual cortex is highly active in terms of blood flow and metabolism, and can shift from a baseline level of activity with eyes closed in the dark to a significantly higher level of activity with eyes open in bright lighting conditions. As shown in Fig. 12.7, the striate cortex demonstrates intense metabolic activity with eyes open when studied by PET imaging of 18F-FDG uptake. The intense glucose uptake activity of this key cortical region dominates the metabolic landscape at all ages when viewed by PET imaging with only a mild decrement seen with normal aging, as shown in Fig. 12.8. Similarly, the electrographic activity of the primary visual cortex dominates the resting brain activity with eyes closed, as shown by the 10 cycle per second alpha rhythm seen on EEG (Fig. 12.9).

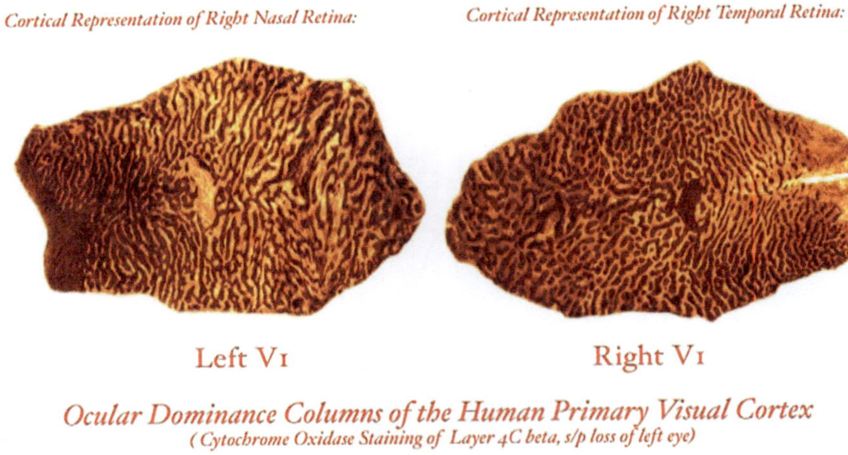

Fig. 12.6 Ocular dominance columns can also be identified by processing the cortex for cytochrome oxidase (CO) after monocular enucleation. The columns of the missing eye appear pale because their metabolic activity is reduced [24]

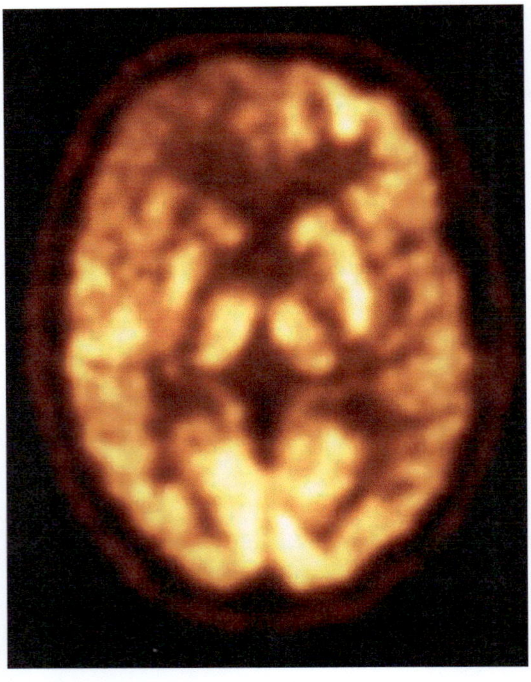

Fig. 12.7 The primary visual cortex is highly active with high 18F-FDG uptake: clinical example of a patient undergoing PET to evaluate post-traumatic changes to the right frontal region; note the normal pattern of metabolic activation for the visual cortex

Interesting yet unfortunate clinical syndromes are noted that affect the visual cortex, and include occlusion of the posterior cerebral artery with secondary infarction of the striate cortex producing homonymous hemianoptic defects (one-half of each visual field is missing on a strictly left-sided or right-sided homonymous basis). Surprisingly, many patients may not be aware of the problem and present with concerns about why they have been involved in more than one motor vehicle accident over a short period of time, or are bumping into doorways; despite having lost a major part of their visual field, affected stroke patients often seem unaware that their residual visual cortex has the ability to falsely fill in the missing details, yet the defects become plainly evident to the examiner testing visual fields individually with one eye closed. Other unusual stroke-related visual phenomenon include pallinopsia, where affected patients hesitatingly admit looking at a single object but then look away and see the object repeat itself in multiple forms across the visual landscape; this typically is seen with lesions of the extra-striate cortex (Brodman areas 18 and 19) within areas of higher and more complex visual processing [7].

When visual field defects arise and progress in patients with atypical progressive dementia characterized by hallucinations, the possibility of Lewy body dementia needs to be considered. Patients with the disorder show loss of executive function and have difficulty with abstract thinking as an early symptom often followed visual hallucinations, which correlate to hypometabolism on brain PET scans [8]. As shown in Fig. 12.10, PET can reveal unilateral significant metabolic

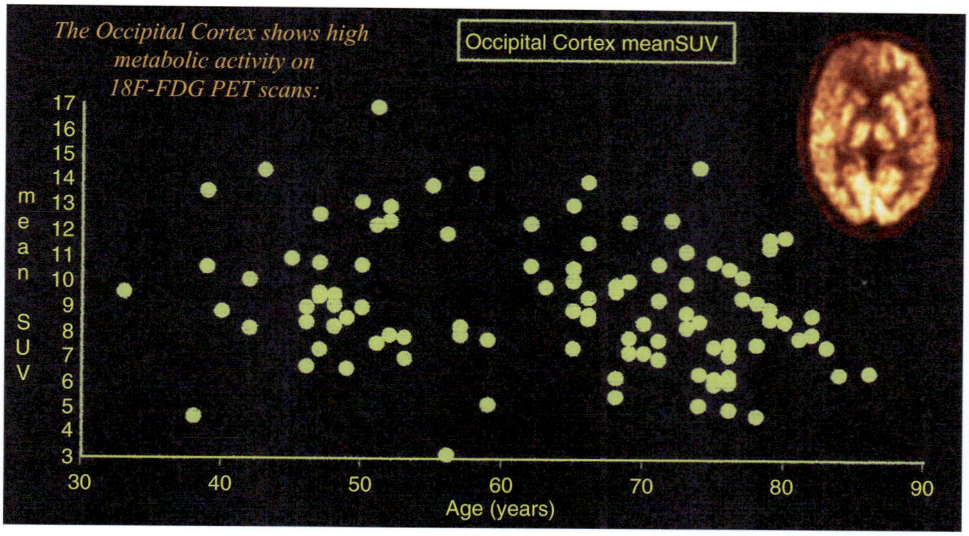

Fig. 12.8 High metabolic rates and correspondingly high FDG uptake levels as reflected by standardized uptake values (SUV) is typical for normal visual cortices with a slight decline with age

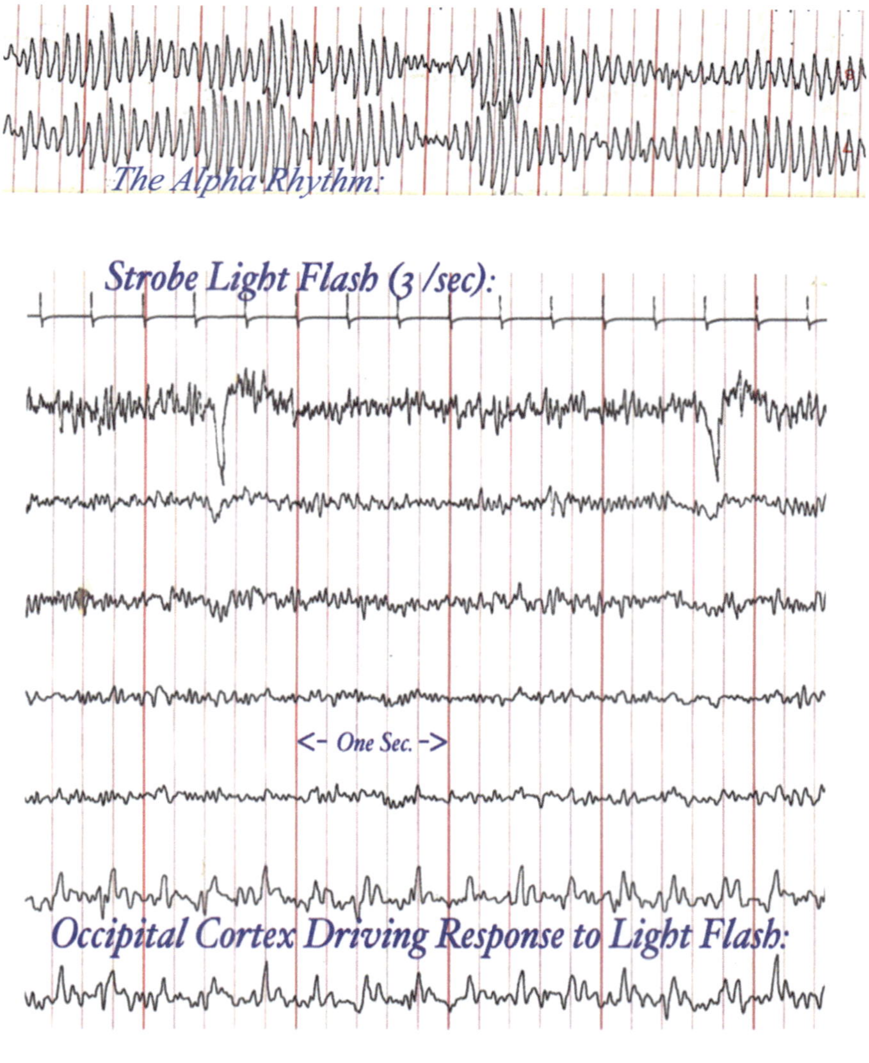

Fig. 12.9 Normal EEG activity for the occipital lobes with demonstration of the posterior dominant alpha rhythm

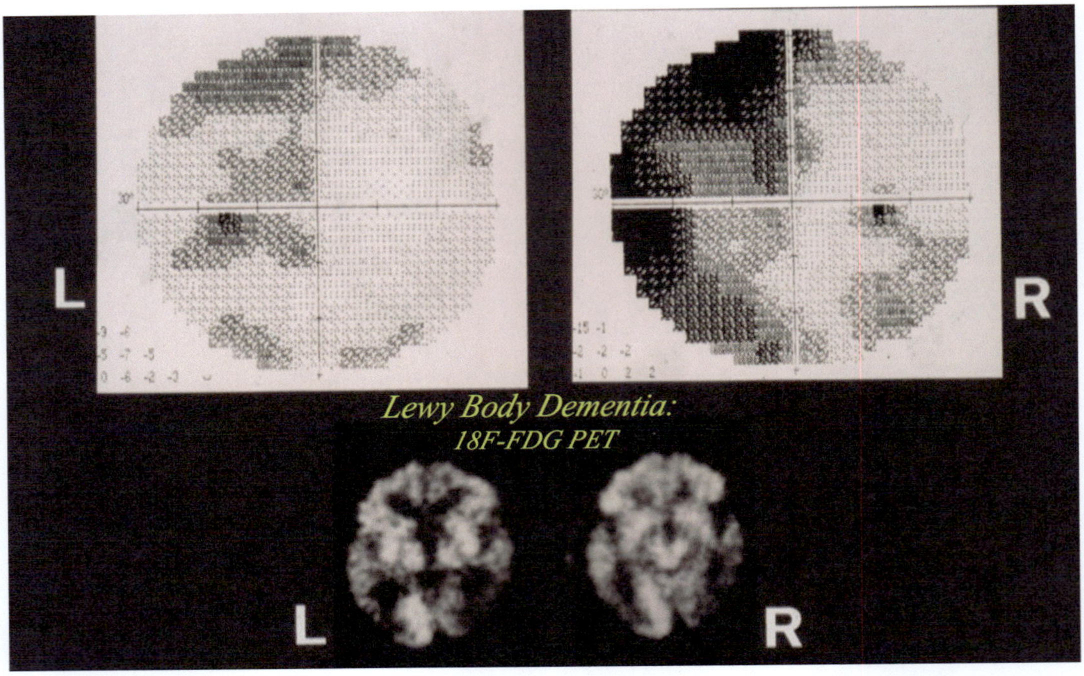

Fig. 12.10 Probable Lewy body disease in a patient with progressive cognitive decline and hemi-neglect of left side of each visual field corresponding to degenerative changes within the right occipital cortex as revealed by PET shown above; note the asymmetry in uptake for the occipital poles with the left being intact but not on the right

depression of the primary visual cortex in patients with cognitive impairment and progressive hemianoptic visual field loss. Postmortem analysis of Lewy body dementia patients reveal characteristic cytoplasmic neuronal inclusions composed of alpha-synuclein aggregates coupled with ubiquitin [9].

12.1 Migraine and the Occipital Cortex

Classic migraine symptoms with prodromal visual auras and light sensitivity are directly referable to the visual cortex. Known to millions of people throughout the world as a stereotypical pattern of premonitory visual symptoms that may be simple in the form of black dots or other complex field defects (scotomata) or bright complex patterns (fortification spectra) with an ensuing severe headache approximately 20 min later; some patients present with acute transient hemianoptic defects. The problem can be overwhelming in many patients, with a clear female predominance noted; most patients are young adults, but may strike at younger ages, but is distinctly unusual to occur de novo in the elderly, where new onset of headache patterns need to be investigated from other causes such as temporal arteritis, or neoplastic.

Genetic factors are important, as two-thirds of affected patients have a family history of migraine [10]. Although the general population displays a 22 % incidence of patent foramen ovale (PFO) on cardiac echocardiograms, a significantly higher proportion have PFO amongst the migraineur population [11]; as pulmonary endothelium metabolize monoamines present in the venous return, the higher prevalence of PFO might suggest provocation by dietary factors that might escape or bypass deamination by lung tissue.

It is critically important to comprehensively evaluate with not only brain MRI but also brain MRA whenever possible, as classic migraine incurs a small but significantly higher risk for stroke than the general population [12]. Furthermore, severe migraine headaches can sometimes take on complicated forms with associated transient unilateral tingling or numbness or weakness, thereby leading to diagnostic confusion in some young adults who may actually have true ischemic acute stroke symptoms attributable to other causes, including concomitant oral contraceptive use. Due to the extreme severity of some true migraines, occasional diagnostic confusion may arise in being able to recognize headache of more serious causes including premonitory "warning leak" events linked to cerebral aneurysm, which in many studies show an incidence of 2 % for unruptured cerebral aneurysm within the general population [13]. Some patients present with familial hemiplegic migraine as a manifestation of a calcium or sodium channel mutation [14], creating diagnostic confusion with true ischemic stroke.

Migraine is a common and disabling disorder with an estimated prevalence of 10–15 % in the general population. About 10 % of these have migraine with aura, most commonly in the form of visual disturbances, such as scintillating scotoma. Leao first described the phenomenon of spreading depression when he found that noxious stimulation of rabbit cerebral cortex produced a spreading decrease in electrical activity, moving at a rate of 2–3 mm/min [15]. This rate corresponds well with the propagation of visual aura. It has been proposed that this cortical spreading depression represents the neurobiological basis for migraine aura whereby neuronal activation and suppression are followed by corresponding vascular changes.

Typical migrainous visual phenomenon are illustrated by hand-drawn depictions by affected patients, as shown in Figs. 12.11 and 12.12, with radiating expanding visual aberrations in a hemianoptic pattern in advance of an ensuing migraine headache, typically occurring 20 min afterwards. Although the overwhelming majority of cases occur within structurally normal occipital cortices, some cases have been described in association with underlying focal cortical pathology referable to the occipital cortex [16]. In this regard, the unusual features of the two illustrated cases display migrainous visual phenomenon within the occipital cortex that is contralateral to any site of posterior circulation pathologic change, invoking the concept of a mirror focus [17] where interconnected left- versus right-sided visual cortical neurons aberrantly discharge in attempts "fill in" missing or altered details from the other side; this concept is hypothetical but

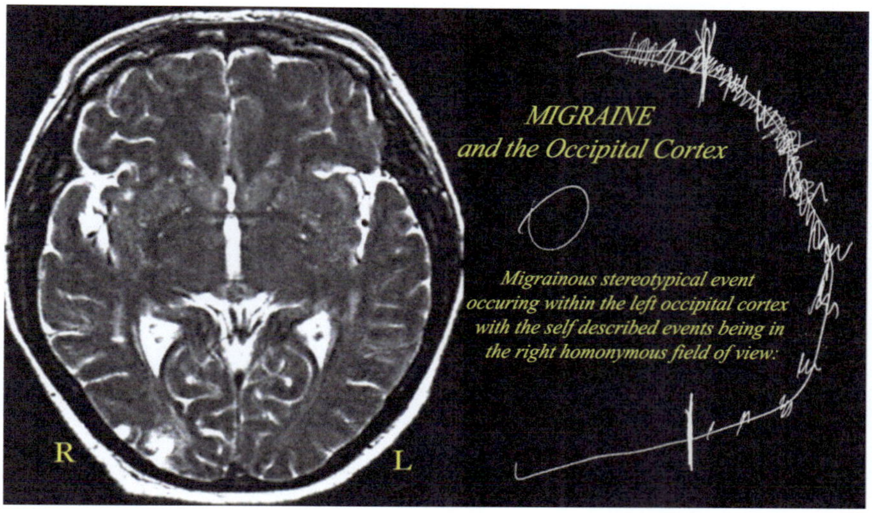

Fig. 12.11 Migrainous visual prodrome: not uncommonly, migrainous visual phenomenon will occur in those with clearly defined occipital cortex lesions, as shown here where the migrainous phenomenon takes place in the hemisphere opposite to where the lesion is; although there is a right occipital cortex lesion shown above in secondary association areas, the migrainous stereotypical event occurs within the left occipital cortex as the self-described events are in the right homonymous field of view

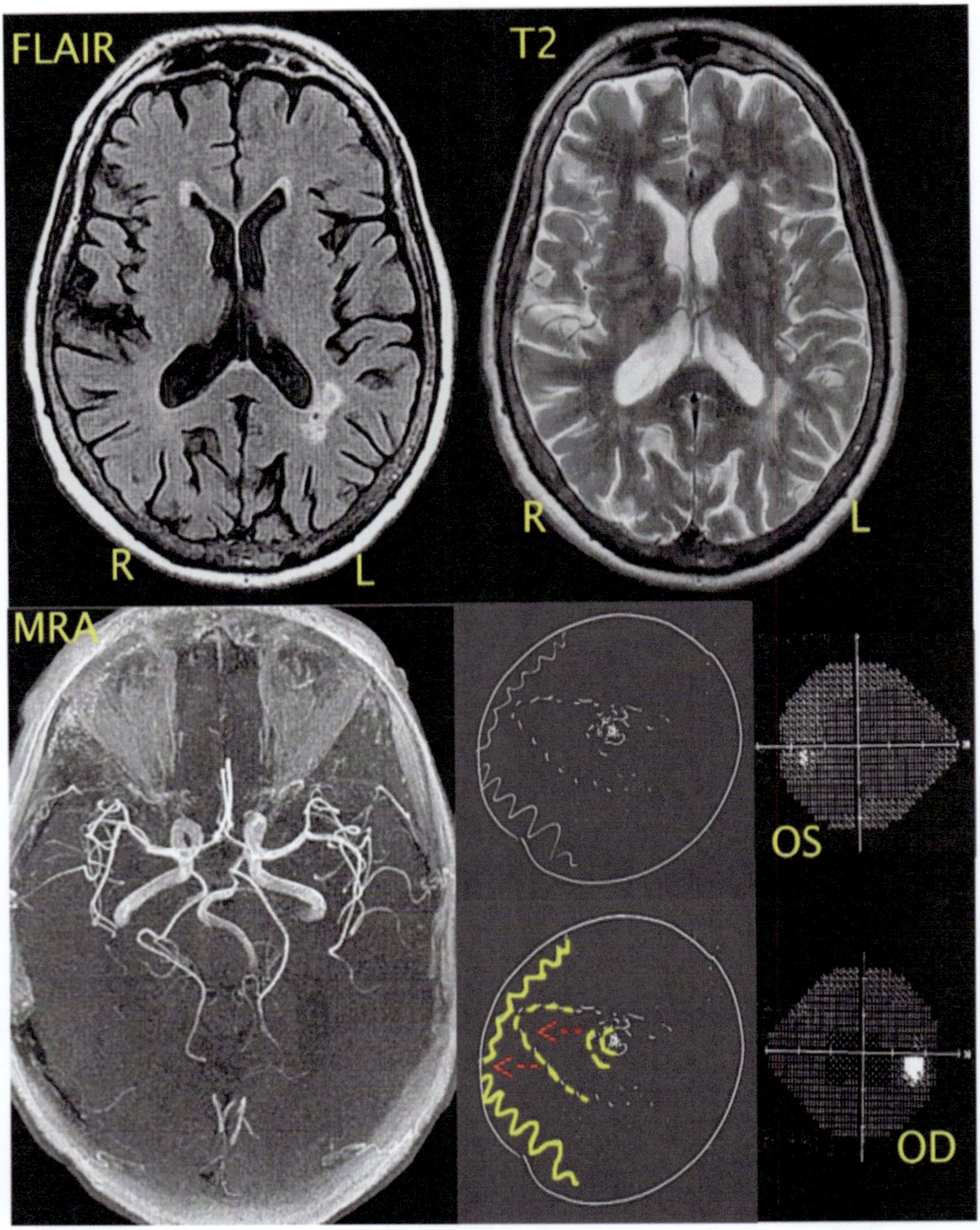

Fig. 12.12 Migrainous visual aura prodrome: Recurrent migrainous events with classical visual phenomenon in setting of prior left-sided closed head injury (note hand-drawn portrayal by patient showing expanding scintillating hemi-field visual event in advance of headache); a "mirror focus" type event is proposed of "filling in" information lost or altered during a migrainous event in this patient with chronic injury to the left occipital radiation fibers who experienced stereotypical events in the left homonymous field of view referable to the right occipital cortex. It is hypothesized that splenial fibers interconnecting mirror areas are likely important in "filling in" the information which is altered or lost during a migrainous event

anecdotally observed as common phenomenon within the visual system, which is remarkably able to seamlessly fuse two hemianoptic representations of the world into one three-dimensional perception of space.

An unusual case of progressively severe daily left-sided migraine headache with prodromal aura referable to a left occipital cortex AVM has been described for a 51-year-old female, “The visual disturbance consists of horizontal, black, squiggly lines in the right visual field, which move downward as new ones are added from the top. It lasts for 10 to 15 min and is followed by headache within 5 to 10 min” [18]. Headaches subsequently improved after gamma knife treatment of the AVM, with an apparent disconnection effect between any residual migrainous auras and recurrent headache. In this regard, it is important to note that migrainous visual auras can sometimes occur as isolated events in some individuals without the ensuing headache (acephalgic migraine).

With regards to treatment, triptan medications that act as serotonin agonists are very effective in migraine (Fig. 12.13) [19]. As shown in Fig. 12.13, triptans share the same basic molecular structure as serotonin (5-hydroxytryptamine, or 5-HT) and therefore display high affinity for 5-HT1B and 5-HT1D receptors. Triptans likely act by causing vasoconstriction of excessively dilated overstretched meningeal and intracranial vessels via activation of 5-HT1B receptors on vascular smooth-muscle cells; triptans also act on presynaptic 5-HT1D neuronal receptors to block the release of vasoactive peptides from the perivascular trigeminal neurons. Triptan medications are not for everyone and are contraindicated in coronary artery disease, poorly controlled hypertension, severe hepatic or renal impairment, or basilar or hemiplegic migraine [19] as well as other complicated forms of migraine strong caution is advised regarding the risks for development of serotonin syndrome in those using selective serotonin-reuptake inhibitors or selective norepinephrine-reuptake inhibitors. Prophylactic medications that may reduce the frequency of recurrent migraines include the use of the anticonvulsants topiramate or valproic acid in the low-dose form.

Atypical headache features, especially in an older patient, should expand considerations to

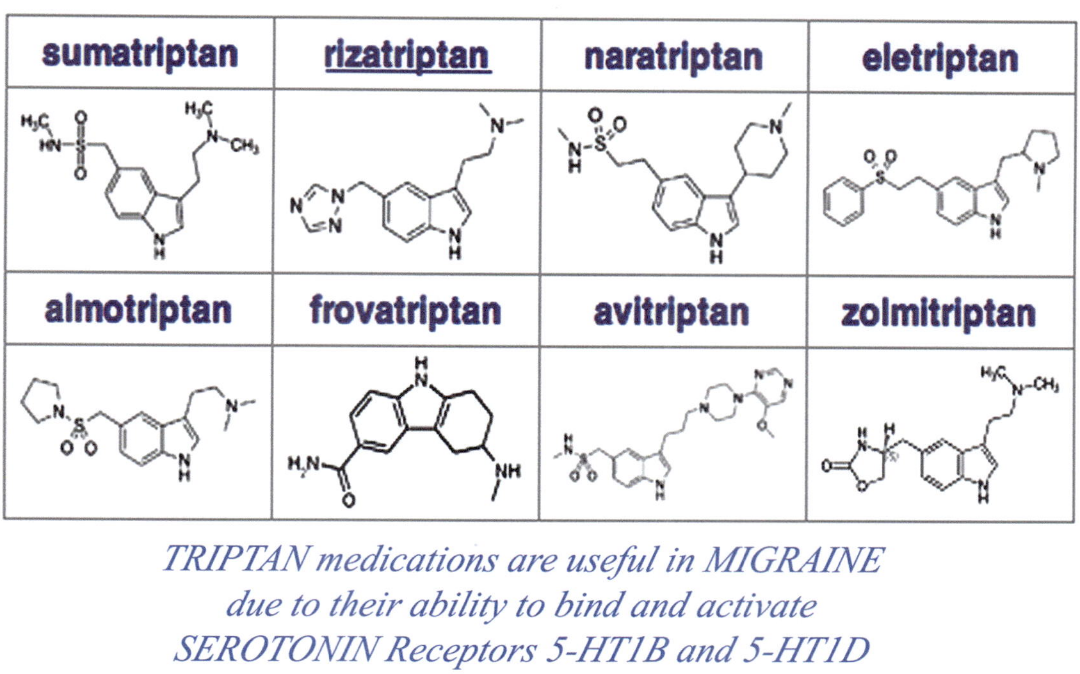

Fig. 12.13 Triptan medications are useful for treating migraine

include temporal arteritis, which is generally associated with an elevated sedimentation rate with jaw claudication and superficial temporal artery prominence with tenderness ([20]—regarding guidelines in the evaluation and treatment of giant cell arteritis). Severe headaches in an overweight female with new progressive visual difficulties should prompt the need to exclude pseudotumor cerebri-associated papilledema by fundoscopy and possible CSF examination to establish a diagnosis of intracranial hypertension via measurement of opening pressures [21]. Headaches that are positional in nature and arise with strain, cough, or other Valsalva procedures may suggest cerebellar tonsil herniation that occurs with the Chiari malformation [22]; other causes for positional headache that is worse with standing include intracranial hypotension due to a CSF leak [23]. In these instances, radionuclide imaging of possible extravasation sites of intrathecally introduced technetium based tracers may be helpful in localizing the leakage of spinal fluid.

References

1. Yu-Wai-Man P, Griffiths PG, Chinnery PF. Mitochondrial optic neuropathies—disease mechanisms and therapeutic strategies. Prog Retin Eye Res. 2011;30(2):81–114.
2. Zabbah S, Rajaei K, Mirzaei A, et al. The impact of the lateral geniculate nucleus and corticogeniculate interactions on efficient coding and higher-order visual object processing. Vision Res. 2014;101:82–93.
3. Guillery R, Sherman SM. Thalamic relay functions and their role in corticocortical communication: generalizations from the visual system. Neuron. 2002;33(2):163–75.
4. Briggs F, Usrey WM. A fast, reciprocal pathway between the lateral geniculate nucleus and visual cortex in the macaque monkey. J Neurosci. 2007;27:5431–6.
5. Wiesel TN, Hubel DH, Lam DM. Autoradiographic demonstration of ocular-dominance columns in the monkey striate cortex by means of transneuronal transport. Brain Res. 1974;79(2):273–9.
6. Gainotti G, Marra C. Differential contribution of right and left temporo-occipital and anterior temporal lesions to face recognition disorders. Front Hum Neurosci. 2011;5:55.
7. Gersztenkorn D, Lee AG. Palinopsia revamped: a systematic review of the literature. Surv Ophthalmol. 2014;60:1–35.
8. Fujishiro H, Iseki E, Kasanuki K, et al. Glucose hypometabolism in primary visual cortex is commonly associated with clinical features of dementia with Lewy bodies regardless of cognitive conditions. Int J Geriatr Psychiatry. 2012;27(11):1138–46.
9. Stuendl A, Kunadt M, Kruse N, et al. Induction of α-synuclein aggregate formation by CSF exosomes from patients with Parkinson's disease and dementia with Lewy bodies. Brain. 2016;139(Pt 2):481–94.
10. Bartleson JD, Cutrer FM. Migraine update. Diagnosis and treatment. Minn Med. 2010;93(5):36–41.
11. Inglessis I, Elmariah S, Rengifo-Moreno PA, et al. Long-term experience and outcomes with transcatheter closure of patent foramen ovale. JACC Cardiovasc Interv. 2013;6(11):1176–83.
12. Guidetti D, Rota E, Morelli N, Immovilli P. Migraine and stroke: "vascular" comorbidity. Front Neurol. 2014;5:193.
13. The UCAS Japan Investigators. The natural course of unruptured cerebral aneurysms in a Japanese Cohort. N Engl J Med. 2012;366:2474–82.
14. Fan C, Wolking S, Lehmann-Horn F, et al. Early-onset familial hemiplegic migraine due to a novel SCN1A mutation. Cephalalgia. 2016, January 12.
15. Engelhardt E, Gomes Mda M. Aristides Leão: a birth centennial homage with comments on his spreading depression. Arq Neuropsiquiatr. 2015;73(6):544–6.
16. Shams PN, Plant GT. Migraine-like visual aura due to focal cerebral lesions: case series and review. Surv Ophthalmol. 2011;56(2):135–61.
17. Kim J, Shin HK, Hwang KJ, et al. Mirror focus in a patient with intractable occipital lobe epilepsy. J Epilepsy Res. 2014;4(1):34–7.
18. Spierings EL. Daily migraine with visual aura associated with an occipital arteriovenous malformation. Headache. 2001;41(2):193–7.
19. Loder E. Triptan therapy in migraine. N Engl J Med. 2010;363:63–70.
20. Bienvenu B, Ly KH, Lambert M, et al. Management of giant cell arteritis: Recommendations of the French Study Group for Large Vessel Vasculitis (GEFA). Rev Med Interne. 2016;37(3):154–65.
21. Dave SB, Subramanian PS. Pseudotumor cerebri: an update on treatment options. Indian J Ophthalmol. 2014;62(10):996–8.
22. Bates JE, Augustine EF. Pearls & Oysters: cough headache secondary to Chiari malformation type I. Neurology. 2014;83(16):e149–51.
23. Lee GK, Abrigo JM, Cheung TC, et al. Spontaneous intracranial hypotension: improving recognition and treatment strategies in the local setting. Hong Kong Med J. 2014;20(6):537–40.
24. Adams DL, Sincich LC, Horton JC. Complete pattern of ocular dominance columns in human primary visual cortex. J Neurosci. 2007;27:10391–403.

13 Infections of the Nervous System

Infections of the nervous system are particularly important to rapidly diagnose and treat as soon as possible to avoid a lethal outcome, as seen in bacterial meningitis, or infective endocarditis (Fig. 13.1) or avoid devastating memory loss and seizures that can occur with viral infections such as herpes encephalitis that can produce long-term damage to the temporal lobes. Fungal infections can present on a slower time frame of weeks to months, and may be difficult to diagnose without high-volume repeated CSF examinations; on the other hand, parasitic diseases of the brain are somewhat more obvious and easier to diagnose such as neurocysticercosis with characteristic cystic lesions that are seen on head CT examinations. Immunocompromised individuals (e.g. HIV infection or post-chemotherapy states) have a characteristic proclivity for certain infections, such as CNS toxoplasmosis or JC polyoma virus-related progressive multifocal leukoencephalopathy (PML). Finally, an extremely rare yet devastating process that can arise spontaneously but have the potential for infectious transmission is Creutzfeldt–Jakob disease due to the misfolded prion protein; unfortunately, there is no treatment available for this and is usually fatal within 1 year after diagnosis. Establishing an infectious agent for those who present with symptoms of encephalitis can be challenging, as one large prospective study revealed only 16 % had a confirmed or probable cause identified; however, about 70 % of these cases were believed to be viral in origin versus bacterial for about 20 % of the group [1].

With regards to treatable infections such as bacterial meningitis, it is important to note that certain bacteria are more prevalent, depending on the age of the patient. For example, neonatal and infantile meningitis cases show higher frequencies for Group B Streptococcus, *Escherichia coli*, and *Listeria monocytogenes*, whereas *Neisseria meningitides* predominates in children, versus *Streptococcus pneumonia* that predominates in adults and the elderly. Meningococcal meningitis is a medical emergency that presents in over 90 % of cases with at least two out of the following four symptoms: stiff neck, high fever, headache, and altered mental status. Risk factors for affected young adults include living closely with others such as college dormitory settings. Despite intensive antibiotics and ICU care, fatalities can occur with significant morbidity; complications of acute fulminant meningitis are known to include coma, bilateral adrenal insufficiency from hemorrhage into the adrenal glands (Waterhouse–Friderichsen syndrome), and disseminated intravascular coagulation [2].

Empiric antibiotic treatment includes intravenous administration of antibiotics with good CNS penetration along with a third-generation cephalosporin, such as ceftriaxone or cefotaxime. *Streptococcus pneumonia* deserves special attention as it is the leading cause of meningitis in the elderly, and a major cause in young adults as well as children older than 2 months.

M.A. Meyer, *Neurologic Disease*, DOI 10.1007/978-3-319-39581-4_13

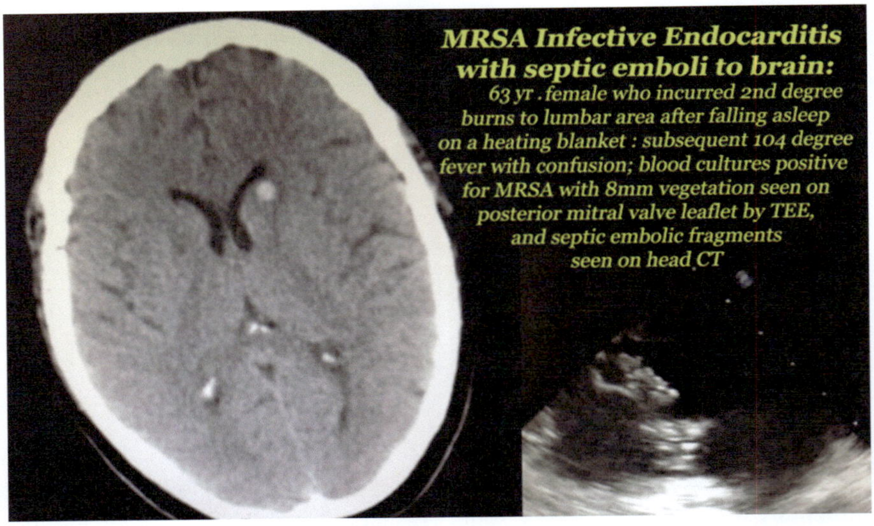

Fig. 13.1 MRSA-related infective endocarditis with septic emboli to the brain

Although 11 out of 12 cases of streptococcal meningitis survive, about 1 out of 4 survivors suffer long-term neurologic adverse effects, including seizures, with mental retardation and deafness noted in children (steroid infusions may reduce the complications of deafness).

For the immunocompromised population, certain organisms predominate, such as HIV-associated meningo-encephalitis due to the slow growing aerobic non-motile acid-fast *Mycobacterium tuberculosis*; on MRI, multiple enhancing lesion may be seen within the brain as discrete tuberculomas [3]. Guidelines for treatment include a 4-drug therapy with isoniazid, rifampin, pyrazinamide, and ethambutol for a period of 2 months, followed by an additional one-half year period of just isoniazid and rifampin. Of these four drugs, the best CNS penetration is found with isoniazid and pyrazinamide.

Another organism that can more commonly infect the brain in immunocompromised states such as HIV includes *Toxoplasma gondii* (Fig. 13.2), which is an obligate intracellular, parasitic protozoan [4]. For congenital cases, e.g. a pregnant woman who may have been exposed to cat litter, the affected infant may present with mental retardation and seizures with blindness and calcifications of the basal ganglia; a classic triad of signs being chorioretinits, hydrocephalus, and ring enhancing calcific lesions seen on CT. A combination of trimethoprim and sulfamethoxazole is useful for prevention against toxoplasmosis in susceptible patients such as those with HIV requires the combination of trimethoprim and sulfamethoxazole; pyrimethamine and sulfadiazine should be initiated once the diagnosis has been established.

Other serious CNS infections include brain abscess, which can frequently present with progressive headaches over days to weeks with lethargy, nausea, vomiting, and new-onset seizures [5]. Although some cases develop by hematogenous spread as in sepsis, over 70 % of cases are thought to arise by direct contiguous spread from sinus infections. Risk factors include recent severe sinus infections, intravenous drug usage, immunocompromised states, steroid usage, and congenital cardiac conditions. Streptococcus are among the most common causative organisms. Readily identified on contrast-enhanced CT or MRI examination, brain abscesses are more commonly found in the frontal and parietal lobes; PET imaging may also help further characterize the lesion (Fig. 13.3) [6]. Surgical indications for excision or aspiration include lesions that are at risk for rupture into the ventricular system or a

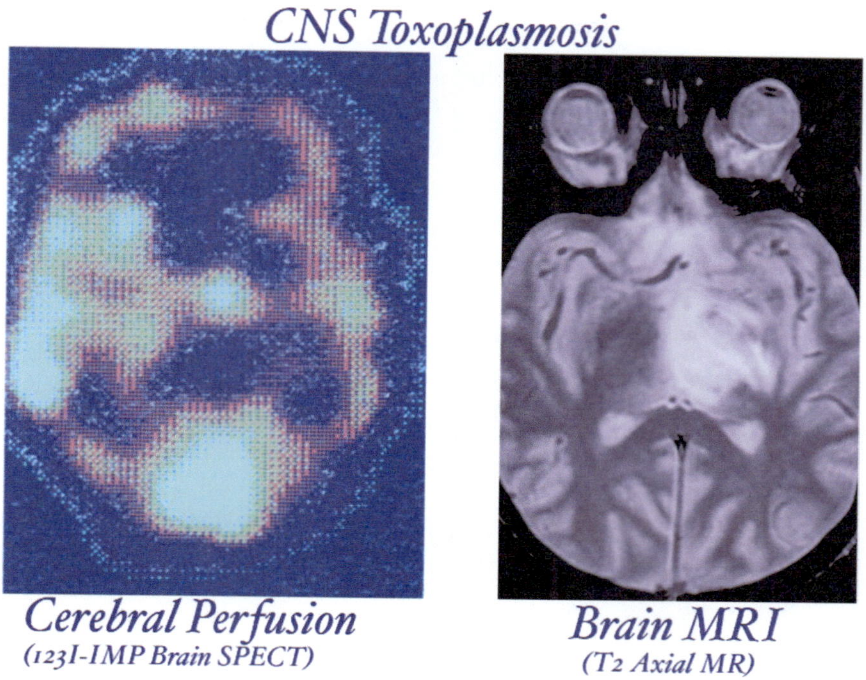

Fig. 13.2 HIV-associated CNS toxoplasmosis affecting the left thalamus

posterior fossa location with mass effect, or when the abscess cavity is large. With regards to antibiotics, a third-generation cephalosporin, such as ceftriaxone is used for streptococcal abscesses, whereas anaerobic abscesses are treated with metronidazole. For those with staphylococcal infections as with IV drug abuse, empiric treatment with vancomycin is indicated as methicillin resistance is a possibility.

Although fungi are rarely isolated as the causative factor for brain abscess within the general population, they are surprisingly frequent in the immunocompromised population; one study from a major cancer center found fungi as the cause in 92 % of cases, with over half being due to *Aspergillus*, with *Candida* being second. For *Candida albicans* brain abscess, intravenous amphoterecin B and flucytosine are recommended, followed by oral agents that have reasonably good brain penetration, such as oral fluconazole [2].

Other fungal infections of the central nervous system include cryptococcal meningitis, which is especially common in the HIV and post-chemotherapy populations. Geography plays a factor as cryptococcal meningitis is more common in the southwestern USA; pigeon droppings carry the organism as well. Intravenous amphoterecin plus flucytosine for 2 weeks are advised, followed by oral fluconazole for at least 10 weeks. Other forms of fungal meningitis include histoplasmosis and blastomycosis which tend to cluster around the Mississippi and Ohio river valleys in the central USA.

Other CNS infections with a characteristic geography include Lyme disease, which is mainly seen in the northeastern USA, and is caused by the spirochete bacteria *Borrelia burgdorferi*, and transmitted after bites from the Ixodes scapularis tick [7]. Days to weeks following the tick bite, the spirochetes spread via hematogenous routes to joints, myocardium, nervous system, and distant skin sites, where symptoms of arthralgias, fever, myalgias, and skin rash develop with the appearance of a characteristic bulls eye pattern; about 25 % of cases have no rash at all. About 1

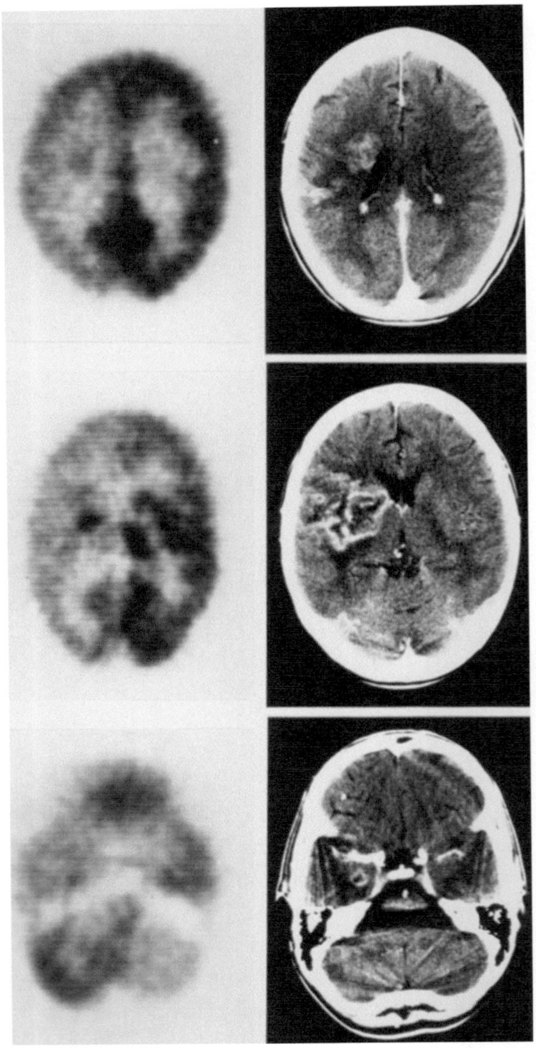

Fig. 13.3 Case example: Bacterial brain abscess: A 29-year-old human immunodeficiency virus-negative intravenous drug abuser with a right hemispheric staphylococcal brain abscess underwent PET imaging of 18F-fluorodeoxyglucose (FDG) brain uptake. Diffuse right cortical hypometabolism was noted, as well as crossed cerebellar diaschisis. Unlike previous PET findings on FDG uptake in a brain abscess, the most intense uptake of FDG was found within the abscess and not in the contrast-enhancing walls

month later after the tick bite, neurologic symptoms appear in about 10–15 % of patients, often with facial palsy, headache, meningismus, plus variable cognitive changes; subcortical white matter lesions can be found on MRI. If left undiagnosed and untreated, the spirochete may persist for months to years, despite the production of *Borrelia*-specific antibodies; however, a 2- to 4-week course of intravenous ceftriaxone is very effective (other recent studies have shown doxycycline to be equally effective).

Another spirochete bacterial infection of the nervous system involves *Treponema pallidum* as the causative agent of neurosyphilis, which can be in one of four forms: asymptomatic, meningovascular, tabes dorsalis, or general paresis [8]. Neurosyphilis usually occurs in about 25–40 % of those who have had chronic, untreated syphilis, but may take about 10–20 years to become clinically apparent. HIV infection is also known to be a significant risk factor for neurosyphilis. Chronic untreated syphilis can invade at multiple levels, from peripheral nerves and spinal cord on up into the brain parenchyma and vasculature; effective treatment includes intravenous penicillin.

In contrast to the slow protracted course of CNS infection by spirochetes, other bacteria such as the gram-positive rods of anthrax can rarely cause a rapidly fatal fulminant hemorrhagic meningoencephalitis [9]. This major neurologic symptom complex of infection by *Bacillus anthracis* has an initial mode of entry that can be via the cutaneous or inhalation route; acute neurologic deterioration has associated findings of dark necrotic pustules on the extremities, gram-positive rods and low glucose in the cerebrospinal fluid, and multifocal areas of intracerebral hemorrhage on CT (Fig. 13.4). The Centers for Disease Control and Prevention notes that ciprofloxacin is a recommended treatment; doxycycline should not be used for anthrax meningoencephalitis because of its poor central nervous system penetration.

Diagnostic imaging tests that can readily localize metabolically active focal bacterial infections that affect the brain and spinal canal include technetium tagged autologous white cells as well as PET imaging of 18F-FDG activity (Figs. 13.3 and 13.5). One recent study found PET to be superior to MRI for postoperative

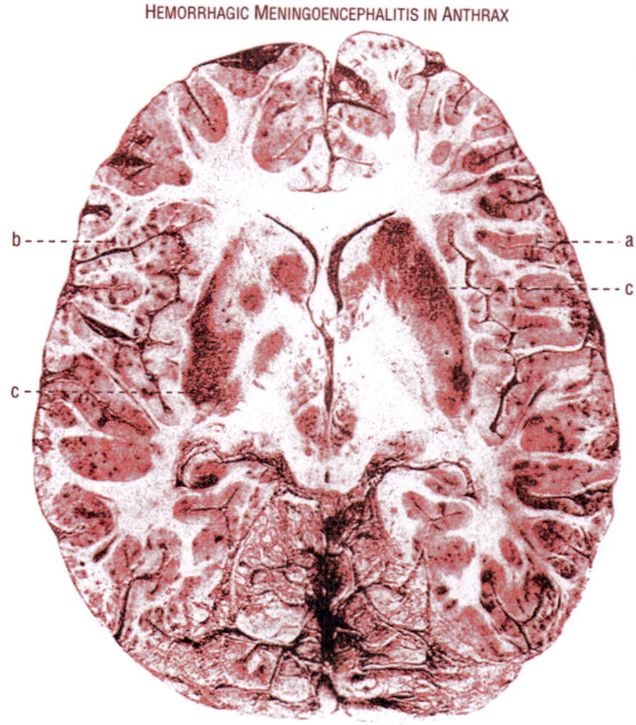

Fig. 13.4 One of the earliest cases of hemorrhagic meningoencephalitis from anthrax, from a 1920 article by House, who noted numerous focal bleeds in the gray matter but "very few hemorrhages of the white matter" [9]

spinal infections; the sensitivity and specificity of PET was 100 % and 79 %, respectively, versus 76 % and 42 % for MRI [10].

Other types of infectious diseases that can rapidly invade the central nervous system and cause serious mortality and morbidity are those arising from viruses (Fig. 13.6) [11], most notably herpes simplex encephalitis [12]. The herpes simplex virus typically affects the temporal lobes, and can rapidly destroy temporal lobe structures, such as the hippocampus, with symptoms including uncontrolled repetitive seizures after a prodromal phase of fever, confusion and headache with long-term complications including profound short term memory loss if treatment is not promptly started that involves high-dose acyclovir for 10–21 days; steroids can be used especially if there is concern about uncal herniation (Fig. 13.7).

A highly serious and often fatal viral infection occurs with rabies [13], which is caused by the lyssavirus Rhabdoviridae, which has a single-stranded negative-sense RNA genome that encodes five proteins: nucleoprotein (N), phosphoprotein (P), matrix protein (M), glycoprotein (G), and the viral RNA polymerase (L). The virus initially replicates within muscle cells close to the site of the bite from an infected animal (usually bat or dog; rarely from rodents) where they bind to acetyl choline receptors at the neuromuscular junction and then travel up the nerve cell axon via retrograde transport via binding of the viral P protein with dynein; after replicating in motor neurons, the virus eventually reaches the brain. Rabies results in the death of up to 55,000 individuals worldwide per year with more than 95 % of rabies deaths occurring in Africa and Asia. Treatment consists of thorough wound cleaning followed by emergent administration of human rabies immune globulin at the site of infection and one shot intramuscularly, followed by five post-exposure vaccinations within the first month.

The major types of equine encephalitis includes Eastern, Western, and Venezualan, and

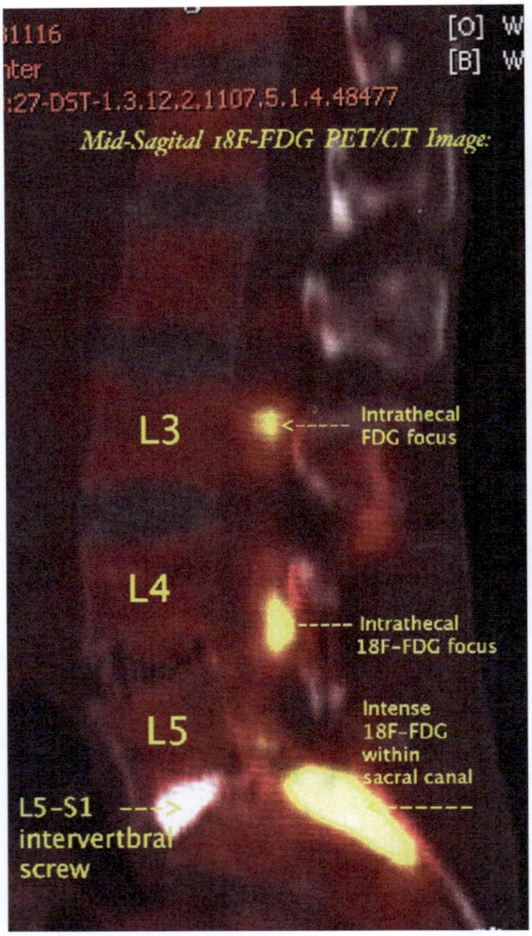

Fig. 13.5 Case example: Bacteroides infection after lumbar spine surgery, as revealed by 18F-FDG PET imaging

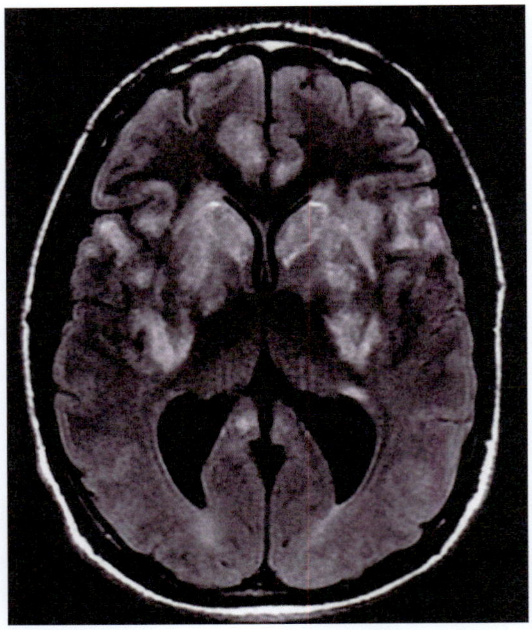

Fig. 13.6 Case example: Viral encephalitis in a young adult: a 21-year-old college student who developed severe Epstein–Barr viral encephalitis. The patient had developed new eye discomfort with his soft contact lenses after starting a new contact lens solution; the problem did not remit despite switching brands of contact lenses. After 3 months of mild chronic discomfort, an extremely severe bilateral viral conjunctivitis developed over 10 days that resolved but then left the patient with myalgias and a stiff neck. Personality changes developed and progressed over the next 2 weeks, leading to being found in an unresponsive state with generalized seizure activity. Intravenous acyclovir was immediately started after a lumbar puncture revealed 35 nucleated cells per cubic microliter with 85 % lymphocytes. Initially, brain MRI was negative but within 6 days, marked limbic and basal ganglia signal changes were found, as also noted on hospital day 16. PCR analysis of a repeat CSF examination revealed low level presence of Epstein–Barr viral DNA. Despite the use of intravenous steroids, subcutaneous interferon beta1a, and the addition of cidofovir, and then switching over to intravenous ganciclovir, no significant clinical improvement was noted

represent a highly serious form of infection, where mortality can range from one in 20 for Western equine encephalitis (WEE), versus one in three for the Eastern forms [14]; unfortunately, there are no specific antiviral medications for these illnesses caused by alphaviruses, which exist as single-stranded positive-sense RNA viruses (Togaviridae family). Generally uncommon, EEE occurs mainly in hot swampy mosquito ridden regions within the southeastern United States and can initially present with a typical flu-like viral infection prodrome followed by rapidly progressive neurologic complications of seizures, coma, and even death. WEE infection tends to be milder, with most recovering fully after a few weeks of being ill. Although a vaccine exists for the VEE virus, none yet exists for EEE or WEE.

Flavivirus encephalitis includes West Nile and Zika virus along with St. Louis, Japanese, Tick-borne and others to form a large group of viruses that have significant morbidity and mortality

Herpes Virus Encephalitis

HSV-1 is the most common cause of viral encephalitis.

Herpes simplex encephalitis remains one of the most devastating infections of the central nervous system, with high morbidity and mortality despite available antiviral therapy.

Imaging evaluation can demonstrate temporal lobe edema/hemorrhage on MRI

Acyclovir is the treatment of choice

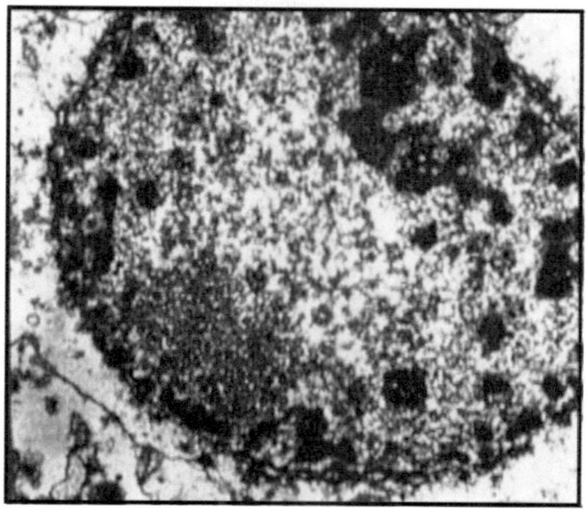

Fig. 13.7 Herpes encephalitis: fact summary; the electron micrograph illustrates intra-nuclear viral particles in the process of assembly and budding

across the globe. Great concern has been focused upon Zika infection of pregnant women, and its adverse effect upon brain development in-utero, with the actual virus being found within microcephalic brain tissue [15]. Zika is a mosquito-borne flavivirus, that was first isolated in 1947 from a monkey living in a Uganda forest but now found throughout South America with Brazil being the most affected country. Aside from its link to microcephaly, the infection for most people is self-limiting, but some rarely go on to develop Guillain–Barré syndrome.

A potentially lethal mosquito borne flavivirus that has neurotropic properties is the West Nile virus (WNV). The virus has a positive sense, single-stranded RNA genome that encodes a single polyprotein, that is then cleaved into three structural proteins (C, prM/M, E) and seven non-structural proteins; invasion of the nervous system may occur via the hematogenous route or by transneural spread via axonal transport mechanisms [16]. Forms of neurologic disease include meningoencephalitis or flaccid paralysis and may even be fatal; in 2012, 286 fatalities were reported amongst 5674 US cases. For neuroinvasive cases, sites of injury include the hippocampus, brainstem, cerebellum, and the anterior horn of the spinal cord; no specific antiviral medication targeted to WNV currently exists.

St. Louis encephalitis virus (SLEV) is a related flavivirus that has been isolated from mosquitoes, birds, and mammals from southern Canada to Argentina [17]. Originally identified during a 1933 St Louis, Missouri outbreak, more than 1000 deaths have subsequently been attributed to the virus; 5 % mortality rate is noted for those younger than 49 years, whereas for those infected by the virus who are over 70 years of age show a 23 % mortality rate. SLEV is transmitted from the bite from a mosquito hosts; infection proceeds over a few weeks with of nonspecific flu-like symptoms, followed by encephalitis and/or a viral meningitis clinical picture. Brain MR examinations show nonspecific edema with seizures occurring in about 10 % of infected patients; occasionally, the Guillain–Barre syndrome may follow primary infection.

Another mosquito borne flavivirus infection is tick-borne encephalitis, which usually occur in the spring and summer months, mostly in Europe and Russia [18]. Clinical symptoms reflect an encephalitic and/or meningitic involvement that

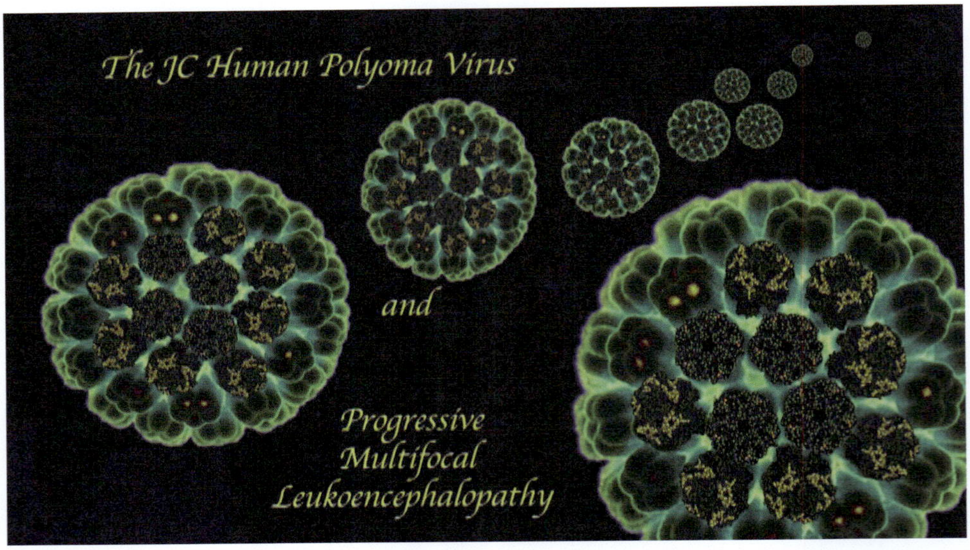

Fig. 13.8 The polyoma JC virus is the causative agent of PML (progressive multifocal leukoencephalopathy). The first case of PML was found in a patient named John Cunningham who was diagnosed with chronic lymphocytic leukemia and Hodgkin's lymphoma in 1958; recently, the incidence has grown to include those with HIV and MS patients treated with natalizumab

may progress to the point of convulsions, and coma. Eastern Russian strains are more virulent, with 10 % fatality rates for European strains versus mortality of 20–60 % for the Russian strains. MRI reveals subcortical diffuse edema with anterior horn signal abnormalities; treatment is largely supportive.

An unusual form of viral encephalitis that occurs within the immunocompromised population is the JC virus-related progressive multifocal leukoencephalopathy (PML), which presents as a destructive demyelinating process within the white matter [19]. The causative polyoma JC virus is neurotropic (Fig. 13.8) and replicates within oligodendroglia as a double-stranded circular DNA virus, causing a lethal burst of the oligodendrocyte as newly replicated viruses are released, only to infect other nearby oligodendroglia. Clinically, the lesions may simulate atypical demyelinating MS lesions and not infrequently occur within the MS population of patients treated with the monoclonal antibody natalizumab that is targeted against integrin membrane proteins; recent studies show an incidence rate of 212 confirmed cases of PML among 99,571 patients treated with natalizumab, equating to 2.1 cases per 1000 treated patients [20]. PML is also surprisingly frequent within the HIV population. Unfortunately, there is no effective medication that specifically targets the JC virus, which causes progressive multifocal leukoencephalopathy; however, for those cases associated with HIV, initiation of retroviral therapy to treat HIV and thereby raise CD4 counts can result in transient improvement, yet still show significant morbidity and mortality (Fig. 13.9).

The most unusual yet very fascinating neurologic disease that can be transmitted in an infectious manner is Creutzfeldt–Jakob disease (CJD) and related prion diseases. The term prion was coined in 1982 by its discoverer Dr Stanley Pruisner as a contraction derived from protein and infection with reference to the term "proteinaceous infectious particle" to describe a self-propagating protein that can impose misfolding and other conformational changes to other similar proteins [21]. The fundamental basis of prion disease relates to the spontaneous conversion of the normal, cellular

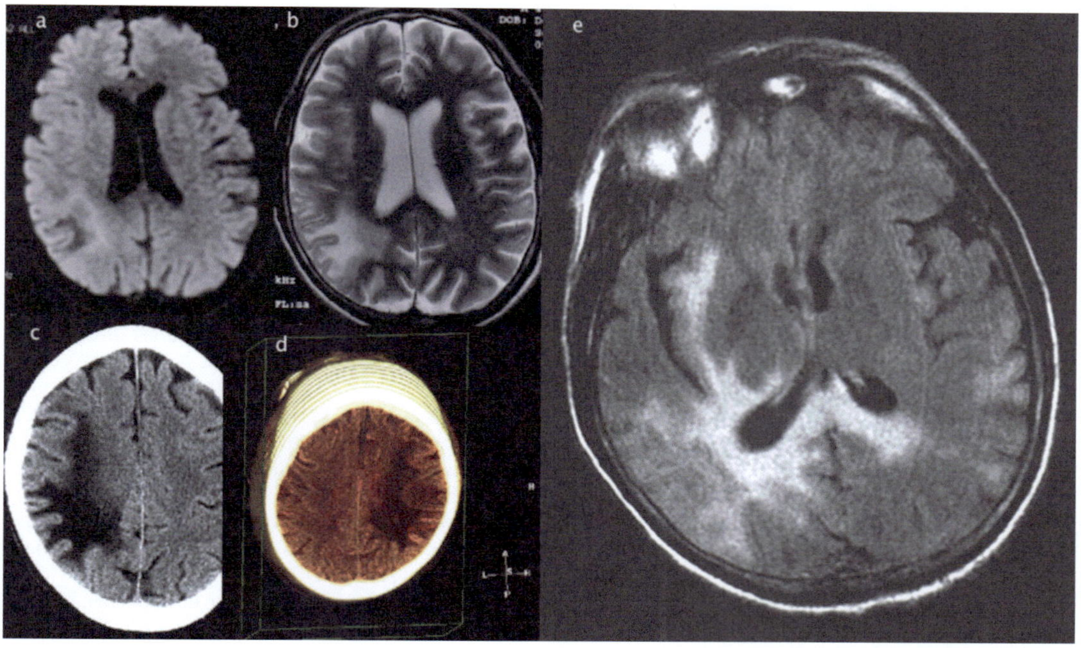

Fig. 13.9 Case example: HIV-related PML as shown by MRI (**a**, **b**) and CT (**c**, **d**) at the time of diagnosis when the patient presented with seizure activity and progressive left-sided weakness, that later progressed to profound dementia with visual neglect (**e**) and death within 18 months

alpha-helical type of the prion protein (PrPc) into the disease-causing protein with a dominant beta-sheet molecular structure (PrPsc). This process forms cytotoxic amyloid deposits, in which the misfolded protein aggregates into tightly packed beta sheets. Prion diseases occur mostly in the sporadic forms (about 87 %), but can occur as well as in genetic (8 %) and transmissible/iatrogenic (5 %) disease forms [22]. Spontaneous misfolding of PrPc into PrPsc is the likely explanation for the sporadic CJD; prions within brain tissue from these unfortunate affected patients can act as infectious agents and transmissible by direct inoculation into the brain of experimental animals resulting in characteristic vacuolating spongiform appearance of brain tissue with gliosis and PrP deposition.

With regards to genetic forms of prion disease, over 40 different PrP gene mutations have been shown to associate with familial prion diseases that include Gerstmann–Sträussler–Scheinker syndrome (GSS), familial (f) CJD, or fatal familial insomnia (FFI), each showing a characteristic spectrum of clinical symptoms.

Infectious forms of prion diseases include kuru related to ritualistic cannibalism in New Guinea, iatrogenic CJD related to neurosurgical procedures involving contaminated dural grafts and depth electrode implantation, and also the variant type (vCJD) transmitted in a fatal form to young adults in Britain that consumed beef products derived from cattle with bovine spongiform encephalopathy otherwise known as "mad cow" disease. With exception of one recently identified case, all of the deceased victims of vCJD were homozygous for methionine at PRNP codon 129 [22].

There is no treatment available for CJD and associated prion diseases. Clinical deterioration is rapid for those afflicted with CJD and most die within a year of diagnosis (Fig. 13.10).

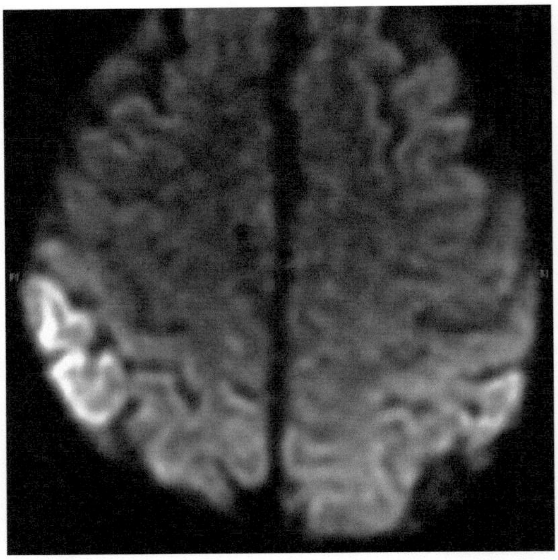

Fig. 13.10 Prion disease case example: A 75-year-old male was eating at a local fast food restaurant and suddenly acted odd and dropped everything from his hands with a blank stare on his face. He was brought emergently to the ER where it was initially thought that he may have had a brainstem stroke, yet MRI was negative for this. He recovered back to baseline within a day or two but then came back again with indeterminate spells of loss of consciousness and confusion, disorientation that progressed rapidly. He had a witnessed generalized seizure and had repeat MRI scans that showed hyper-intense changes in the right posterior parietal cortex. No clear diagnosis was evident at first but Creutzfeldt–Jakob disease was suspected, with CSF and repeat MR diffusion imaging confirming this as Creutzfeldt–Jakob disease (CJD); the illness was ultimately fatal 4 months later with intervening rapid functional decline noted

References

1. Glaser CA, Honarmand S, Anderson LJ, et al. Beyond viruses: clinical profiles and etiologies associated with encephalitis. Clin Infect Dis. 2006;43(12):1565–77.
2. Parikh V, Tucci V, Galwankar S. Infections of the nervous system. Int J Crit Illn Inj Sci. 2012;2(2):82–97.
3. Murphy K, Brunberg JA. Miliary tuberculosis involving the central nervous system. N Engl J Med. 1996;334:769.
4. Blanchard N, Dunay IR, Schlüter D. Persistence of Toxoplasma gondii in the central nervous system: a fine-tuned balance between the parasite, the brain and the immune system. Parasite Immunol. 2015;37(3):150–8.
5. Muzumdar D, Jhawar S, Goel A. Brain abscess: an overview. Int J Surg. 2011;9(2):136–44.
6. Meyer MA, Frey K, Schwaiger M. Discordance between F-18 fluorodeoxyglucose uptake and contrast enhancement in a brain abscess. Clin Nucl Med. 1993;18(8):682–4.
7. Donta ST. Issues in the diagnosis and treatment of lyme disease. Open Neurol J. 2012;6:140–5.
8. Czarnowska-Cubała M, Wiglusz MS, Cubała WJ, et al. MR findings in neurosyphilis—a literature review with a focus on a practical approach to neuroimaging. Psychiatr Danub. 2013;Suppl 2:S153–7.
9. Meyer MA. Neurologic complications of anthrax: a review of the literature. Arch Neurol. 2003;60(4):483–8.
10. Nakahara M, Ito M, Hattori N, et al. 18F-FDG-PET/CT better localizes active spinal infection than MRI for successful minimally invasive surgery. Acta Radiol. 2015;56(7):829–36.
11. Big C, Reineck LA, Aronoff DM. Viral infections of the central nervous system: a case-based review. Clin Med Res. 2009;7(4):142–6.
12. Jouan Y, Grammatico-Guillon L, Espitalier F, et al. Long-term outcome of severe herpes simplex encephalitis: a population-based observational study. Crit Care. 2015;19:345.
13. Mani RS, Madhusudana SN. Laboratory diagnosis of human rabies: recent advances. Scientific World Journal. 2013;2013:569712.
14. Mukerji SS, Lam AD, Wilson MR. Eastern equine encephalitis treated with intravenous immunoglobulins. Neurohospitalist. 2016;6(1):29–31.
15. Mlakar J, Korva M, Tul N, et al. Zika Virus associated with microcephaly. N Engl J Med. 2016;374:951–8.
16. Samuel MA, Wang H, Siddharthan V, et al. Axonal transport mediates West Nile virus entry into the central nervous system and induces acute flaccid paralysis. Proc Natl Acad Sci U S A. 2007;104(43):17140–5.
17. May FJ, Li L, Zhang S, et al. Genetic variation of St. Louis encephalitis virus. J Gen Virol. 2008;89(Pt 8):1901–10.
18. Bogovic P, Strle F. Tick-borne encephalitis: a review of epidemiology, clinical characteristics, and management. World J Clin Cases. 2015;3(5):430–41.
19. Lindå H, von Heijne A, Major EO, et al. Progressive multifocal leukoencephalopathy after natalizumab monotherapy. N Engl J Med. 2009;361:1081–7.
20. Bloomgren G, Richman S, Hotermans C, et al. Risk of natalizumab-associated progressive multifocal leukoencephalopathy. N Engl J Med. 2012;366(20):1870–80.
21. Colby DW, Pruisner SB. Prions cold spring. Harb Perspect Biol. 2011;3(1):a006833.
22. Saba R, Booth SA. The genetics of susceptibility to variant Creutzfeldt-Jakob disease. Public Health Genomics. 2013;16(1–2):17–24.

14 Neoplastic Diseases

Neoplastic disorders of the nervous system represent a particularly difficult area of medicine as the outcomes are generally not very good for those with a high-grade primary neoplastic disorder of the nervous system. In particular, glioblastoma has a very poor and limited survival rate despite intensive radiation therapy and chemotherapy [1]—this tragic problem represents one of the main challenges in neurological research with a need to come up with a safe and effective treatment (Fig. 14.1). Curiously, there is a small group of patients who still survive at 5 years (about 2 %) but likely with significant morbidity; there are occasional case reports of patients who are long-term survivors, which raises questions about the accuracy of the original diagnosis.

In this regard, a growing body of evidence has now found that some patients are formally diagnosed from biopsy samples or tissue from surgically resection as having a high-grade glioma, yet then with further investigation are instead noted to have progressive multifocal leukoencephalopathy as unusual viral infection from the JC virus, which unfortunately is also fatal in many cases with little that can be done for these individuals. By staining tissue for the large T antigen of the JC virus, the alternate diagnosis of a JC virus-related infection can be made when the presumption was otherwise thought to be a malignant glioma [2]. Furthermore, PCR analysis of gliomas reveal a link to other viruses as well for other patients, including CMV [3]. In this regard, a recent study with antiviral medications resulted in an improved survival curve for the group of glioma patients that were studied [4]. Viral pathogenesis of glioma has been proposed by Meyer [5].

With regard to viral pathogenesis of glioma, DNA tumor viruses may play in tumor formation. Wakefield et al. [6] provide evidence that further supports prior research findings that link cytomegalovirus to glioma, as CMV antigens pp65 and IE1-72 as well as CMV nucleic acids have been found in pediatric glioblastomas. Other DNA viruses, such as JC virus, have been implicated in glioma pathogenesis [7]. In this regard, it is also important to note that detection of atypical nuclei and high-proliferation indexes in a brain biopsy led to, in at least one instance, the misdiagnosis of a grade III astrocytoma; subsequent polymerase-chain-reaction studies led to a diagnosis of progressive multifocal leukoencephalopathy related to JC virus [2]. Further research is therefore needed to understand the link between DNA viruses and glioma.

Of the 22,500 new cases of malignant primary brain tumors that are diagnosed in adults in the US annually, about 70 % are malignant gliomas [1]; anaplastic astrocytomas account for 10–15 %, and anaplastic oligodendrogliomas and anaplastic oligoastrocytomas comprise 10 % (uncommon neoplasms such as anaplastic gangliogliomas and ependymomas comprise the remainder). For glioblastoma, the median age at the time of diagnosis is 64 years, yet for anaplastic gliomas, this is earlier at age 45. A family history of gliomas is

M.A. Meyer, *Neurologic Disease*, DOI 10.1007/978-3-319-39581-4_14

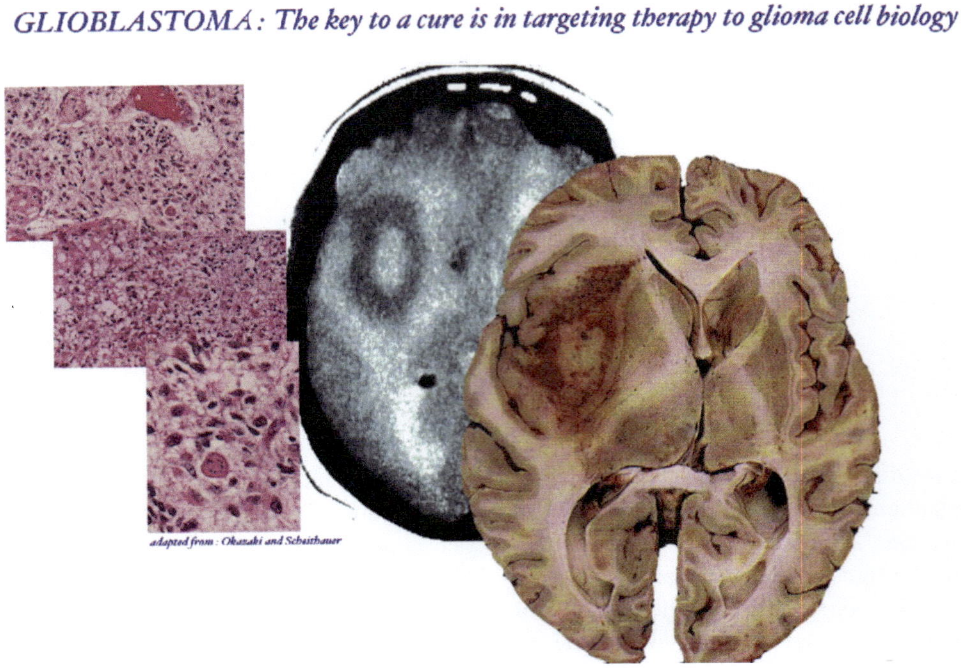

Fig. 14.1 Axial post-mortem section through the brain of a patient with a left frontal-parietal glioblastoma centered in the left insular cortex with matching pre-mortem CT shown here on an inverted gray scale along with histologic images revealing bizarre multinucleated giant cells that can be encountered in glioblastoma; this deadly form of brain neoplasia represents a biologic puzzle where the key may lie in targeting treatment to glioma cell biology

noted in 5 % of all glioma cases, which is often linked to familial neurofibromatosis or the Li–Fraumeni syndrome (p53 mutations that predispose to cancer), and Turcot's syndrome characterized by intestinal polyposis and brain tumors.

A relatively large part of neuro-oncology is dealing with the neurological complications of systemic cancer originating outside the nervous system. These complications include not only direct metastatic spread to brain and/or spinal cord, but may include neurological toxicity from chemotherapy. For example, vincristine effectively disrupts microtubules within dividing cancer cells, but unfortunately also disrupts those within peripheral nerve fibers and can produce severe neuropathy symptoms of distal tingling and numbness. Radiation also has its long-term effects as well, with the unfortunate late development of radiation necrosis within the brain for which there is little that can be done. Another set of complications that can occur with metastatic cancer is a terminal complication of seeding within the cerebrospinal fluid, where it can infiltrate throughout the nervous system and implant upon leptomeningeal surfaces. Although more common with leukemia and lymphoma patients, this can occur with solid tumors as well such as breast cancer and may require intrathecal chemotherapy.

New therapies are being tried with the use of immune sensitization of dendritic cells to the patients' own brain tumor biopsy specimen [8]—this clinical trial is one of many that are now in progress and is designed to compare this against the control group of patients who will receive the standard of care, including radiation and Temodar therapy. Despite these ongoing efforts, life expectancy for glioblastoma patients still remains in the 12- to 15-month range after diagnosis.

One potential avenue of research is to focus a biologic therapy against the extreme motility of glioma cells that enable extensive early invasion into health tissue (Fig. 14.2).

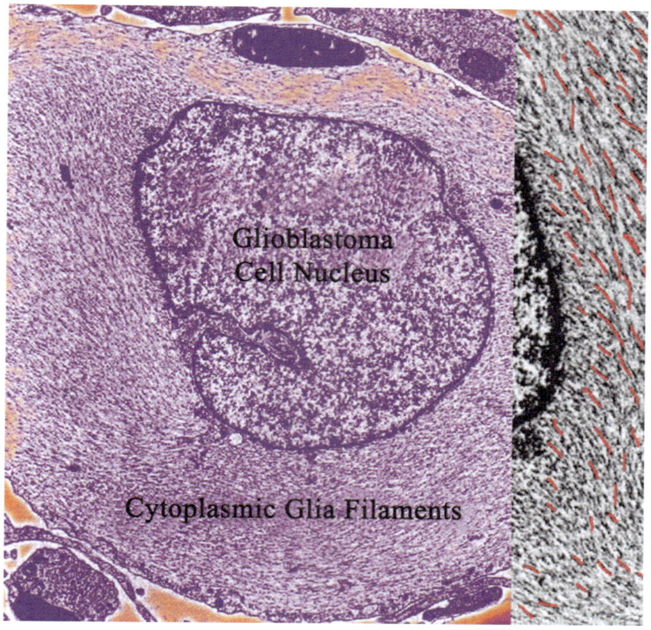

Fig. 14.2 Electron microscopy of glioma cells reveal massive over-production of cytoplasmic filaments that likely contributes to their motility and invasiveness

In order to make advances in treatment, a better understanding is needed on a molecular level to better define those genes which are overexpressed in glioma, as exemplified in a recently published study (Fig. 14.3) [9]. Gene expression within human glioblastomas were analyzed from data on 20,083 genes entered into the on-line Human Protein Atlas. In selecting genes that are strongly expressed within normal human brain tissue, 58 genes were identified from a search of the 20,083 entries that were rated as showing 90 % or greater intensity of expression within normal brain tissues. Of these 58, a subset of 48 genes was identified that not only had expression data for human glioblastomas but also for the human glioblastoma cell line U-251. Four of these 48 selected genes were found to be strongly expressed within the cytoplasm when assessed by both histologic sampling of high-grade glioma patient cases as well as U-251 glioblastoma cell line immunofluoresence analysis. These four human genes are: AGBL2 (ATP/GTP binding protein-like 2), BLOC1S6 (biogenesis of lysosomal organelles complex-1, subunit 6), MAP1A (microtubule-associated protein 1A), and ZSWIM5 (zinc finger, SWIM-type containing 5, also known as KIAA1511).

Chemotherapy options for glioma are illustrated in Fig. 14.4. MGMT is an important repair enzyme that contributes to resistance to temozolomide (Fig. 14.5). In a companion study to the EORTC–NCIC study reported by Stupp and colleagues [10], tumor specimens from the patients were examined for epigenetic silencing of the MGMT gene. MGMT promoter methylation silences the gene, thus decreasing DNA repair activity and increasing the susceptibility of the tumor cells to temozolomide. Patients with glioblastoma and MGMT promoter methylation (45 % of the total) who were treated with temozolomide had a median survival of 21.7 months and a 2-year survival rate of 46 %. In contrast, patients without MGMT promoter methylation who were treated with temozolomide had a significantly shorter median survival of only 12.7 months and a 2-year survival rate of 13.8 %.

As shown in Fig. 14.6, low-grade astrocytomas (grade 2 at lower right) are typically hypometabolic, but most high-grade gliomas show an elevated FDG uptake as shown in Fig. 14.7. Extreme forms of hypermetabolism is characteristically seen with PET imaging of primary CNS lymphoma lesions (Fig. 14.6).

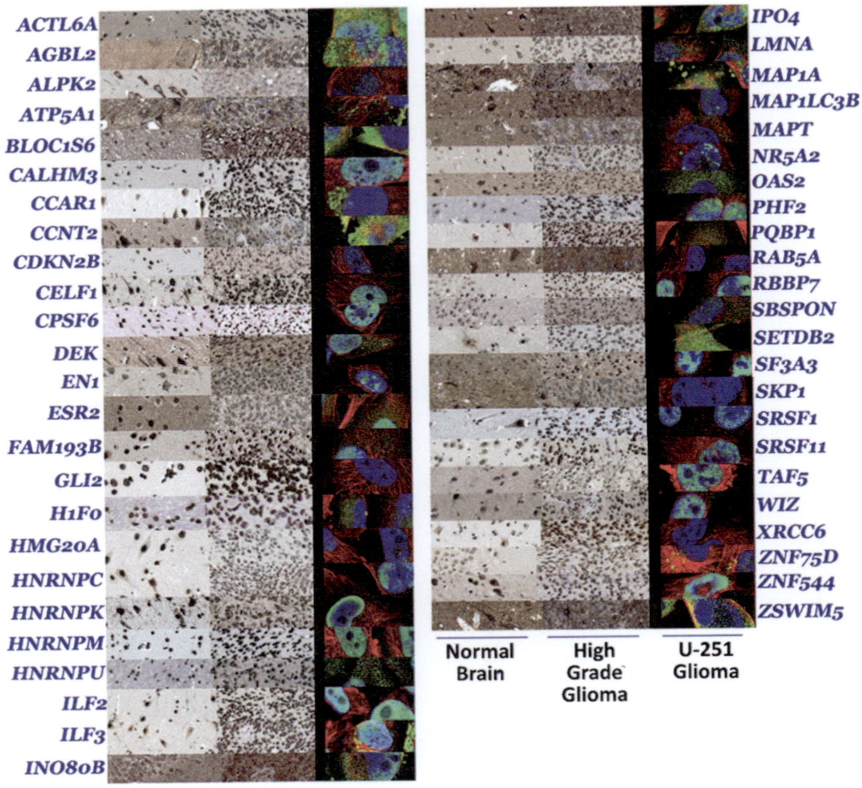

Fig. 14.3 Gene expression within human glioblastomas were analyzed from data on 20,083 genes entered into the on-line Human Protein Atlas; 48 genes were identified that not only had intense expression data for human glioblastomas (*center panel*) but also for the human glioblastoma cell line U-251 (*right panel*). Four of these 48 selected genes were found to be strongly expressed within the cytoplasm when assessed by both histologic sampling of high-grade glioma patient cases as well as U-251 glioblastoma cell line immunofluoresence analysis. These four human genes are: AGBL2, BLOC1S6, MAP1A, and ZSWIM5. Data extracted and analyzed by Michael A. Meyer, MD from The Human Protein Atlas http://www.proteinatlas.org/ [9]

Fig. 14.4 Commonly used chemotherapeutic agents include BCNU as an implantable wafer as well as orally administered temozolamide

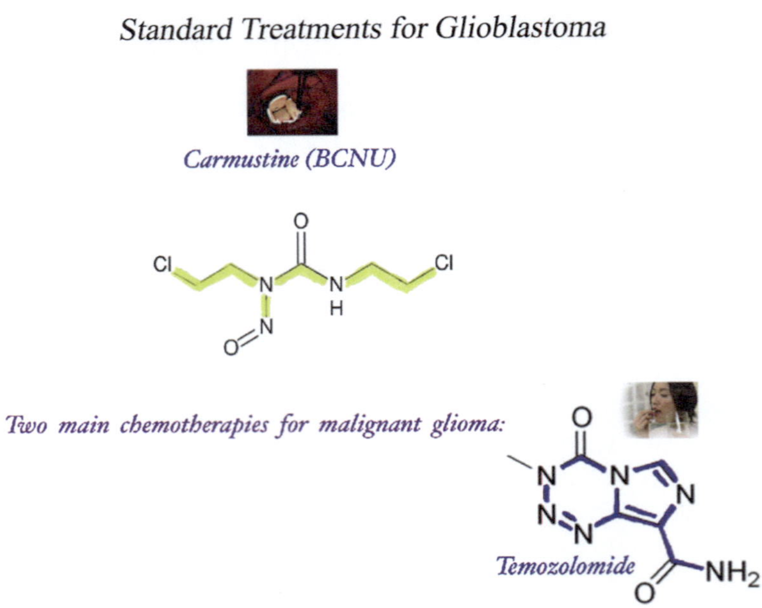

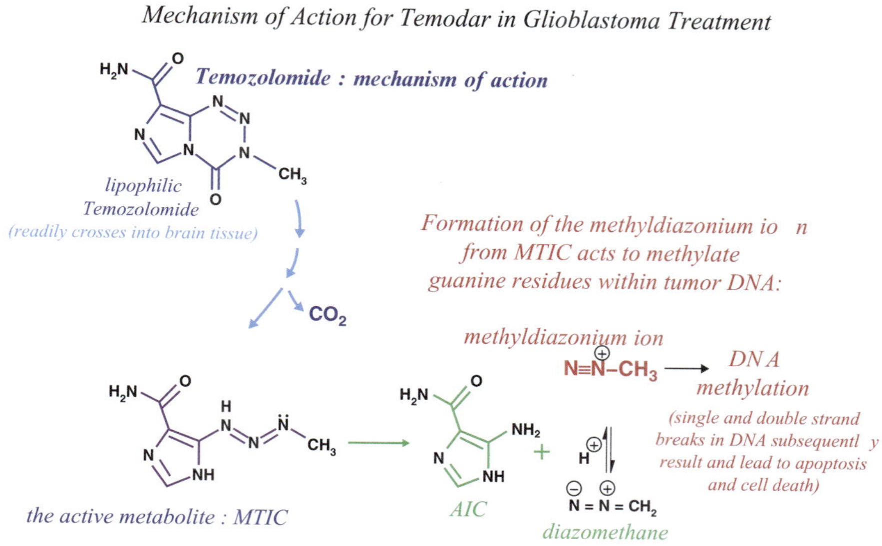

Fig. 14.5 Mechanism of action for temozolamide to induce single and double-strand breaks within glioma cell DNA by the methylation action of the MTIC active metabolite

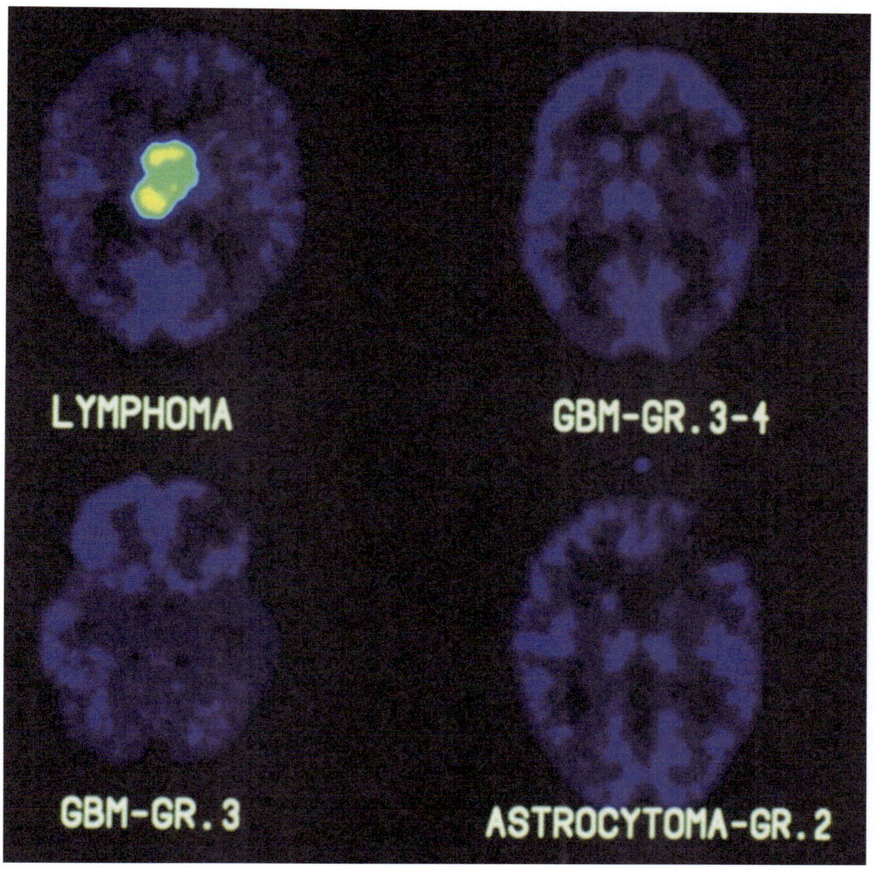

Fig. 14.6 Intense metabolic activity is characteristic of CNS lymphoma as seen on 18F-FDG PET imaging

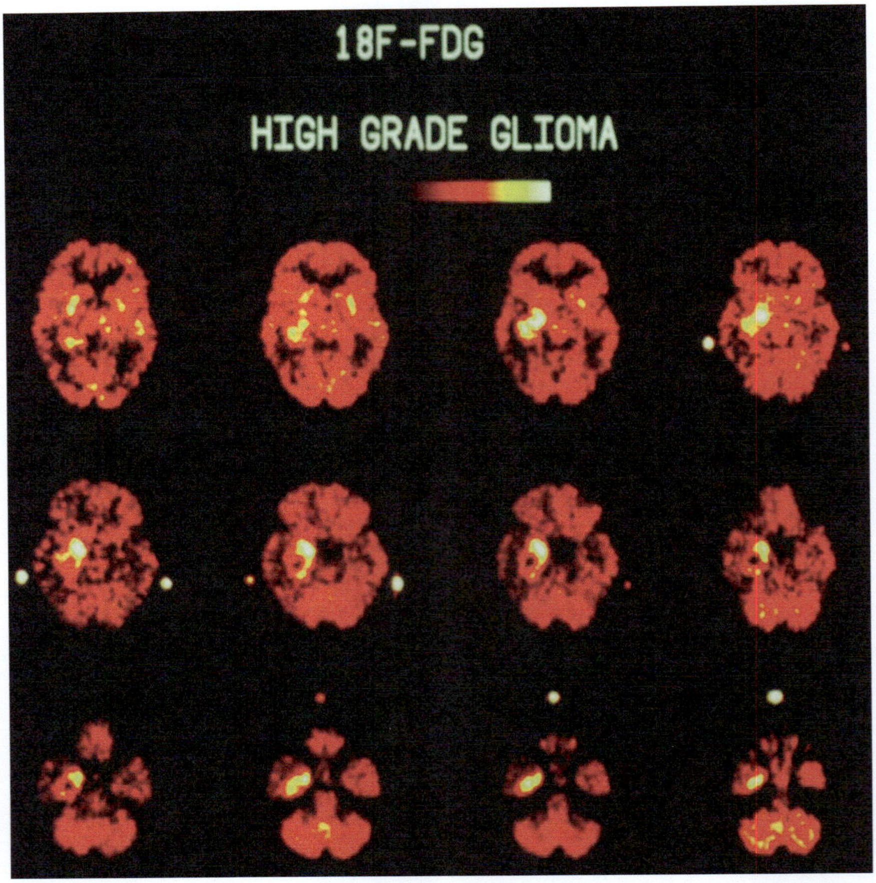

Fig. 14.7 Intense metabolic activity within the medial rim of a right temporal glioma that displays a necrotic center, revealed as a central void of tracer uptake

Clinical Examples
Another clinical example is shown in Fig. 14.8 at the time of diagnosis of a bifrontal glioma presenting with headaches and forgetfulness; the PET examination is taken before surgery that was later followed by radiation and chemotherapy.

Whole body imaging helps greatly in cases of metastatic disease, where the extra-cerebral tumor burden can be easily assessed, as in the case example shown in Fig. 14.9 for lung cancer with a solitary metastatic focus to the left frontal lobe. As shown in Fig. 14.10, lung cancer can present initially with neurologic symptoms from metastatic disease; the case example is that of a 48-year-old smoker who presented to ER with progressive headaches and confusion developing over last 1 month; craniotomy performed for resection of metastatic focus (pathology consistent with adenocarcinoma of the lung).

Three-dimensional rendering techniques are also helpful in determining minimal estimates of tumor volume as assessed by gadolinium enhancement, which is significantly smaller than the area of edema as shown in Fig. 14.11, with biopsy studies showing glioma infiltration occurring well beyond the areas of obvious edema.

In many cases, the level of infiltration is extreme as shown in Fig. 14.12 of a fatal brain stem glioma with pallisading of glioma cells

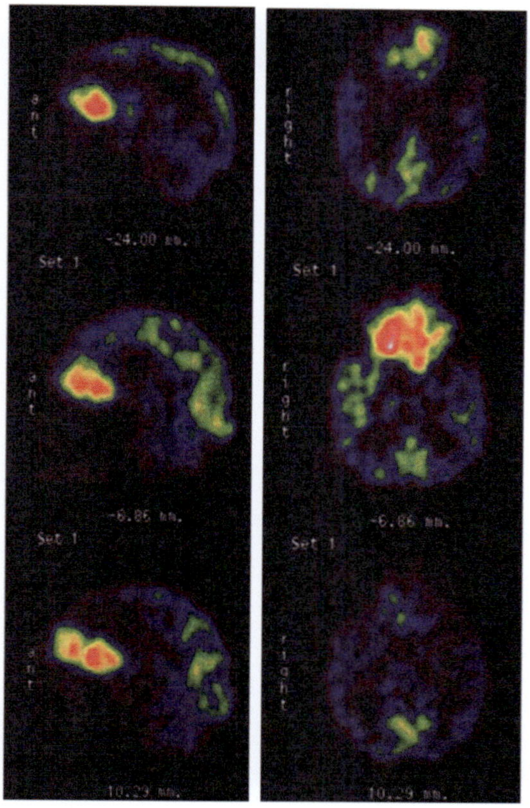

Fig. 14.8 Pre-operative PET images of a frontal lobe glioblastoma in a 54-year-old with headaches and forgetfulness. 18F-FDG PET (sagittal at *left*, axial at *right*) SUV max = 12, mean SUV = 9.25

along the infoldings of neuronal structures within the inferior olive.

Long-term survival is certainly likely and possible with patients who have grade 2 pathologies or those that merge grade with grade 3 features; with aggressive combined approach of using surgery, radiation, and medical therapies that include not only Temodar but also Avastin, lack of recurrence can be documented not only by PET measures of metabolism with 18F-FDG but also by markers of thymidine incorporation using 11C-FLT (flourothymidine), as shown in Fig. 14.13.

A similar approach of aggressive treatment for recurrent oligodendroglioma is well illustrated in Fig. 14.14 by the following case of a young adult who presented with right hand incoordination many years after gamma knife radiation therapy; the incorporation of PET lead to life saving identification of tumor recurrence leading to resection in someone who otherwise was suspected to have radiation necrosis.

In summary, PET is very helpful in identifying tumor recurrence even when there are no obvious symptoms at the time of a routine surveillance contrast-enhanced CT (please see lower left panel of Fig. 14.15) or can confirm signs of global radiation necrosis developing in a long-term glioma survivor with rapidly progressive dementia, as shown in Fig. 14.16.

14.1 Radiation Necrosis

An unusual case is shown in Figs. 14.16 and 14.17 for a woman who survived over 20 years after initial surgery and radiation for glioblastoma, only to incur a rapidly progressive dementia in her early 40s.

Glioma growth is typically very rapid, as shown by the illustrated case example (Fig. 14.18) using contrast-enhanced MRI in a 75-year-old with new onset of right facial numbness and weakness.

At the other spectrum of growth is the primary meningeal neoplasm known as meningioma, which usually grows very slowly and in most cases is biologically benign; in the case shown in Fig. 14.19, a typical CT appearance to a contrast enhancing left parietal dural-based meningioma is seen in a 44-year-old presenting with a new onset of nocturnal seizure coupled by a seizure like event of speech arrest. Meningiomas are known to expand only slightly over time, and grow slowly over the time span of years; there are exceptions however, and rarely may be malignant. Meningiomas commonly display estrogen receptors [11], and correspondingly are overall clearly more common in women than men.

14.2 Genetic Defects and Primary Neoplasms

Special pediatric neoplastic disorders include tuberous sclerosis, which can be multifocal but also be associated with hyper-metabolic subep-

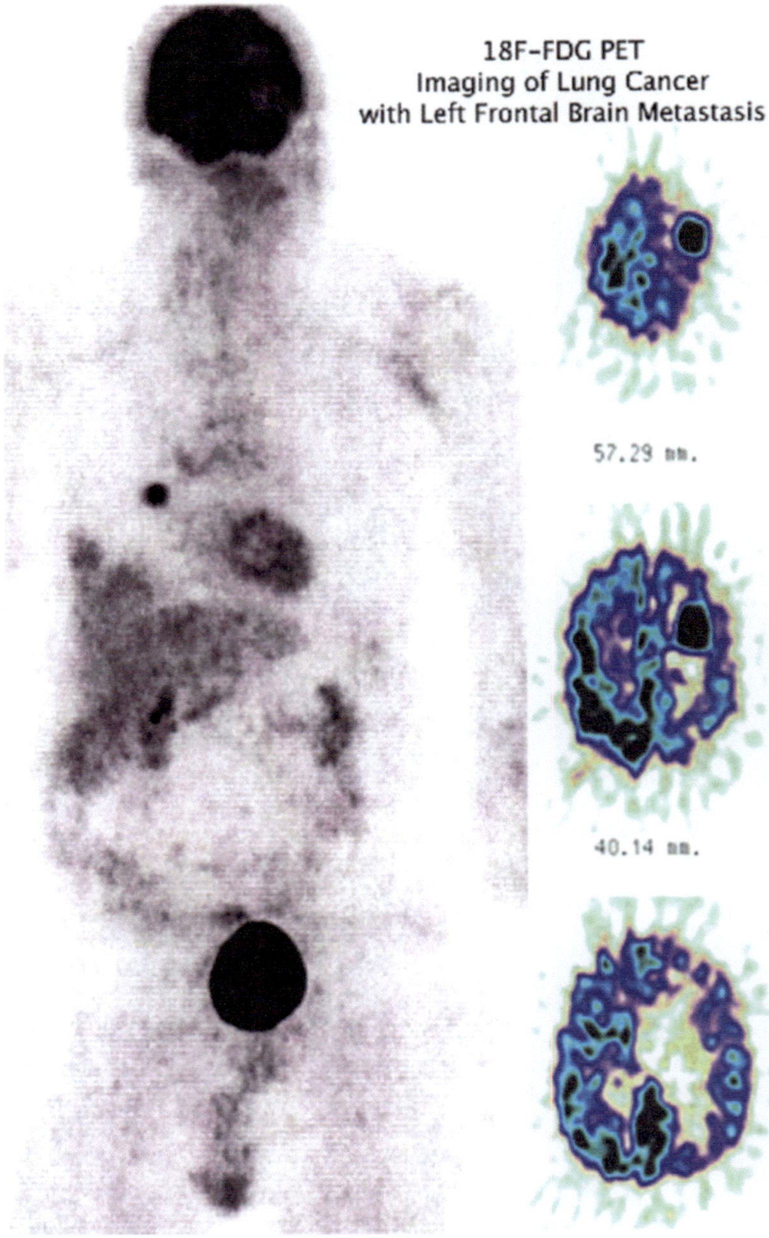

Fig. 14.9 Whole body PET imaging reveals a left frontal metastatic lesion from a primary focus of lung cancer within the medial right lower lung field

endymal malignant giant cell astrocytomas [12]. In the case example shown in Fig. 14.20, PET imaging was able to exclude this in a child with known tuberous sclerosis and presented with recent ictal blindness; PET revealed focal metabolic defects characteristic to cortical tubers. Facial angiofibromas, periungual fibromas, and a shagreen patch, respectively, are characteristic of tuberous sclerosis, an autosomal dominant disorder in which mutations in tumor suppressor gene TSC1 or TSC2 result in the formation of benign hamartomas throughout the body.

Neurofibromatosis type I (NF1) is a genetic disease found in about 100,000 individuals in the US that is linked to the development of benign neurofibromas and malignant tumors of the central

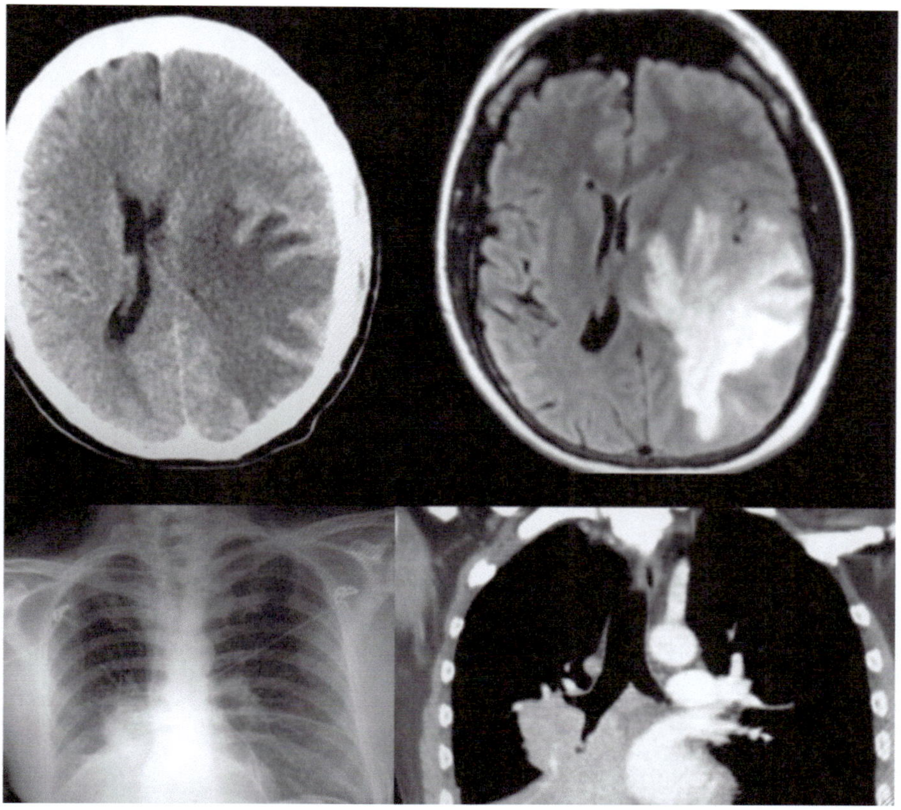

Fig. 14.10 Lung cancer can present initially with neurologic symptoms from metastatic disease; CT at *upper left* and MR at *upper right* reveals an edematous metastatic focus with left to right shift in a 48-year-old smoker who presented to ER with progressive headaches and confusion developing over last 1 month; craniotomy performed for resection of metastatic focus revealed pathology consistent with adenocarcinoma of the lung

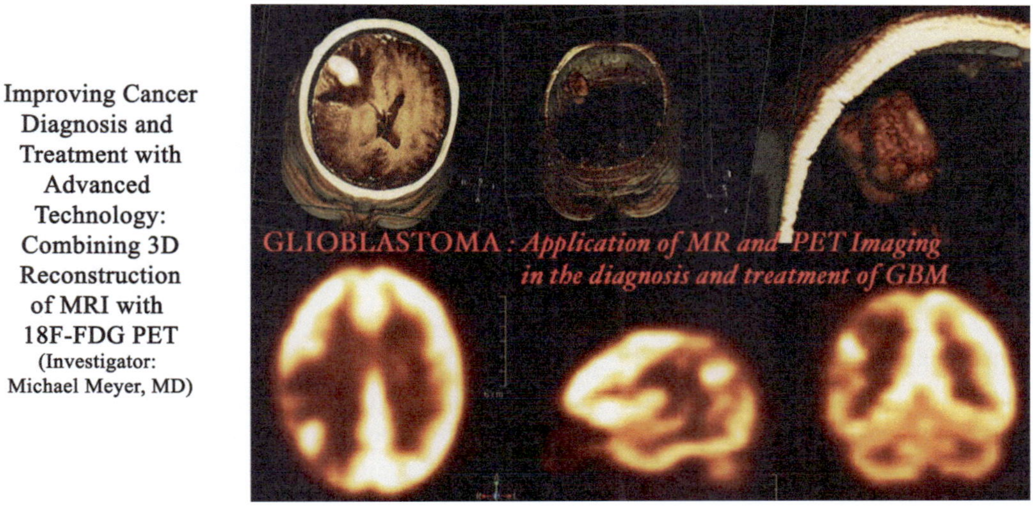

Fig. 14.11 Gadolinium enhancement coincident with location of hypermetabolism within a right posterior parietal glioblastoma

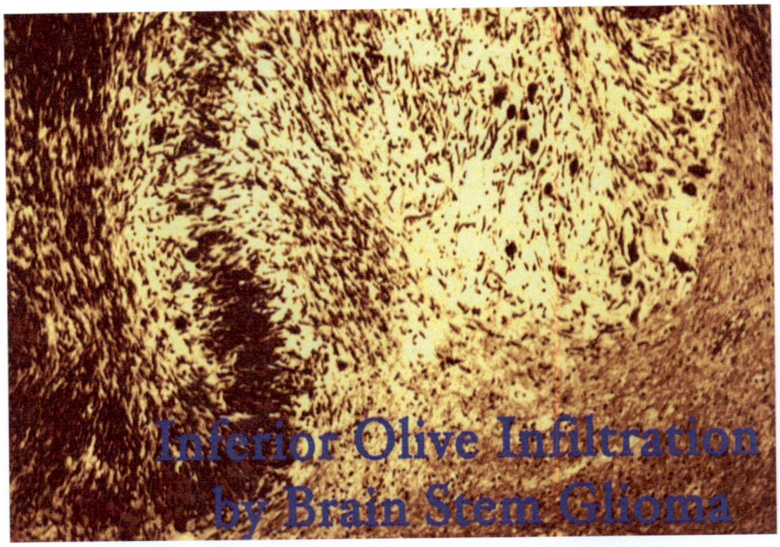

Fig. 14.12 In some cases, the level of glioma cell infiltration is extreme as shown here for a fatal brain stem glioma with pallisading of glioma cells along the infoldings of neuronal structures within the inferior olive

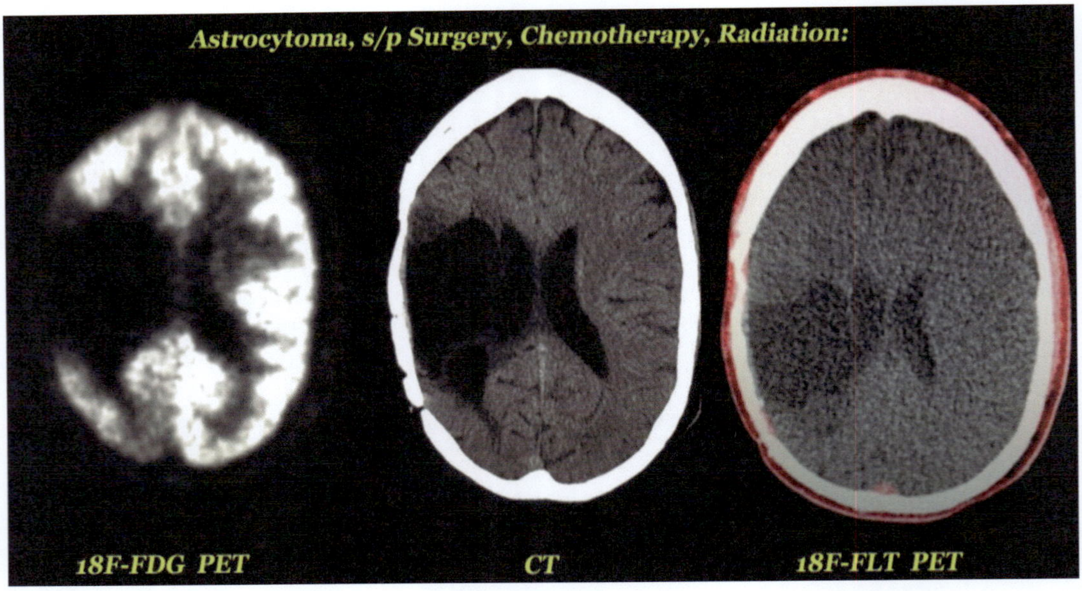

Fig. 14.13 Through an aggressive combined approach of using surgery, radiation, and medical therapies that include not only Temodar but also Avastin, lack of recurrence can be documented not only by PET measures of metabolism with 18F-FDG but also by markers of thymidine incorporation using 11C-FLT (flourothymidine)

and peripheral nervous system (Figs. 14.21 and 14.22) [13]. Café-au-lait spots or axillary freckling can be seen in most affected patients by age 8, with other findings include Lisch nodules within the iris; genetic testing reveals a mutation in the gene that encodes neurofibromin, which normally acts to regulate cell proliferation and differentiation of neural crest cells.

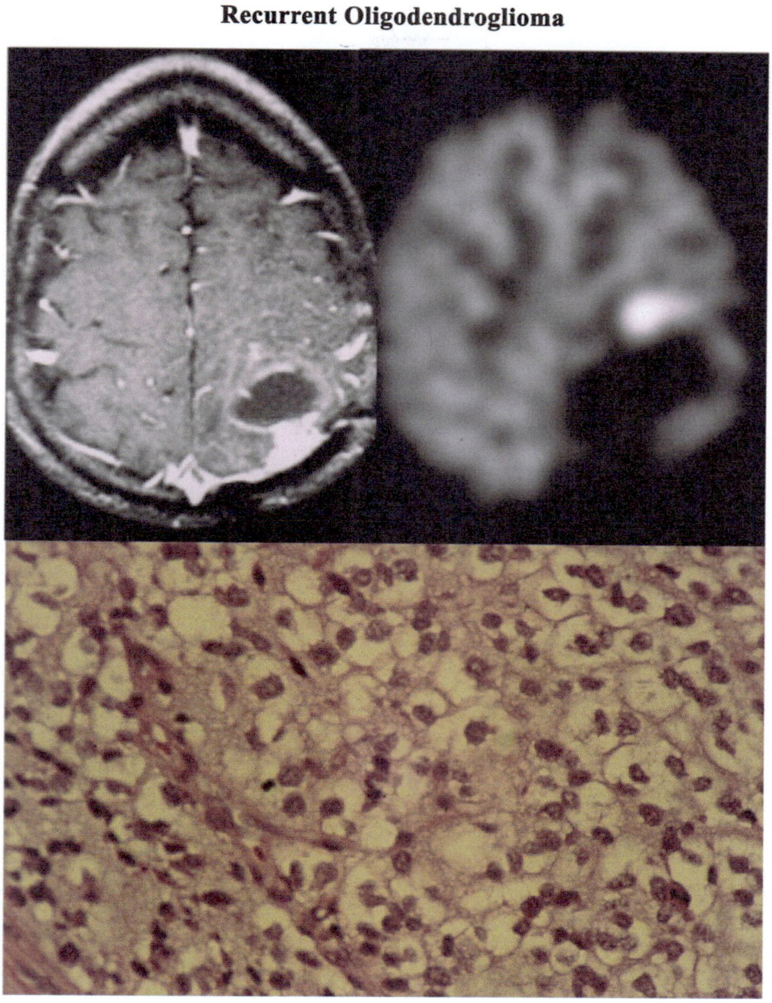

Fig. 14.14 Recurrent oligodendroglioma. Aggressive treatment approach for recurrent oligodendroglioma is well illustrated here for the case of a young adult who presented with right hand incoordination many years after gamma knife radiation therapy; the incorporation of PET at upper right lead to life saving identification of tumor recurrence, leading to surgical resection with clinical improvement (histology shown in *lower panel*)

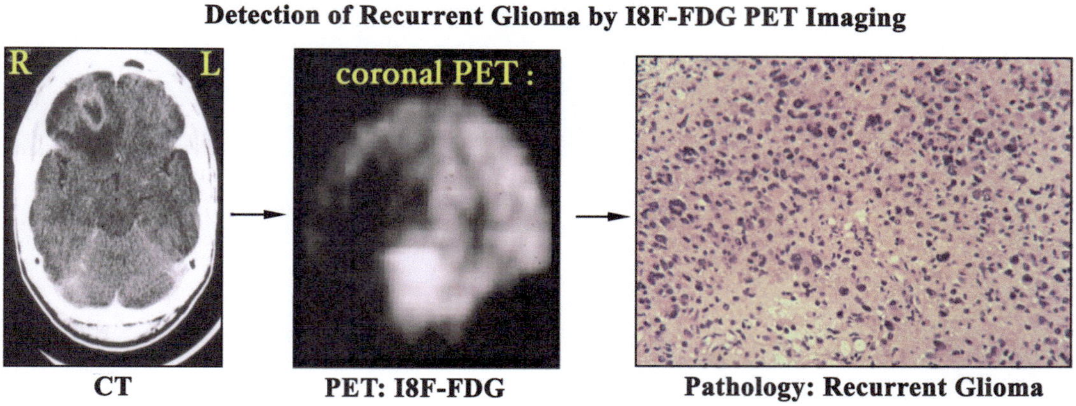

Fig. 14.15 Routine surveillance follow-up contrast-enhanced CT examination was indeterminant for radiation necrosis versus recurrent tumor; PET imaging suggested the latter, prompting surgery and confirmed by histologic examination (*right panel*)

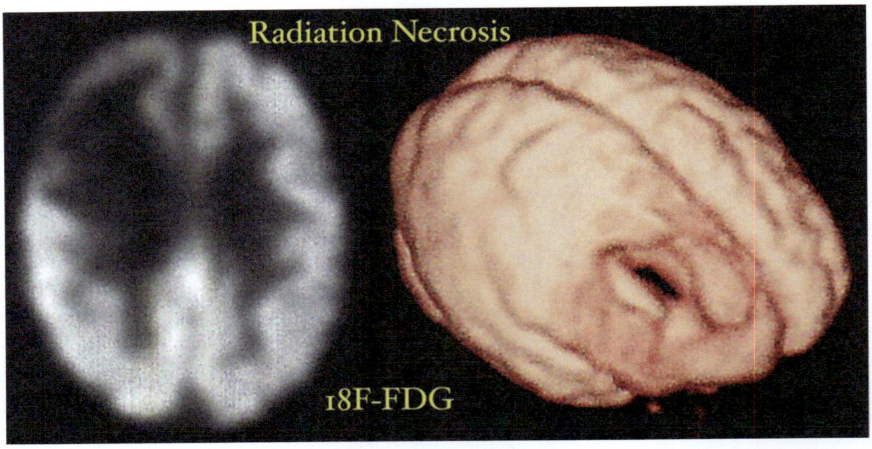

Fig. 14.16 An unusual case is shown here for a woman who survived over 20 years after initial surgery and radiation for glioblastoma, only to incur a rapidly progressive dementia in her early 40s; PET revealed evidence for radiation necrosis in the right frontal area (axial section at *left* with 3D surface rendering at *right*)

Fig. 14.17 MRI examination of same patient shown in Fig. 14.16 supports the impression of radiation necrosis

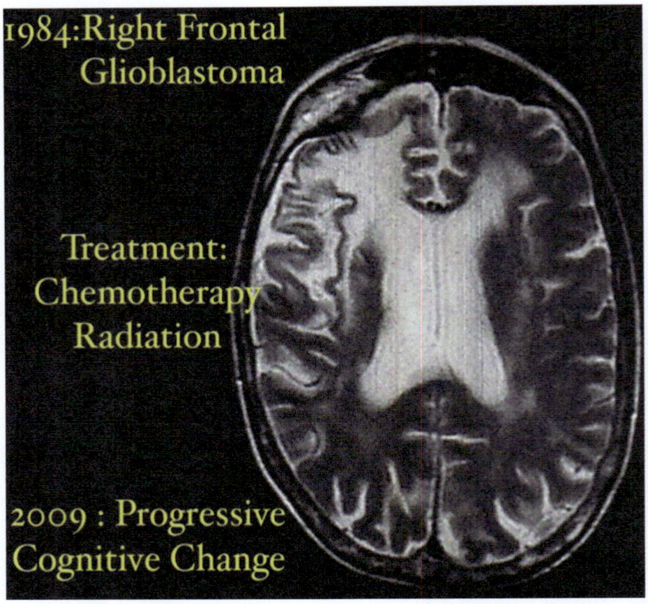

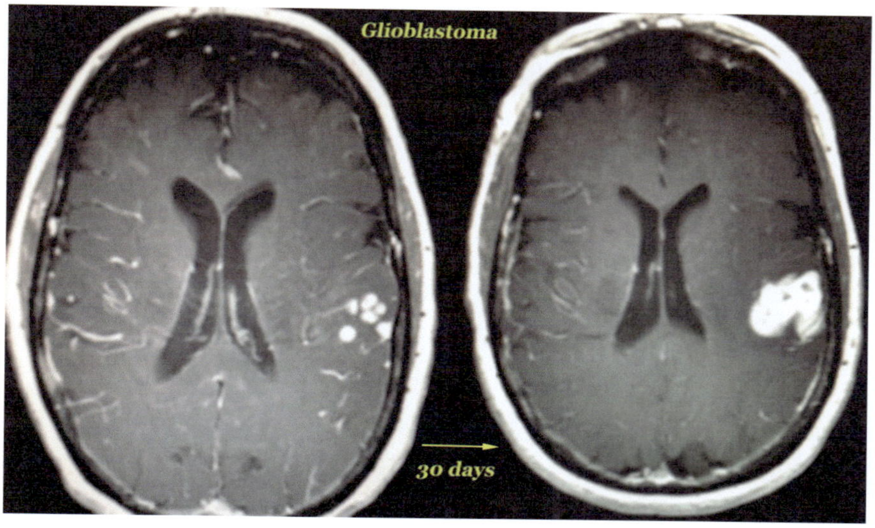

Fig. 14.18 Glioma growth is typically very rapid, as shown by this case example using contrast enhanced MRI in a 75-year-old with new onset of right facial numbness and weakness; impressive tumor growth and vascular proliferation are evident over a pre-operative period of only 30 days

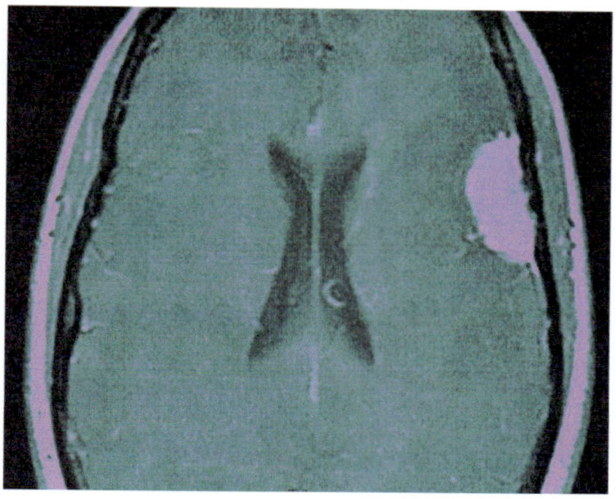

Fig. 14.19 Typical CT appearance to a contrast enhancing left parietal dural-based meningioma is seen in a 44-year-old presenting with a new onset of nocturnal seizure coupled by a seizure like event of speech arrest

Due to the chromosome 17-associated neurofibromin mutation, individuals with NF1 may develop both a variety of benign and malignant forms of peripheral nerve sheath tumors, including optic nerve gliomas (Fig. 14.22). Plexiform neurofibromas may undergo malignant transformation into malignant peripheral nerve sheath tumors; in such cases, whole body PET imaging is a sensitive and specific imaging modality to evaluate the biologic behavior of these NF1-associated nerve sheath tumors (Fig. 14.21) [14].

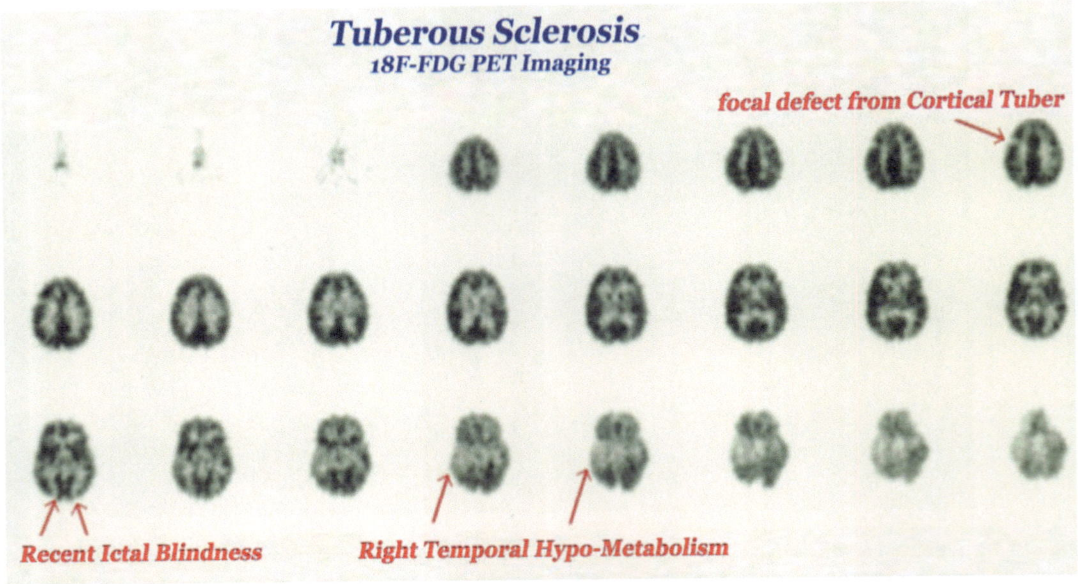

Fig. 14.20 PET imaging in a child with tuberous sclerosis helps exclude hyper-metabolic subependymal malignant giant cell astrocytoma. In the case example, PET imaging in a child with known tuberous sclerosis and recent ictal blindness revealed focal metabolic defects characteristic to cortical tubers

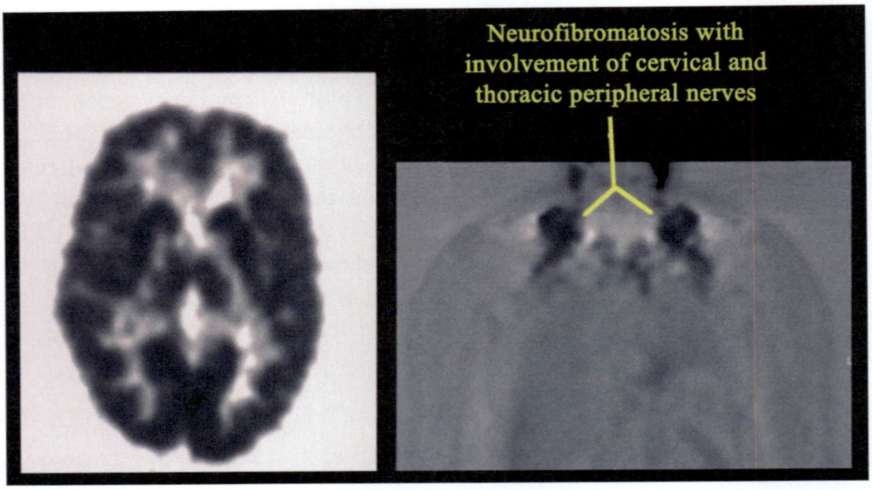

Fig. 14.21 PET imaging in a patient with neurofibromatosis revealed no intracranial lesions (panel at *left*) yet clearly revealed hypermetabolic neurofibromas affecting bilateral cervical and upper thoracic nerves (coronal image at *right*)

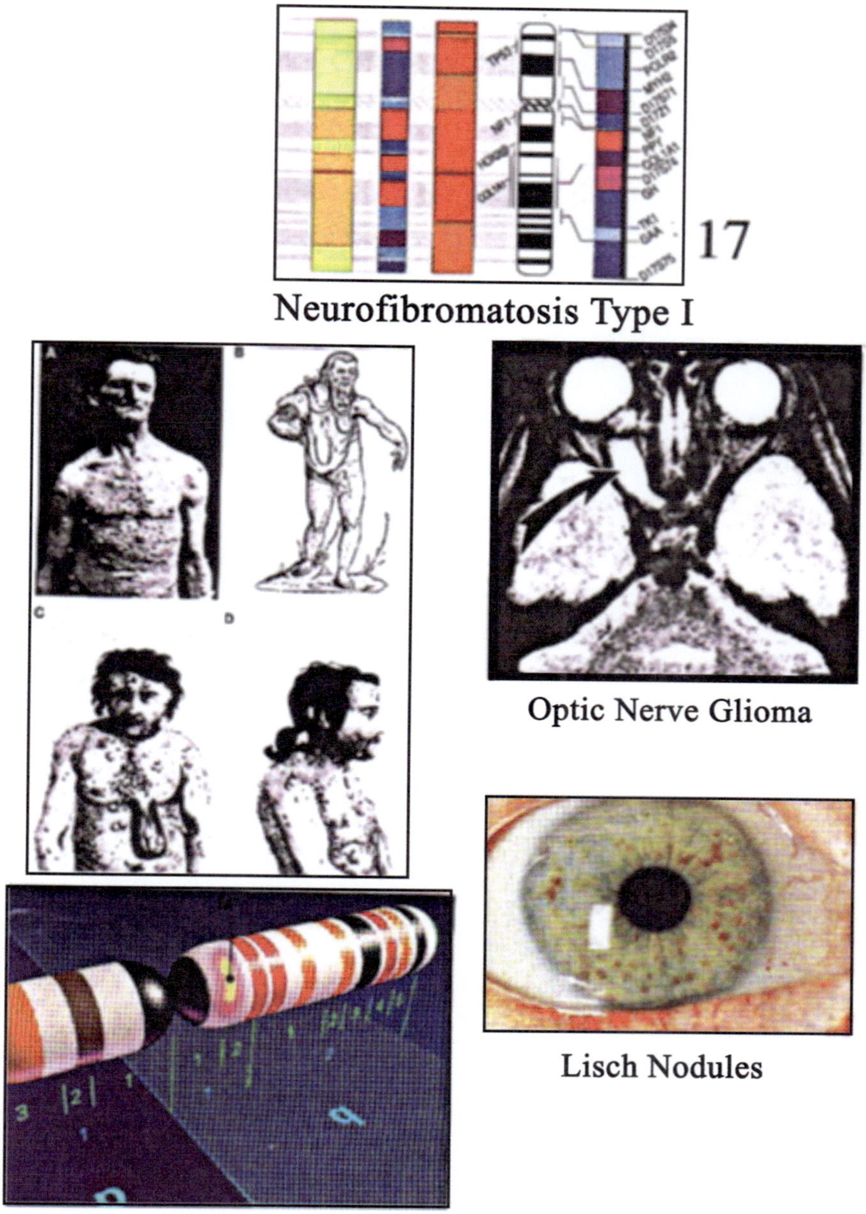

Fig. 14.22 Composite image portraying the genetic mutation on chromosome 17 that produces the clinical changes characteristic to neurofibromatosis type 1 (NF1)

References

1. Wen PY, Kesari S. Malignant gliomas in adults. N Engl J Med. 2008;359:492–507.
2. Van Assche G, Van Ranst M, Sciot R, et al. Progressive multifocal leukoencephalopathy after natalizumab therapy for Crohn's disease. N Engl J Med. 2005;353(4):362–8.
3. Solomon IH, Ramkissoon SH, Milner Jr DA, Folkerth RD. Cytomegalovirus and glioblastoma: a review of evidence for their association and indications for testing and treatment. J Neuropathol Exp Neurol. 2014;73(11):994–8.

4. Soderberg-Naucler C, Rahbar A, Stragliotto G. Survival in patients with glioblastoma receiving valganciclovir. N Engl J Med. 2013;369:985–6.
5. Meyer MA. Malignant gliomas in adults. N Engl J Med. 2008;359(17):18505.
6. Wakefield A, Pignata A, Ghazi A, et al. Is CMV a target in pediatric glioblastoma? Expression of CMV proteins, pp 65 and IE1–72 and CMV nucleic acids in a cohort of pediatric glioblastoma patients. J Neurooncol. 2015;125(2):307–15.
7. Brassesco MS, Darrigo Jr LG, Valera ET, et al. Giant-cell glioblastoma of childhood associated with HIV-1 and JC virus coinfection. Childs Nerv Syst. 2013; 29(8):1387–90.
8. Hsu M, Sedighim S, Wang T, et al. TCR sequencing can identify and track glioma-infiltrating T cells after DC vaccination. Cancer Immunol Res. 2016;4:412–8.
9. Meyer MA. Highly expressed genes in human high grade gliomas: immunohistochemical analysis of data from the human protein atlas. Neurol Int. 2014; 6(2):5348.
10. Hegi ME, Diserens AC, Gorlia T, et al. MGMT gene silencing and benefit from temozolomide in glioblastoma. N Engl J Med. 2005;352(10):997–1003.
11. Ghasimi S, Haapasalo H, Eray M, et al. Immunohistochemical analysis of LRIG proteins in meningiomas: correlation between estrogen receptor status and LRIG expression. J Neurooncol. 2012; 108(3):435–41.
12. Krueger DA, Northrup H, International Tuberous Sclerosis Complex Consensus Group. Tuberous sclerosis complex surveillance and management: recommendations of the 2012 International Tuberous Sclerosis Complex Consensus Conference. Pediatr Neurol. 2013;49(4):255–65.
13. Abramowicz A, Gos M. Neurofibromin in neurofibromatosis type 1—mutations in NF1gene as a cause of disease. Dev Period Med. 2014;18(3):297–306.
14. Salamon J, Mautner VF, Adam G, Derlin T. Multimodal imaging in neurofibromatosis type 1-associated nerve sheath tumors. Rofo. 2015;187(12): 1084–92.

Traumatic and Toxic Effects on the Nervous System 15

This chapter reviews the effects of trauma and toxins upon the central and peripheral nervous system. With regards to chronic, repeated head trauma, an emerging concept relates to long-term functional impairments of dementia and Parkinsonian symptoms associated with neurofibrillary changes as a progressive tauopathy. Traumatic brain injury is critically important to discuss, as it is a major cause of death and disability worldwide, resulting in enormous health care costs and lost productivity. In considering statistics from the US alone, traumatic brain injury (TBI) affects over 1.7 million, and linked to 50,000 deaths annually, at an estimated cost of over $60 billion; traumatic brain injury is a primary cause of death worldwide for those under 45 years old. Given the newly recognized link between repeated head trauma and the future onset of neurodegenerative disorders, including Alzheimer's disease and related tauopathies, more intensive research and study is needed on the prevention and treatment of TBI.

Diffuse axonal injury is an emerging concept related to the traumatic disruption of the axonal cytoskeleton, causing an interference with normal retrograde and anterograde transport mechanisms as the pathologic correlate to the cognitive and functional disruption that occurs after a concussive non-hemorrhagic injury to the brain. Myelinated nerve fibers seem to be more resistant and tolerant to the effects of trauma; in-vivo studies have shown that the finer and more delicate unmyelinated axons were found more likely to incur irreversible post-traumatic dysfunction [1, 2].

As far back as 1928, the relationship between repeated head trauma and progressive dementia has become progressively more clear ([3]—original description of dementia pugilistica in boxers). As shown in deceased football players who had a progressive post-traumatic dementia, abnormal intracellular accumulations of hyperphosphorylated microtubule-associated tau protein in the form of tangles have been noted along with Alzheimer-like beta-amyloid plaques, forming the concept of chronic traumatic encephalopathy as a cumulative late effect from repeated minor head injuries (CTE) [4].

With regards to major events of head injury, therapeutic hypothermia has been explored as possibly protective [5]. Induced hypothermia is viewed as a convenient way to possibly reduce apoptosis and other secondary effects of brain tissue damage by decreasing the metabolic rate and excito-toxic effects as well as reduce inflammation and minimize ATP energy depletion; hypothermia reduces free radical production while limiting intracellular calcium influx that would otherwise trigger programmed cell death (apoptosis). Despite that mild hypothermia (33 °C) has a widely accepted role in post-resuscitative care and perinatal asphyxia [6], it remains controversial in head trauma. Although a 2012 review of 13 randomized clinical trials on intracranial

M.A. Meyer, *Neurologic Disease*, DOI 10.1007/978-3-319-39581-4_15

hypertension management in head trauma patients showed significant reductions in intracranial pressure with the use of hypothermia, it remains controversial how this may translate into improved functional outcomes [7].

Traumatic carotid artery dissections are relatively uncommon and may be difficult to diagnose in the setting of multi-organ major trauma. Although the majority of carotid artery dissections occur spontaneously, about 1 in 25 cases are associated with severe trauma. Whereas spontaneous carotid dissections are typically seen in older age groups, traumatic dissections are more common amongst young patients [8]. These concepts relating to post-traumatic vascular injury can also be illustrated in the form of case examples, including post-traumatic dissection of the internal carotid resulting in left MCA occlusion that was urgently reversed by intra-arterial directed thrombolytic therapy (Fig. 15.1). As shown in Fig. 15.1, post-traumatic carotid dissection has the potential to cause devastating hemispheric ischemia, as shown for the case of a 25-year-old male status post-trauma-related jaw fracture with facial injuries including a post-traumatic ICA dissection with sudden hemi-paresis while recovering in hospital. Urgent revascularization was achieved via intra-arterial directed thrombolytic therapy (panel B at right, with good functional outcome and only a small subcortical ischemic infarct evident on CT in panel C).

Large subdural hygromas can sometimes be found as the late effects of head trauma, and occurs as a late effect of liquefaction of a subdural bleed; as shown in Fig. 15.2, this can also be the late and delayed result from tearing of bridging veins that may occur after shunting, such as the illustrated case of a patient with a ventriculo-peritoneal shunt for normal pressure hydrocephalus.

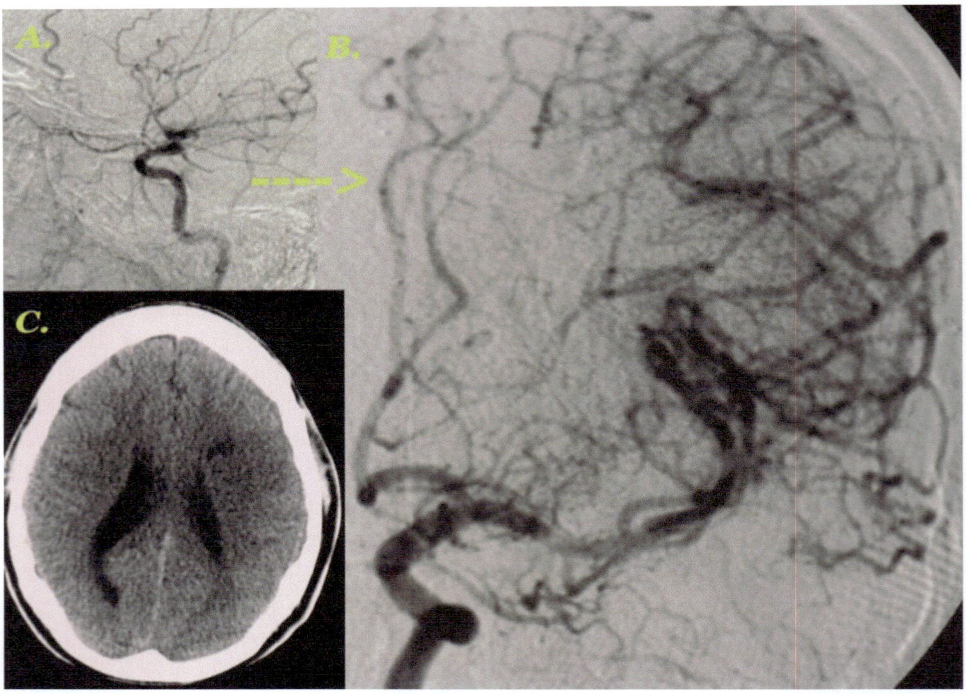

Fig. 15.1 A 25-year-old male s/p trauma-related jaw fracture with facial injuries including a post-traumatic ICA dissection with sudden hemi-paresis while recovering in hospital, causing embolic occlusion acutely of the left MCA (**a**). Urgent revascularization was achieved via intra-arterial directed thrombolytic therapy (**b** at *right*, with good functional outcome and only a small subcortical ischemic infarct evident on CT in **c**)

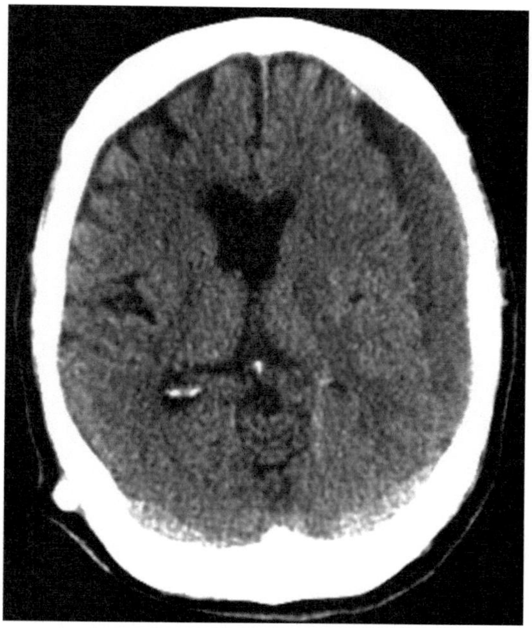

Fig. 15.2 Large subdural hygroma as a late effect of liquefaction of a subdural bleed secondary to tearing of bridging veins that may occur after shunting, such as the illustrated case of a patient with a ventriculo-peritoneal shunt for normal pressure hydrocephalus

In contrast to the large post-traumatic subdural fluid collection that is easily identified on CT, there are many cases with more subtle findings that can be easily overlooked if MRI is not employed in the trauma evaluation as well. The diagnostic value of using MRI to clarify uncertain or subtle CT findings in trauma patients is well illustrated in Fig. 15.3.

Brain PET imaging can help identify functional long-term effects of head trauma, as shown in Fig. 15.4.

As noted in the autopsy studies by Courville [9], the inferior frontal and temporal lobes are frequently injured in closed head trauma, as illustrated in Fig. 15.5.

15.1 Toxins and the Nervous System: Alcohol, Mercury, Lead, Medications

As shown in Fig. 15.6, chronic alcohol use heavily damages the cerebellum with atrophy of the cerebellar hemispheres evident on both CT and MRI, with abnormal loss of Purkinje cells evident

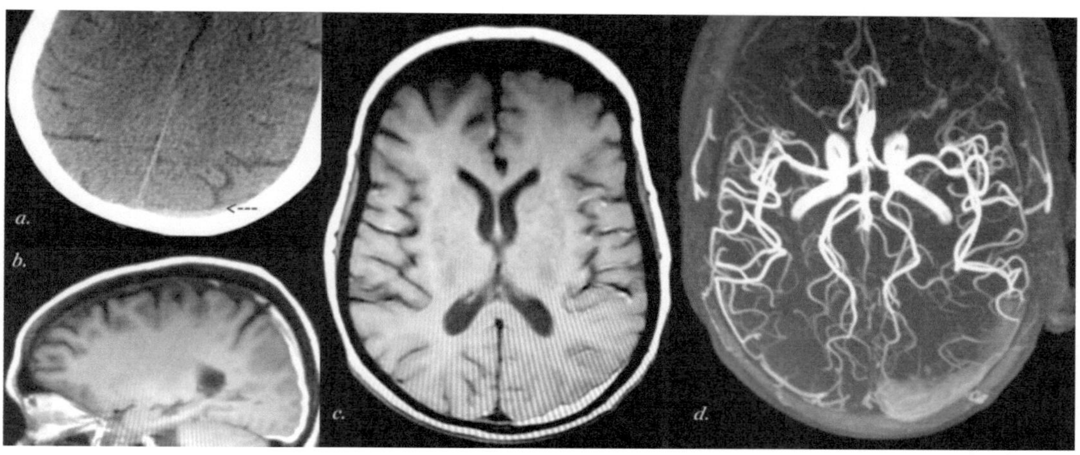

Fig. 15.3 Slip and fall accident with head trauma in a 64-year-old female complaining of persistent headache; left occipital-parietal hematoma evident on MR (**b**, **c**) but seen only as a subtle crescent of high density change on CT (**a**). As there was no mass effect, and the subdural fluid collection is small, medical management was elected with slow improvement thereafter. Note the bright signal effect of blood products within the left occipital-parietal region on the brain MRA (**d**)

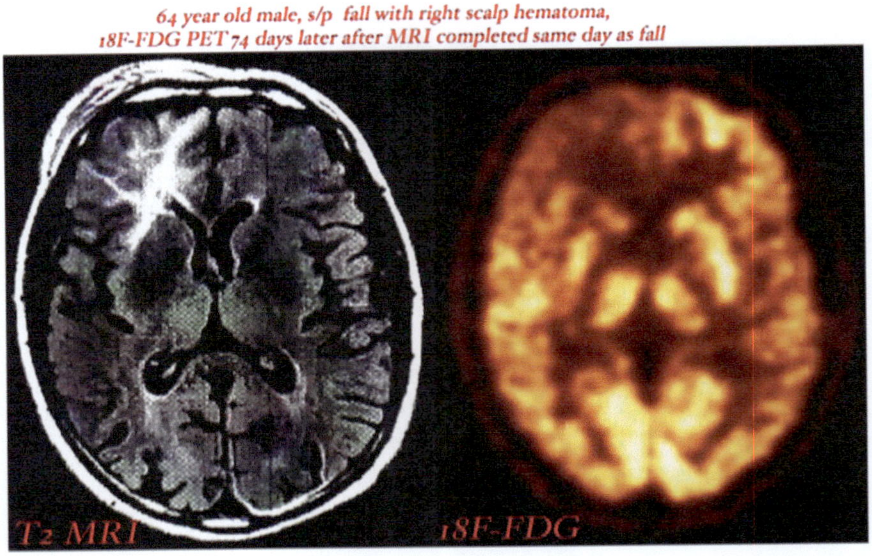

Fig. 15.4 PET brain imaging is useful for identifying the functional long-term effects of head trauma, where extensive right frontal hypometabolism is noted, concordant with an area of presumed subcortical gliosis seen on MRI

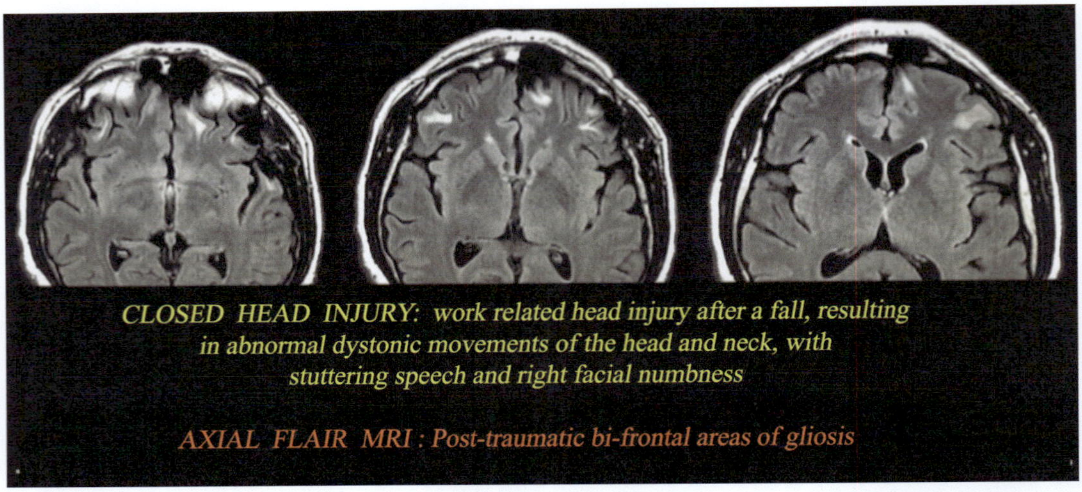

Fig. 15.5 Due to contre-coup jarring of the brain with sudden acceleration/deceleration effects from closed head injury, the inferior frontal lobes are frequently affected, as shown in this case of a work-related head injury that resulted in multifocal areas of subcortical frontal lobe gliosis linked to long-term cognitive changes with stuttering speech and abnormal dystonic movements

on post-mortem histologic examination. Although alcohol is commonly related to chronic cerebellar degeneration (Fig. 15.6), there are other causes to consider including long-term phenytoin use.

Severe nervous system toxicity can result with ingestion of methylmercury, as had occurred in 1956 in the Minamata Bay industrial accident in Japan (Fig. 15.7). The neurotoxicology of the accident has been well reviewed by Eto [10], "……Minamata disease, or methylmercury poisoning, was first discovered in 1956 around Minamata Bay, Kumamoto Prefecture, Japan. A similar epidemic occurred in 1965 along the Agano River, Niigata

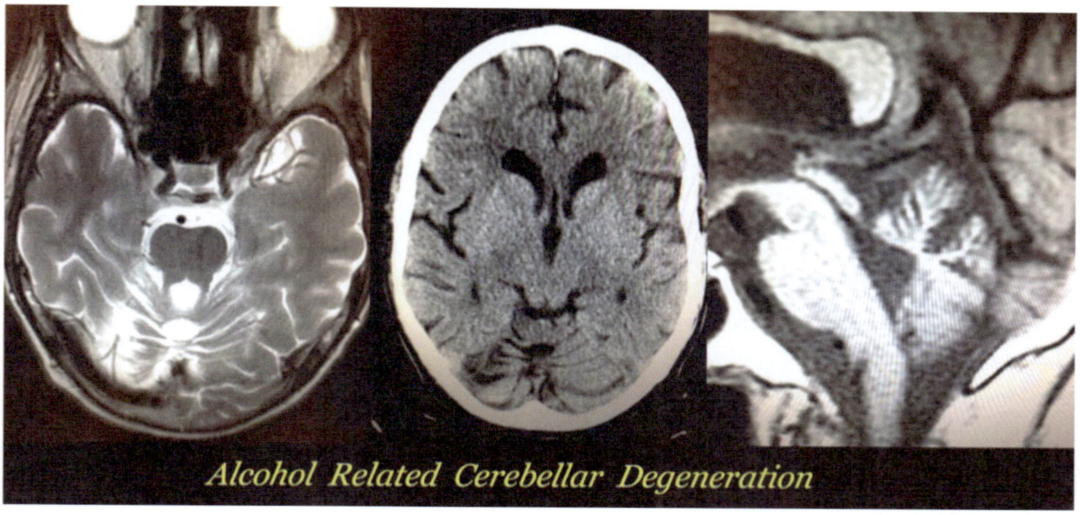

Fig. 15.6 Long-term superior cerebellar vermian atrophy secondary to chronic heavy use of alcohol over many years as shown by CT (*center*) and MRI (*left* and *right panels*)

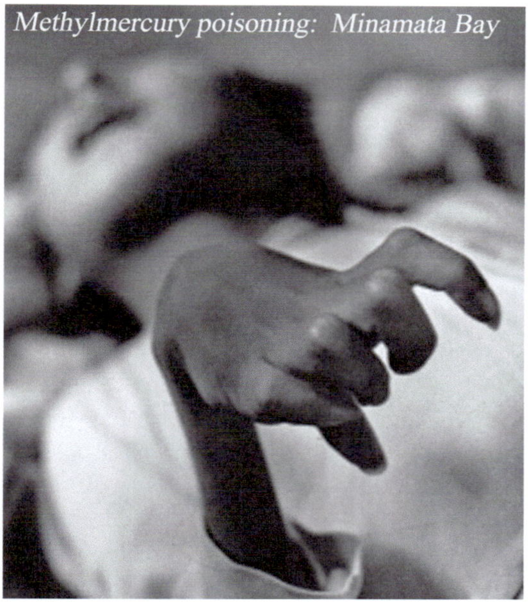

Fig. 15.7 Severe long-term permanent neurotoxic damage in a survivor of methylmercury exposure in the Minamata Bay industrial accident event, Minamata, Japan (reproduced with permission of the Aileen Archive)

Prefecture, Japan. ..... Nervous system lesions associated with Minamata disease have a characteristic distribution. In the cerebral cortex, the calcarine cortex was found to be involved in all cases of Minamata disease, particularly along the calcarine fissure. The destruction of nerve tissue was prominent in the anterior portions of the calcarine cortex. Occasionally, the centrifugal route from the visual and visual association areas (internal sagittal stratum) showed secondary degeneration in prolonged cases after acute onset. Postcentral, precentral, and temporal transverse cortices showed similar changes, though they were less severe. Intense lesions in the precentral cortex caused the development of secondary bilateral degeneration of the pyramidal tracts. In the cerebellum, the lesions occurred deeper in the hemisphere. The granule cell population was most affected. In the peripheral nerves, sensory nerves were more affected than motor nerves. Secondary degeneration of Goll's tracts was occasionally seen in prolonged or chronic cases."

Even a tiny amount of dimethylmercury exposure can produce fatal neurotoxic effects, as illustrated in the unfortunate autopsy case of a 48-year-old chemistry professor. As outlined by Nierenberg et al. [11], the patient recalled that in August 1996, while transferring liquid dimethylmercury from a container to a capillary tube, she spilled several drops from the tip of the pipette onto the dorsum of her gloved hand. She presented to the hospital 4 months later with moderate upper-extremity dysmetria, dystaxic handwriting, a widely based gait, and ".....scanning speech; her blood mercury level was 4000 micrograms per liter, or 80 times the toxic threshold". Despite chelation therapy, she rapidly declined and expired. At autopsy, "… the cortex of the cerebral hemispheres was diffusely thinned, to 3 mm. The visual cortex around the calcarine fissure was grossly gliotic, as was the superior surface of the superior temporal gyri. The cerebellum showed diffuse atrophy of both vermal and hemispheric folia. Microscopical study showed extensive neuronal loss and gliosis bilaterally within the primary visual and auditory cortices, with milder loss of neurons and gliosis in the motor and sensory cortices. There was widespread loss of cerebellar granular-cell neurons, Purkinje cells, and basket-cell neurons, with evidence of loss of parallel fibers in the molecular layer. Bergmann gliosis was well developed and widespread."

The literary expression "mad as a hatter" reflected the dementia commonly encountered in those who participated in the making of hats with one step in the process involving the use of mercury, producing toxic symptomatic exposure-related cognitive changes.

On a related historical note is the exposure incurred by Sir Isaac Newton in his alchemy experiments. To investigate his known history for "nervous breakdowns" and psychiatric instability, a 1979 post-mortem analysis of hair and bone revealed very high levels of both mercury and lead (see: "Mercury poisoning: a probable cause of Isaac Newton's physical and mental ills") [12].

The fall of the Roman Empire has also been linked to lead poisoning within wine as explained by Esinger [13], "… the colica Pictonum or colic of Poitou, under these and many other names, was a frequent, widespread, and deadly disease from Roman times until the eighteenth century. Its unique pathognomonic, notably a severe colic succeeded by paralysis and other central nervous system dysfunction, makes it possible to identify the disease with certainty as chronic lead disease, usually caused by the ingestion of lead-adulterated wines. The custom of sweetening and preserving sour wines with lead-containing additives is traced to the Romans."

Lead poisoning continues to this day to be a public health concern; fortunately, lead levels are declining overall. The National Health and Nutrition Examination Survey estimated the prevalence of high blood lead levels (>10 μg/dL) among US children in the 1988–1991 time frame to be 8.6 % versus 1.4 % in the 1999–2004 time frame, equating to an 84 % decline [14]. Lead is especially toxic to the developing brain, and alters neuronal migration and differentiation, interferes with neurotransmitter release and energy metabolism, as well as triggering apoptosis via interfering with calcium release from the mitochondria resulting in formation of the permeability transition pore, thereby triggering the process of programmed cell death [14].

Medications comprise an important source of toxic effects upon the nervous system. One of many examples is illustrated in Fig. 15.8, where the immunosuppressive agent cyclosporine can often produce tremor, but in certain cases there may be neuropsychiatric effects as well with flat affect and withdrawn behavior noted with severe tremor; in the illustrated example, striking hypermetabolism was seen within the basal ganglia bilaterally (see Fig. 15.8, lower panel). Both cyclosporine and tacrolimus may produce neurotoxic side effects that varies from tremor and acute encephalopathy to status epilepticus and even coma in extreme cases; white matter lesions can be seen in some cases that seem to represent vasogenic edema [15].

Fig. 15.8 Brain 18F-FDG PET images in the axial (*left*), sagittal (*center*), and coronal planes reveal cyclosporine-associated neurotoxic effects in a bone marrow transplant patient displaying neuropsychiatric changes with flat affect and withdrawn behavior along with severe tremor; in the illustrated example, striking hyper-metabolism was seen within the basal ganglia bilaterally

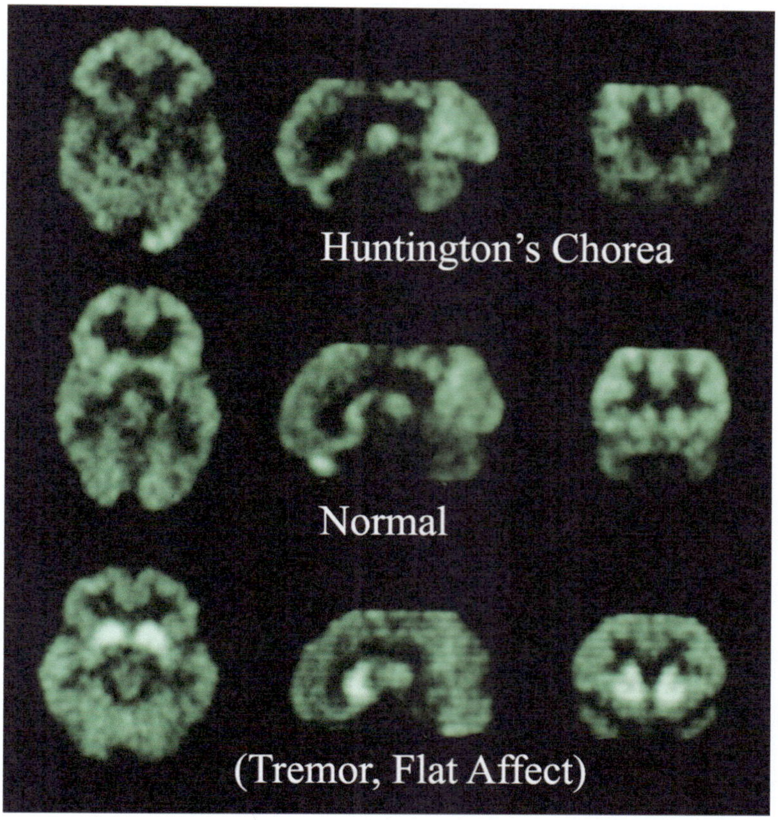

References

1. Johnson VE, Stewart W, Smith DH. Axonal pathology in traumatic brain injury. Exp Neurol. 2013;246:35–43.
2. Staal JA, Vickers JC. Selective vulnerability of non-myelinated axons to stretch injury in an in vitro co-culture system. J Neurotrauma. 2011;28(5):841–7.
3. Martland H. Punch drunk. J Am Med Assoc. 1928;91:1103–7.
4. Omalu BI, DeKosky ST, Hamilton RL, et al. Chronic traumatic encephalopathy in a national football league player: part II. Neurosurgery. 2006;59(5):1086–92.
5. Andresen M, Gazmuri JT, Marín A, et al. Therapeutic hypothermia for acute brain injuries. Scand J Trauma Resusc Emerg Med. 2015;23:42.
6. Nielsen N, Wetterslev J, Cronberg T, et al. Targeted temperature management at 33°C versus 36°C after cardiac arrest. N Engl J Med. 2013;369(23):2197–206.
7. Sadaka F, Veremakis C. Therapeutic hypothermia for the management of intracranial hypertension in severe traumatic brain injury: a systematic review. Brain Inj. 2012;26(7–8):899–908.
8. Crönlein M, Sandmann GH, Beirer M, et al. Traumatic bilateral carotid artery dissection following severe blunt trauma: a case report on the difficulties in diagnosis and therapy of an often overlooked life-threatening injury. Eur J Med Res. 2015;20:62.
9. Rand CW, Courville CB. Histologic changes in the brain in cases of fatal injury to the head; alterations in nerve cells. Arch Neurol Psychiatry. 1946;55:79–110.
10. Eto K. Pathology of Minamata disease. Toxicol Pathol. 1997;25(6):614–23.
11. Nierenberg DW, Nordgren RE, Chang MB, et al. Delayed cerebellar disease and death after accidental exposure to dimethylmercury. New Engl J Med. 1998;338(23):1672–6.
12. Johnson LW, Wolbarsht ML. Mercury poisoning: a probable cause of Isaac Newton's physical and mental ills. Notes Rec R Soc Lond. 1979;34(1):1–9.
13. Eisinger J. Lead and wine. Eberhard Gockel and the colica Pictonum. Med Hist. 1982;26(3):279–302.
14. Mason LH, Harp JP, Han DY. Pb neurotoxicity: neuropsychological effects of lead toxicity. Biomed Res Int. 2014;2014:840547.
15. Wijdicks EF. Neurotoxicity of immunosuppressive drugs. Liver Transpl. 2001;7(11):937–42.

Conclusions

16

16.1 Introduction

The future of neuroscience lies in basic science discoveries—understanding the molecular mechanisms of memory within the human brain will likely lead to new therapies to delay or hopefully halt cognitive decline in Alzheimer's disease patients. A fundamental understanding about how proteins become misfolded and then self-aggregate to form the nidus of new neurotoxic aggregates will likely lead to new therapies for currently incurable degenerative neurologic diseases such as Huntington's disease or spinocerebellar ataxias. The time frame in which these future advances are made may be close at hand; hopefully, this text may inspire dedicated individuals to help make the "lab bench to bedside" transformations for one of many of the currently untreatable illnesses that affect the nervous system.

With regards to the tragic decline that occurs in degenerative muscle diseases, such as Duchenne muscular dystrophy, there is very promising research going forward into clinical trials that explores the unique aspects of exon skipping so that functional proteins of abbreviated length can be "stitched together" and still preserve protective levels of dystrophin. By analogy, there are other neurologic illnesses that have similar genetic defects that can also hopefully be "skipped over" by exon skipping oligonucleotides, leading to functional proteins that are abbreviated in size but still do the job they are designed to accomplish. Of additional note, there are unfortunate enzymatic deficiencies such as Krabbe's globoid leukodystrophy or metachromatic leukodystrophy that may respond to bone marrow transplantation—it is felt that progress to date with this unique approach may be related to competent engrafted progenitor cells that migrate into the brain and differentiate into microglia.

With regards to stroke, great new advances have been made with intravenous as well as by catheter-directed thrombolytic therapy with tPA as well as direct catheter disruption versus retrieval of thrombus. New imaging modalities are in development for imaging the site and mechanism to the acute vascular occlusion with greater precision, with technology needed still that can identify tissue viability for the prediction in advance who is more likely to benefit from re-perfusion therapy and likewise identify those who might suffer life-threatening reperfusion hemorrhage into nonviable tissue—perhaps PET may hold the key for this.

Exciting advances in basic science work to map brain activity in real time at a cellular level using optogenetic techniques in the transparent zebrafish; in real time, the actual activity of individual neurons can now be visualized within the transparent brain of the zebrafish, and even selectively stimulated with optical techniques [1, 2].

Postmortem techniques have also now been developed to make the mammalian brain transparent to visualize labeled neurons and astrocytes

M.A. Meyer, *Neurologic Disease*, DOI 10.1007/978-3-319-39581-4_16

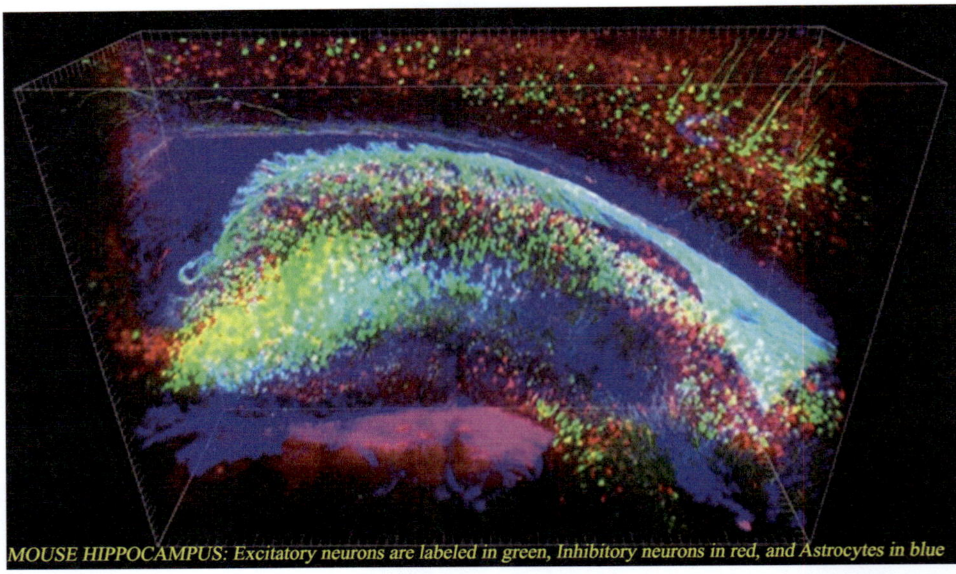

Fig. 16.1 Mouse hippocampus stained with fluorescent antibodies: excitatory neurons are labeled in *green*, inhibitory neurons in *red*, and astrocytes in *blue* (reproduced with permission of Dr. Karl Deisseroth)

in a three-dimensional manner. Using a technique they term CLARITY investigators were able to transform brain tissue into a nanoporous hydrogel-hybridized network of hydrophilic polymers that is optically transparent and macromolecule-permeable, thereby gaining unique insight to the neuronal circuitry within large volumes of brain tissue (Fig. 16.1) [3].

One of the greatest advances to come will be in the unraveling of the molecular mechanism to neuronal apoptosis and finding ways to overcome the process and halt neuronal death. Consider the tragedy of post-anoxic encephalopathy—although we can make some impact on this with therapeutic hypothermia, a molecular treatment to halt the process of apoptosis is needed to prevent post-anoxic death of neurons—this may be the greatest challenge to modern neurology, as this would also directly apply to minimizing brain damage with ischemic acute stroke. RNAi or RNA interference is another technique in development that holds great promise in treating not only acute stroke and brain ischemia but also other forms of neurologic disease by modifying adverse gene transcription.

Finally, it is important to understand the amazing potential of the human mind that is inherent in all us—as it is well known that certain individuals (savants) have gained amazing skills through injuries to the brain suggest the potential for these and other amazing cognitive abilities remain within all of us.

References

1. Fajardo O, Zhu P, Friedrich RW. Control of a specific motor program by a small brain area in zebrafish. Front Neural Circuits. 2013;7:67.
2. Arrenberg AB, Driever W. Integrating anatomy and function for zebrafish circuit analysis. Front Neural Circuits. 2013;7:74.
3. Chung K, Wallace J, Kim SY, et al. Structural and molecular interrogation of intact biological systems. Nature. 2013;497(7449):332–7.

Index

M.A. Meyer, *Neurologic Disease*, DOI 10.1007/978-3-319-39581-4

MIX
Papier aus verantwortungsvollen Quellen
Paper from responsible sources
FSC® C105338

If you have any concerns about our products,
you can contact us on
ProductSafety@springernature.com

In case Publisher is established outside the EU,
the EU authorized representative is:
Springer Nature Customer Service Center GmbH
Europaplatz 3, 69115 Heidelberg, Germany

Printed by Libri Plureos GmbH
in Hamburg, Germany